U0348385

七年之"养",探索创新,共向未来

首都医科大学宣武医院一体化PET/MR成果集

主　编◎卢　洁

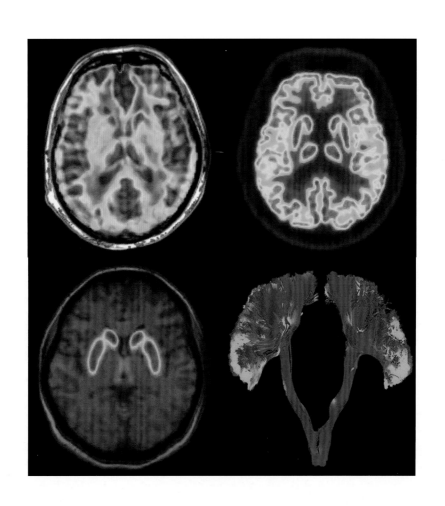

科学技术文献出版社
SCIENTIFIC AND TECHNICAL DOCUMENTATION PRESS
·北京·

图书在版编目（CIP）数据

首都医科大学宣武医院一体化 PET/MR 成果集／卢洁主编 . —北京：科学技术文献出版社，2023.6

ISBN 978-7-5235-0284-6

Ⅰ . ①首… Ⅱ . ①卢… Ⅲ . 计算机 X 线扫描体层摄影②磁共振成像 Ⅳ . ① R814. 42 ② R445. 2

中国国家版本馆 CIP 数据核字（2023）第 095787 号

首都医科大学宣武医院一体化PET/MR成果集

策划编辑：张　蓉　责任编辑：张　蓉　段思帆　责任校对：张吲哚　责任出版：张志平

出　版　者	科学技术文献出版社
地　　　址	北京市复兴路15号　邮编 100038
编　务　部	（010）58882938，58882087（传真）
发　行　部	（010）58882868，58882870（传真）
邮　购　部	（010）58882873
官　方　网　址	www.stdp.com.cn
发　行　者	科学技术文献出版社发行　全国各地新华书店经销
印　刷　者	北京地大彩印有限公司
版　　　次	2023年6月第1版　2023年6月第1次印刷
开　　　本	889×1194　1/16
字　　　数	407千
印　　　张	16.75
书　　　号	ISBN 978-7-5235-0284-6
定　　　价	185.00元

PET/MR 主编简介

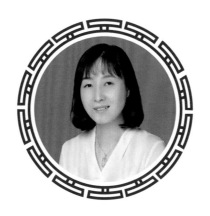

卢 洁

主任医师，教授，博士研究生导师

首都医科大学宣武医院副院长、放射与核医学科主任，国家神经疾病医学中心副主任

神经变性病教育部重点实验室副主任、磁共振成像脑信息学北京市重点实验室主任

学术成果：

以第一作者或通讯作者发表 SCI 收录论文 200 余篇，代表作发表在 *Neuron*、*Nature Communications*、*Radiology*、*Brain*、*Neurology*、*EJNMMI* 等国际权威期刊；主持国家自然科学基金重点项目、国家自然科学基金优秀青年科学基金项目、科技部"十四五"及"十三五"国家重点研发计划、北京自然科学基金重点项目等 19 项课题；主编（译）专著 10 部；授权专利 10 项；专家共识 13 项；获华夏医学科技奖一等奖、北京市留学人员创新创业特别贡献奖、国家"万人计划"科技创新领军人才、茅以升北京青年科技奖、中国产学研合作创新奖、中华医学会放射学分会杰出青年奖、北京医学会首都青年医学创新与转化大赛一等奖等多项学术奖励。

学术兼职：

中华医学会放射学分会全国委员、中国医学影像技术研究会放射学分会副主任委员、北京医学会放射学分会副主任委员、北京医师协会放射医师分会副会长等；担任 *EJNMMI*、*Neuroimage* 等国际期刊编委。

PET/MR
编者名单

主 编

卢 洁

编 者

张海琴（首都医科大学宣武医院）

张 春（首都医科大学宣武医院）

张 苗（首都医科大学宣武医院）

崔碧霄（首都医科大学宣武医院）

闫少珍（首都医科大学宣武医院）

PET/MR
前　言

时光荏苒，日月如梭，我院自 2015 年安装亚洲首台一体化 TOF PET/MR 至今已有七年，回首过往的探索经历，团队围绕一体化 PET/MR 的优势，结合我院神经系统和老年疾病特色，开展了一系列临床科研工作。我们的团队也逐渐成长壮大，每一位成员都为团队注入新活力，贡献新成果。

通过七年的坚持和努力，我们从最初对 PET/MR 的懵懂逐渐走向了解，付出终将会有收获，每个成果都是对艰辛付出的肯定。截至 2022 年 12 月，团队共发表 35 篇 SCI 收录文章，33 篇国内统计源期刊收录文章，主要涉及阿尔茨海默病、帕金森病、癫痫、脑肿瘤、脑血管病等；撰写 33 篇摘要进行国际核医学与分子影像年会（Society of Nuclear Medicine and Molecular Imaging，SNMMI）、北美放射学年会（Radiological Society of North American，RSNA）等国际会议交流；出版 7 部 PET/MR 专 / 译著；获批 28 项国家级、北京市级科研课题基金资助；培养 20 余名硕士研究生、博士研究生及博士后；举办 7 届全国 PET/MR 脑功能成像学习班，搭建多学科交流平台。

本成果集主要记录我院一体化 PET/MR 七年的成果，以图文并茂形式进行呈现和总结，为今后继续进行深入的科研和临床应用奠定基础。在此感谢全国各位专家和同道给予的帮助和支持！感谢临床各科室的通力合作！感谢团队成员的辛勤付出！七年之"养"，不忘初心，不负韶华，我们愿与广大同道携手前行，探索创新，共向未来，为一体化 PET/MR 更好服务患者而努力！

首都医科大学宣武医院
2023 年 1 月 29 日

PET/MR 目 录

PET/MR

第一章

一体化 PET/MR 科研成果

近年来多模态影像设备迅速发展，尤其一体化 PET/MR 技术的完善和应用，在医学影像学历程中具有里程碑意义。首都医科大学宣武医院 2015 年安装 GE 公司一体化 TOF PET/MR，2019 年安装联影公司一体化 TOF PET/MR，作为国内先行的探路者，团队克服了重重困难，逐渐有所收获，2016 年第一个国际会议发言，2016 年第一项科技部重点研发项目，2017 年第一项国家自然科学基金项目，2017 年第一部国内专著，2018 年第一项发明专利，2019 年第一篇 EJNMMI 文章发表……经过七年不懈的努力和探索，截至 2022 年 12 月，团队共发表 35 篇 SCI 收录文章，33 篇国内统计源期刊文章；撰写 33 篇摘要进行国内国际会议交流；出版 7 部 PET/MR 专 / 译著；获批 28 项国家级、北京市级科研课题基金资助。

PET/MR 第一节 SCI 收录文章

一体化 PET/MR 相关 SCI 收录文章共 35 篇，其中 30 篇为神经系统和老年疾病（包括认知障碍疾病 9 篇、癫痫 8 篇、脑胶质瘤 4 篇、脑血管病 3 篇、帕金森病 2 篇、脑影像技术 4 篇），5 篇发表于核医学顶级期刊 *Eur J Nucl Med Mol Imaging*。

1.SCI 收录文章列表

[1] GUO K, WANG J, WANG Z, et al.Morphometric analysis program and quantitative positron emission tomography in presurgical localization in MRI-negative epilepsies: a simultaneous PET/MRI study.Eur J Nucl Med Mol Imaging, 2022, 49(6): 1930-1938.

[2] WANG J, YANG H, CUI B, et al.Effects of MRI protocols on brain FDG uptake in simultaneous PET/MR imaging.Eur J Nucl Med Mol Imaging, 2022, 49(8): 2812-2820.

[3] GUO K, WANG J, CUI B, et al.[^{18}F] FDG PET/MRI and magnetoencephalography may improve presurgical localization of temporal lobe epilepsy.Eur Radiol, 2022, 32(5): 3024-3034.

[4] WANG J, GUO K, CUI B, et al.Individual [^{18}F] FDG PET and functional MRI based on simultaneous PET/MRI may predict seizure recurrence after temporal lobe epilepsy surgery.Eur Radiol, 2022, 32(6): 3880-3888.

[5] WANG M, CUI B, SHAN Y, et al.Non-invasive glucose metabolism quantification method based on unilateral ICA image derived input function by hybrid PET/MR in ischemic cerebrovascular disease. IEEE J Biomed Health Inform, 2022, 26(10): 5122-5129.

[6] CUI B, SHAN Y, ZHANG T, et al.Crossed cerebellar diaschisis-related supratentorial hemodynamic and metabolic status measured by PET/MR in assessing postoperative prognosis in chronic ischemic cerebrovascular disease patients with bypass surgery.Ann Nucl Med, 2022；36(9): 812-822.

[7] SONG S, SHAN Y, WANG L, et al.MGMT promoter methylation status shows no effect on [^{18}F] FET uptake and CBF in gliomas: a stereotactic image-based histological validation study.Eur Radiol, 2022, 32(8): 5577-5587.

[8] LI W, ZHAO Z, LIU M, et al.Multimodal classification of Alzheimer's disease and amnestic mild

cognitive impairment: integrated ^{18}F-FDG PET and DTI study.J Alzheimers Dis, 2022, 85(3): 1063-1075.

[9] ZANG Z, SONG T, LI J, et al.Modulation effect of substantia nigra iron deposition and functional connectivity on putamen glucose metabolism in Parkinson's disease.Hum Brain Mapp, 2022, 43(12): 3735-3744.

[10] ZANG Z, SONG T, LI J, et al.Simultaneous PET/fMRI revealed increased motor area input to subthalamic nucleus in Parkinson's disease.Cereb Cortex, 2022, 33(1): 167-175.

[11] SHAN Y, WANG Z, SONG S, et al.Integrated positron emission tomography/magnetic resonance imaging for resting-state functional and metabolic imaging in human brain: what is correlated and what is impacted.Front Neurosci, 2022, 16: 824152.

[12] TIAN D, YANG H, LI Y, et al.The effect of Q. Clear reconstruction on quantification and spatial resolution of ^{18}F-FDG PET in simultaneous PET/MR.EJNMMI Phys, 2022, 9(1): 1.

[13] DONG QY, LI TR, JIANG XY, et al.Glucose metabolism in the right middle temporal gyrus could be a potential biomarker for subjective cognitive decline: a study of a Han population.Alzheimers Res Ther, 2021, 13(1): 74.

[14] CHEN Y, WANG J, CUI C, et al.Evaluating the association between brain atrophy, hypometabolism, and cognitive decline in Alzheimer's disease: a PET/MRI study.Aging (Albany NY), 2021, 13(5): 7228-7246.

[15] DU W, DING C, JIANG J, et al.Women exhibit lower global left frontal cortex connectivity among cognitively unimpaired elderly individuals: a pilot study from SILCODE.J Alzheimers Dis, 2021, 83(2): 653-663.

[16] CHU M, LIU L, WANG J, et al.Investigating the roles of anterior cingulate in behavioral variant frontotemporal dementia: a PET/MRI study.J Alzheimers Dis, 2021, 84(4): 1771-1779.

[17] DING C, DU W, ZHANG Q, et al.Coupling relationship between glucose and oxygen metabolisms to differentiate preclinical Alzheimer's disease and normal individuals.Hum Brain Mapp, 2021, 42(15): 5051-5062.

[18] CHENG Y, SONG S, WEI Y, et al.Glioma imaging by O-(2-^{18}F-Fluoroethyl)-L-tyrosine PET and diffusion-weighted MRI and correlation with molecular phenotypes, validated by PET/MR-guided biopsies.Front Oncol, 2021, 11: 743655.

[19] SONG S, WANG L, YANG H, et al.Static ^{18}F-FET PET and DSC-PWI based on hybrid PET/MR for the prediction of gliomas defined by IDH and 1p/19q status.Eur Radiol, 2021, 31(6): 4087-4096.

[20] GUO K, CUI B, SHANG K, et al.Assessment of localization accuracy and postsurgical prediction of simultaneous ^{18}F-FDG PET/MRI in refractory epilepsy patients.Eur Radiol, 2021, 31(9): 6974-6982.

[21] LI X, YU T, REN Z, et al.Localization of the epileptogenic zone by multimodal neuroimaging and high-frequency oscillation.Front Hum Neurosci, 2021, 15: 677840.

[22] WANG J, SUN H, CUI B, et al.The relationship among glucose metabolism, cerebral blood flow, and functional activity: a hybrid PET/fMRI study.Mol Neurobiol, 2021, 58(6): 2862-2873.

[23] CUI B, ZHANG T, MA Y, et al.Simultaneous PET-MRI imaging of cerebral blood flow and glucose metabolism in the symptomatic unilateral internal carotid artery/middle cerebral artery steno-occlusive disease.Eur J Nucl Med Mol Imaging, 2020, 47(7): 1668-1677.

[24] YAN S, ZHENG C, CUI B, et al.Multiparametric imaging hippocampal neurodegeneration and functional connectivity with simultaneous PET/MRI in Alzheimer's disease.Eur J Nucl Med Mol Imaging, 2020, 47(10): 2440-2452.

[25] LI TR, WU Y, JIANG JJ, et al.Radiomics analysis of magnetic resonance imaging facilitates the identification of preclinical Alzheimer's disease: an exploratory study.Front Cell Dev Biol, 2020, 8: 605734.

[26] LU H, JING D, CHEN Y, et al.Metabolic changes detected by ^{18}F-FDG PET in the preclinical stage of familial Creutzfeldt-Jakob disease.J Alzheimers Dis, 2020, 77(4): 1513-1521.

[27] SONG S, CHENG Y, MA J, et al.Simultaneous FET-PET and contrast-enhanced MRI based on hybrid PET/MR improves delineation of tumor spatial biodistribution in gliomas: a biopsy validation study. Eur J Nucl Med Mol Imaging, 2020, 47(6): 1458-1467.

[28] WANG J, SHAN Y, DAI J, et al.Altered coupling between resting-state glucose metabolism and functional activity in epilepsy.Ann Clin Transl Neurol, 2020, 7(10): 1831-1842.

[29] ZHANG L, SONG T, MENG Z, et al.Correlation between apparent diffusion coefficients and metabolic parameters in hypopharyngeal squamous cell carcinoma: A prospective study with integrated PET/ MRI.Eur J Radiol, 2020, 129: 109070.

[30] HUANG C, SONG T, MUKHERJI SK, et al.Comparative study between integrated positron emission tomography/magnetic resonance and positron emission tomography/computed tomography in the T and N Staging of hypopharyngeal cancer: an initial result.J Comput Assist Tomogr, 2020, 44(4): 540-545.

[31] WANG YH, AN Y, FAN XT, et al.Comparison between simultaneously acquired arterial spin labeling and ^{18}F-FDG PET in mesial temporal lobe epilepsy assisted by a PET/MR system and SEEG. Neuroimage Clin, 2018, 19: 824-830.

[32] SONG T, CUI B, YANG H, et al.Diffusion-weighted imaging as a part of PET/MR for small lesion detection in patients with primary abdominal and pelvic cancer, with or without TOF reconstruction technique.Abdom Radiol (NY), 2019, 44(7): 2639-2647.

[33] SHANG K, WANG J, FAN X, et al.Clinical value of hybrid TOF-PET/MR imaging-based multiparametric imaging in localizing seizure focus in patients with MRI-negative temporal lobe epilepsy.AJNR Am J Neuroradiol, 2018, 39(10): 1791-1798.

[34] HE Y, XIE F, YE J, et al.1-(4-[^{18}F] Fluorobenzyl)-4-[(tetrahydrofuran-2-yl)methyl] piperazine: a novel suitable radioligand with low lipophilicity for imaging σ 1 receptors in the brain.J Med Chem, 2017, 60(10): 4161-4172.

[35] SHANG K, CUI B, MA J, et al.Clinical evaluation of whole-body oncologic PET with time-of-flight and point-spread function for the hybrid PET/MR system.Eur J Radiol, 2017, 93: 70-75.

2.SCI 收录文章研究简介及原文首页

📋 **文章 1**

GUO K, WANG J, WANG Z, et al.Morphometric analysis program and quantitative positron emission tomography in presurgical localization in MRI-negative epilepsies: a simultaneous PET/MRI study.Eur J Nucl Med Mol Imaging, 2022, 49(6): 1930-1938.

【研究简介】

研究背景：MRI 阴性的局灶性癫痫患者识别癫痫区（epileptogenic zone，EZ）有助于制订手术治疗方案，发作间期 ^{18}F-FDG PET 局灶性低代谢病灶与 EZ 相关，基于统计参数图（statistical parametric mapping，SPM）的定量 PET（QPET）分析提供客观数据，MRI 形态测量分析方法（morphometric analysis program，MAP）技术可以显示 MRI 阴性局灶性皮质发表不良的细微异常，有助于提高 ^{18}F-FDG PET 的病灶定位。

资料与方法：71 例 MRI 阴性的癫痫患者采用一体化 PET/MR 同步获得 ^{18}F-FDG PET 和 MRI 图像，以手术切除病理学诊断和随访术后癫痫发作是否缓解（Engel Ⅰ 级和 Engel Ⅱ - Ⅳ级）作为定位"金标准"，分析和比较 MAP、QPET、QPET/MAP 和 QPET+MAP 的定位效能，并分析影像定位与手术切除部位一致性与患者预后是否相关。

研究结果：71 例 MRI 阴性的癫痫患者 MAP 的定位灵敏性、特异度、PPV 和 NPV 分别为 64.4%、69.2%、78.3% 和 52.9%。QPET 的定位灵敏性、特异度、PPV、NPV 分别为 73.3%、65.4%、78.6% 和 58.6%。与单独的 QPET 和 MAP 相比，QPET+MAP 定位 EZ 的灵敏性降低（53.3%）、特异度增加（88.5%），而 QPET/MAP 定位的灵敏性增加（86.7%）但特异度降低（46.2%）（图 1-1-1）。当 MAP、QPET、QPET/MAP 和 QPET+MAP 确定的 EZ 与手术切除部位一致时，患者预后良好，QPET+MAP 表现最佳（$P < 0.001$）（图 1-1-2）。

研究结论：一体化 PET/MR 同机扫描获得 ^{18}F-FDG 和 MRI 图像，QPET+MAP 可以提高诊断测试的特异度，而 QPET/MAP 可以增加诊断测试的灵敏性，联合 PET/MR 扫描及图像后处理技术定位致痫灶与手术切除范围一致时，手术效果良好。

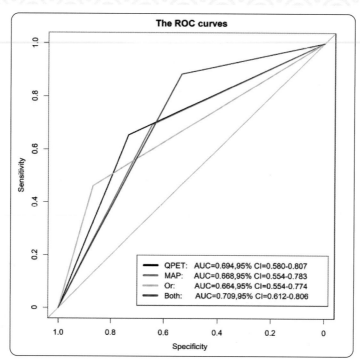

图 1-1-1　MAP、QPET、QPET/MAP 和 QPET+MAP 图像定位癫痫患者致痫灶的 ROC 图

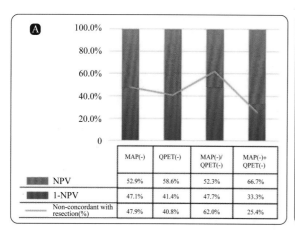

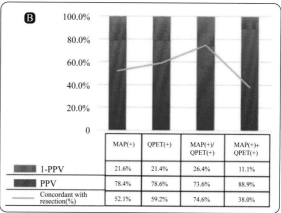

图 1-1-2　癫痫患者 QPET 和 MAP 定位致痫灶结果与临床预后的相关性

European Journal of Nuclear Medicine and Molecular Imaging
https://doi.org/10.1007/s00259-021-05657-w

ORIGINAL ARTICLE

Morphometric analysis program and quantitative positron emission tomography in presurgical localization in MRI-negative epilepsies: a simultaneous PET/MRI study

Kun Guo[1] · Jingjuan Wang[1] · Zhenming Wang[1] · Yihe Wang[2] · Bixiao Cui[1] · Guoguang Zhao[2] · Jie Lu[1,3]

Received: 28 August 2021 / Accepted: 12 December 2021
© The Author(s), under exclusive licence to Springer-Verlag GmbH Germany, part of Springer Nature 2021

Abstract

Purpose To evaluate morphometric analysis program (MAP) and quantitative positron emission tomography (QPET) in epileptogenic zone (EZ) identification using a simultaneous positron emission tomography/magnetic resonance imaging (PET/MRI) system in MRI-negative epilepsies.

Methods Seventy-one localization-related MRI-negative epilepsies who underwent preoperative simultaneous PET/MRI examination and surgical resection were enrolled retrospectively. MAP was performed on a T1-weighted volumetric sequence, and QPET was analyzed using statistical parametric mapping (SPM) with comparison to age- and gender-matched normal controls. The sensitivity, specificity, positive predictive value (PPV), and negative predictive value (NPV) of MAP, QPET, MAP + QPET, and MAP/QPET in EZ localization were assessed. The correlations between surgical outcome and modalities concordant with cortical resection were analyzed.

Results Forty-five (63.4%) patients had Engel I seizure outcomes. The sensitivity, specificity, PPV, and NPV of MAP were 64.4%, 69.2%, 78.3%, and 52.9%, respectively. The sensitivity, specificity, PPV, NPV of QPET were 73.3%, 65.4%, 78.6%, and 58.6%, respectively. MAP + QPET, defined as two tests concordant with cortical resection, had reduced sensitivity (53.3%) but increased specificity (88.5%) relative to individual tests. MAP/QPET, defined as one or both tests concordant with cortical resection, had increased sensitivity (86.7%) but reduced specificity (46.2%) relative to individual tests. The regions determined by MAP, QPET, MAP + QPET, or MAP/QPET concordant with cortical resection were significantly associated with the seizure-free outcome.

Conclusion QPET has a superior sensitivity than MAP, while the combined MAP + QPET obtained from a simultaneous PET/MRI scanner may improve the specificity of the diagnostic tests in EZ localization coupled with the preferable surgical outcome in MRI-negative epilepsies.

Keywords Epilepsy · PET/MRI · MAP · Quantitative PET · Localization

Kun Guo and Jingjuan Wang contributed equally to this article

This article is part of the Topical Collection on Neurology

✉ Jie Lu
imaginglu@hotmail.com

1 Department of Radiology and Nuclear Medicine, Xuanwu Hospital Capital Medical University, Beijing 100053, China

2 Department of Neurosurgery, Xuanwu Hospital, Capital Medical University, Beijing, China

3 Key Laboratory of Magnetic Resonance Imaging and Brain Informatics, Beijing, China

Introduction

For magnetic resonance imaging (MRI)-negative intractable focal epilepsy patients, identifying a subtle abnormality that was previously undetected helps to provide an opportunity for surgical treatment. Longitudinal studies in MRI-negative focal epilepsy patients showed that resected surgery offers the potential for long-term seizure control [1, 2], which encouraged researchers to use postprocessing imaging analysis to identify more potential epileptogenic zone (EZ).

In morphometric analysis program (MAP), one of many MRI postprocessing imaging analyses, several researchers have demonstrated that MAP could be helped detect subtle abnormalities of focal cortical dysplasia (FCD) in

Published online: 23 December 2021

WANG J, YANG H, CUI B, et al.Effects of MRI protocols on brain FDG uptake in simultaneous PET/MR imaging.Eur J Nucl Med Mol Imaging, 2022, 49(8): 2812-2820.

【研究简介】

研究背景： 一体化 ^{18}F-FDG PET/MR 成像技术可以同时获取代谢、功能和组织信息，但 MRI 扫描可能会对 PET 成像造成潜在影响，包括电磁波效应及生理性影响等，这些影响的相关研究较少。

资料与方法： 本研究设计了 3 组成像协议比较 MRI 扫描在不同阶段对 ^{18}F-FDG 摄取的影响（图 1-1-3），分别是 continuous MRI——全程 MRI 和 PET 同步扫描；late MRI-MRI 和 PET 扫描始于 ^{18}F-FDG 注射后 40 分钟；no MRI——全程无 MRI 扫描；PET 扫描始于 ^{18}F-FDG 注射后 40 分钟。将 70 例健康志愿者分组为 continuous/late/no MRI=30/30/10 例，3 组被试年龄及性别无显著差异。另外，10 例癫痫患者采用 continuous MRI 评估 MRI 扫描对 ^{18}F-FDG PET 的影响。

研究结果： 研究发现 continuous MRI 扫描 ^{18}F-FDG 的 SUV（standard uptake value）显著高于 late MRI（$P < 0.001$）和 no MRI（$P=0.041$），但 late MRI 和 no MRI 的 SUV 无显著差异（$P=0.096$）。continuous MRI 扫描在初级听觉皮层、壳核 SUVR（standard uptake value ratio）较高，枕叶和小脑区 SUVR 较低（图 1-1-4）。此外，癫痫患者大脑代谢区域可能受 MRI 扫描的影响（图 1-1-5）。

研究结论： 一体化 PET/MR 扫描的 MRI 扫描对 ^{18}F-FDG PET 摄取存在影响，^{18}F-FDG 注射后立即进行 MRI 扫描时最显著，但注射 ^{18}F-FDG 40 分钟后再进行 MRI 扫描，影响基本可以忽略，因此临床患者的 PET/MR 研究需要考虑 MRI 扫描的影响。

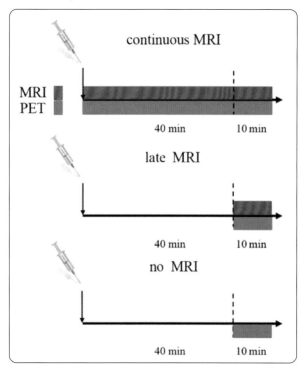

图 1-1-3　continuous/late/no MRI 3 种成像扫描方案示意

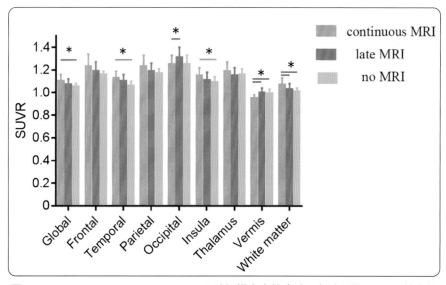

图 1-1-4　continuous/late/no MRI 3 种扫描方案的全脑和各脑区的 SUVR 值比较

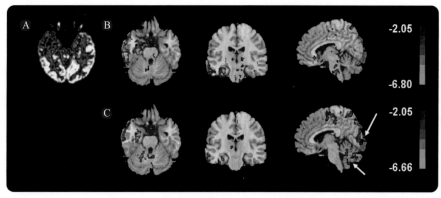

图 1-1-5　颞叶癫痫患者 SUVR 与健康组比较

European Journal of Nuclear Medicine and Molecular Imaging
https://doi.org/10.1007/s00259-022-05703-1

ORIGINAL ARTICLE

Effects of MRI protocols on brain FDG uptake in simultaneous PET/MR imaging

Jingjuan Wang[1] · Hongwei Yang[1] · Bixiao Cui[1] · Baoci Shan[2,3] · Jie Lu[1,4]

Received: 22 July 2021 / Accepted: 23 January 2022
© The Author(s), under exclusive licence to Springer-Verlag GmbH Germany, part of Springer Nature 2022

Abstract

Purpose To investigate the potential effects of MRI protocols on brain FDG uptake in simultaneous PET/MR imaging.

Methods Seventy healthy subjects and ten patients with temporal lobe epilepsy were enrolled. Healthy subjects were divided to three groups to undergo different PET/MR scan protocols: "continuous MRI" with MRI stimulation presented during the whole scan, "late MRI" with MRI stimulation started after 40 min glucose uptake, and "no MRI" without MRI stimulation at all. Region-wise and voxel-wise differences in FDG uptake among the three protocols were compared. All epilepsy patients were scanned with the "continuous MRI" scan protocol. The effects of MRI protocol stimulation on pathological interpretation were evaluated.

Results Highest global averaged metabolism was found in the normal dataset with continuous MRI scan protocol ($P < 0.05$). Specifically, we observed higher FDG uptake in the primary auditory cortex, putamen, and lower FDG uptake in the occipital lobe and cerebellum during the "continuous MRI" scan protocol. However, MRI protocol stimulation after 40 min glucose uptake did not cause any significant differences in FDG uptake. Respectively compared to the normal dataset, patients with epilepsy showed consistent hypometabolism in the temporal lobe. Besides, significant metabolism changes in the primary auditory cortex, vermis, and occipital lobe were found in the "late MRI" protocol.

Conclusion The effects of MRI protocol on brain FDG uptake were varied. The effects, including from other practical setting, were conspicuous for scans where MRI protocol started immediately after glucose uptake, but would dramatically decrease to negligible 40 min later. Hence, it would be necessary for pathology studies to collect data from a normal control group using the same scan protocol for unbiased evaluation.

Keywords PET/MR · Glucose metabolism · Physiological interference · MRI acoustic noise · Brain

This article is part of the Topical Collection on Technology

✉ Baoci Shan
shanbc@ihep.ac.cn

✉ Jie Lu
imaginglu@hotmail.com

1   Department of Radiology and Nuclear Medicine, Xuanwu Hospital Capital Medical University, 45 Changchun Street, Xicheng District, Beijing 100053, China

2   Engineering Research Center of Radiographic Techniques and Equipment, Institute of High Energy Physics, Chinese Academy of Sciences, Beijing 100049, China

3   School of Nuclear Science and Technology, University of Chinese Academy of Sciences, Beijing, China

4   Key Laboratory of Magnetic Resonance Imaging and Brain Informatics, Beijing, China

Introduction

Simultaneous ^{18}F-fluorodeoxyglucose positron emission tomography/magnetic resonance imaging (^{18}F-FDG PET/MRI) has been increasingly applied in clinical and scientific research in the recent decade because of its superiority in simultaneously acquiring both the glucose metabolic information and the functional and structural information [1]. Multiparametric PET/MR quantitative imaging has played important roles in localizing epileptogenic zone [2], assessing the surgical outcomes [3, 4], grading of tumors [5], et al. In addition, structural MRI provides the opportunity for methodological novelty, for example, PET motion tracking [6], attenuation estimation [7], partial volume effects correction [8], and image-based arterial input function estimation [9].

Published online: 07 February 2022

 Springer

GUO K, WANG J, CUI B, et al.[^{18}F] FDG PET/MRI and magnetoencephalography may improve presurgical localization of temporal lobe epilepsy.Eur Radiol, 2022, 32(5): 3024-3034.

【研究简介】

研究背景：颞叶癫痫（temporal lobe epilepsy，TLE）是最常见的癫痫类型。对于药物难治性颞叶癫痫患者，外科手术可显著减少癫痫发作或使患者无癫痫发作。癫痫手术的成功取决于术前精准识别致痫区。^{18}F-FDG PET/MR 多参数成像可为致痫区定位提供更高的灵敏性，但特异度有限。脑磁图（magnetoencephalography，MEG）是临床非侵袭性致痫区定位诊断技术，具有高时空分辨率，对棘波精确定位，但 MEG 在颞叶内侧较深区域的定位具有挑战性，因此多模态信息有助于定位颞叶癫痫患者的致痫区。

资料与方法：本研究纳入 73 例接受 PET/MR 和 MEG 检查的颞叶癫痫患者，同时招募 20 例健康志愿者。^{18}F-FDG PET/MR 图像由两名影像医师阅片定位致痫区，其中 ^{18}F-FDG PET 图像运用 SPM 软件处理定位低代谢灶。MEG 峰源融合至 T_1WI 上定位致痫区。以手术切除病理和术后 1 年随访结果为"金标准"，评估 ^{18}F-FDG PET/MR、MEG 和联合 ^{18}F-FDG PET/MR/MEG 定位致痫区的临床价值。

研究结果：在 73 例颞叶癫痫患者中，46.6% 的患者 MRI 明确显示结构异常，且与手术切除一致；67.1% 的患者 SPM-PET 低代谢区与手术切除一致，进行 MRI 配准后一致性增加至 82.2%；71.2% 的患者 MEG 定位结果与手术切除一致；94.5% 的患者使用联合 ^{18}F-FDG PET/MR/MEG 可准确定位致痫区（图 1-1-6），灵敏性、特异度和准确度分别为 100%、44.4% 和 93.2%，与手术切除的一致性显著优于单独 PET/MR 或 MEG，PET/MR/MEG 定位结果与手术切除一致的患者预后良好（表 1-1-1）。

研究结论：^{18}F-FDG PET/MR 与 MEG 联合可提高颞叶癫痫患者致痫区的检出率，从而指导手术决策。

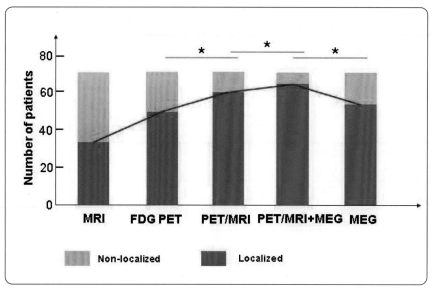

图 1-1-6 　MRI、[18]F-FDG PET、PET/MRI、PET/MRI/MEG、MEG 定位致病区的患者数量

表 1-1-1 　内侧颞叶癫痫患者手术结果与 PET/MRI、MEG、PET/MRI/MEG 与皮质切除一致 / 不一致的相关性分析

	Engel Ⅰ（n=64）	Engel Ⅱ~Ⅳ（n=9）	P
MRI			0.002
Concordant with resection	34	0	
Non-Concordant with resection	30	9	
^{18}F-FDG PET			0.005
Concordant with resection	47	2	
Non-Concordant with resection	17	7	
^{18}F-FDG PET/MRI			< 0.001
Concordant with resection	58	2	
Non-Concordant with resection	6	7	
^{18}F-FDG PET/MRI/MEG			< 0.001
Concordant with resection	64	5	
Non-Concordant with resection	0	4	
MEG			0.022
Concordant with resection	49	3	
Non-Concordant with resection	15	6	

European Radiology
https://doi.org/10.1007/s00330-021-08336-4

NUCLEAR MEDICINE

[18F]FDG PET/MRI and magnetoencephalography may improve presurgical localization of temporal lobe epilepsy

Kun Guo[1] · Jingjuan Wang[1] · Bixiao Cui[1] · Yihe Wang[2] · Yaqin Hou[1] · Guoguang Zhao[2] · Jie Lu[1,3]

Received: 29 April 2021 / Revised: 10 August 2021 / Accepted: 25 August 2021
© European Society of Radiology 2021, corrected publication 2022

Abstract

Objectives To evaluate the clinical value of the combination of [18F]FDG PET/MRI and magnetoencephalography (MEG) ([18F]FDG PET/MRI/MEG) in localizing the epileptogenic zone (EZ) in temporal lobe epilepsy (TLE) patients.

Methods Seventy-three patients with localization-related TLE who underwent [18F]FDG PET/MRI and MEG were enrolled retrospectively. PET/MRI images were interpreted by two radiologists; the focal hypometabolism on PET was identified using statistical parametric mapping (SPM). MEG spike sources were co-registered onto T1-weighted sequence and analyzed by Neuromag software. The clinical value of [18F]FDG PET/MRI, MEG, and PET/MRI/MEG in locating the EZ was assessed using cortical resection and surgical outcomes as criteria. The correlations between surgical outcomes and modalities concordant or non-concordant with cortical resection were analyzed.

Results For 46.6% (34/73) of patients, MRI showed definitely structural abnormality concordant with surgical resection. SPM results of [18F]FDG PET showed focal temporal lobe hypometabolism concordant with surgical resection in 67.1% (49/73) of patients, while the concordant cases increased to 82.2% (60/73) patients with simultaneous MRI co-registration. MEG was concordant with surgical resection in 71.2% (52/73) of patients. The lobar localization was defined in 94.5% (69/73) of patients by the [18F]FDG PET/MRI/MEG. The results of PET/MRI/MEG concordance with surgical resection were significantly higher than that of PET/MRI or MEG ($\chi^2 = 13.948$, $p < 0.001$; $\chi^2 = 5.393$, $p = 0.020$). The results of PET/MRI/MEG cortical resection concordance with surgical outcome were shown to be better than PET/MRI or MEG ($\chi^2 = 6.695$, $p = 0.012$; $\chi^2 = 16.991$, $p < 0.0001$).

Conclusions Presurgical evaluation by [18F]FDG PET/MRI/MEG could improve the identification of the EZ in TLE and may further guide surgical decision-making.

Key Points
- *Lobar localization was defined in 94.5% of patients by the [18F]FDG PET/MRI/MEG.*
- *The results of PET/MRI/MEG concordance with surgical resection were significantly higher than that of PET/MRI or MEG alone.*
- *The results of PET/MRI/MEG cortical resection concordance with surgical outcome were shown to be better than that of PET/MRI or MEG alone.*

Keywords Epilepsy · Positron emission tomography · Magnetic resonance imaging · Magnetoencephalography · Surgery

Abbreviations

[18F]FDG	18F-Fluorodeoxyglucose
EZ	Epileptogenic zone
FCD	Focal cortical dysplasia
HS	Hippocampal sclerosis
MEG	Magnetoencephalography
MRI	Magnetic resonance imaging
PET	Positron emission tomography
SPM	Statistical parametric mapping
TLE	Temporal lobe epilepsy

Kun Guo and Jingjuan Wang contributed equally to this article.

✉ Jie Lu
imaginglu@hotmail.com

1 Department of Radiology and Nuclear Medicine, Xuanwu Hospital Capital Medical University, Beijing 100053, China

2 Department of Neurosurgery, Xuanwu Hospital, Capital Medical University, Beijing, China

3 Key Laboratory of Magnetic Resonance Imaging and Brain Informatics, Beijing, China

Springer

WANG J, GUO K, CUI B, et al.Individual [^{18}F] FDG PET and functional MRI based on simultaneous PET/MRI may predict seizure recurrence after temporal lobe epilepsy surgery.Eur Radiol, 2022, 32(6): 3880-3888.

【研究简介】

研究背景： 颞叶癫痫是最常见的局灶性癫痫类型，海马硬化（hippocampal sclerosis，HS）是内侧颞叶癫痫（medial temporal lobe epilepsy，mTLE）的常见病理特征。前颞叶切除术（anterior temporal lobectomy，ATL）是难治性 mTLE-HS 的主要治疗方法，但 30% 的患者于术后 1 年出现癫痫发作，可能与脑内致痫网络有关，因此术前评价致痫网络有助于预测手术结果，改善患者预后。

资料与方法： 本研究纳入 39 例单侧 mTLE-HS 行前颞叶切除术患者，一体化 ^{18}F-FDG PET/MR 可同时获得发作间期葡萄糖代谢和功能 MRI（functional magnetic resonance imaging，fMRI）图像的低频波动振幅（amplitude of low frequency fluctuation，ALFF）归一化指数 fALFF，以量化癫痫活动网络，并使用机器学习预测术分析 ^{18}F-FDG PET 和 fALFF 异常与 mTLE-HS 患者的手术结果之间的关系（图 1-1-7）。

研究结果： 39 例单侧 mTLE-HS 行前颞叶切除术患者，根据术后 1 年随访结果分成癫痫复发（$n=17$）和无癫痫发作（$n=22$）两组，其中 90.9%（20/22）无癫痫发作患者的同侧海马网络出现 FDG 代谢异常，而 81.8%（18/22）显示 fALFF 异常。而所有癫痫复发患者均显示同侧海马低代谢，41.2%（7/17）对侧海马网络低代谢，82.3%（14/17）同侧海马 fALFF 信号异常（图 1-1-8）。机器学习分类模型显示对侧海马网络 ^{18}F-FDG、fALFF 异常和发病年龄可有效预测术后癫痫复发。在验证集中，^{18}F-FDG 和 fALFF 预测模型的效能 [ROC 曲线的曲线下面积（area under the curve，AUC）=0.905] 高于单独 ^{18}F-FDG（AUC=0.762）和 fALFF（AUC=0.810）（图 1-1-9）。

研究结论： 基于一体化 PET/MR 获得的 ^{18}F-FDG 代谢信息、fMRI 等多模态多参数优势，结合机器学习分类模型，可有效预测术后癫痫复发，为颞叶癫痫患者的预后改善提供更有针对性的治疗策略，进一步助力实现颞叶癫痫精准诊疗。

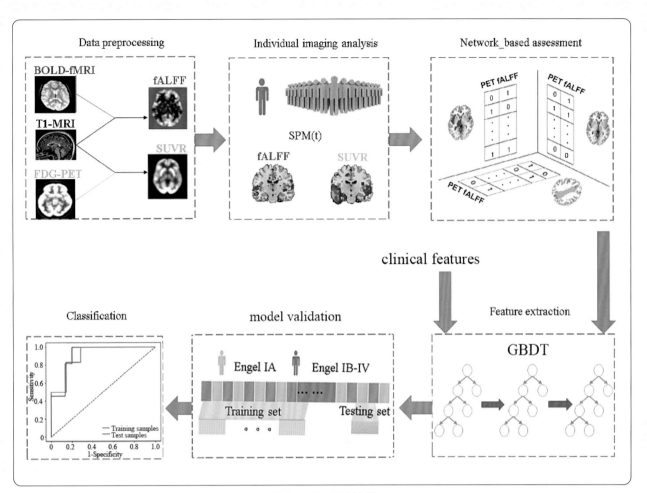

图 1-1-7 研究流程

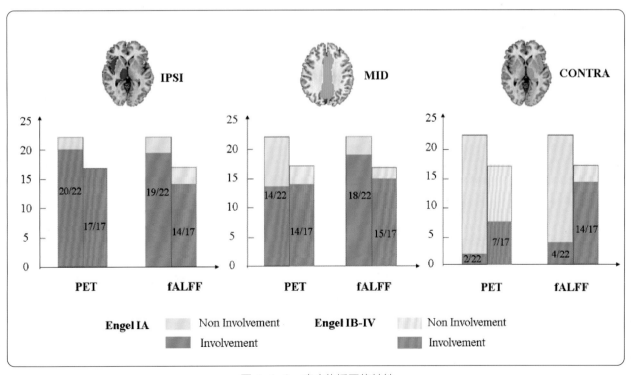

图 1-1-8 癫痫传播网络特性

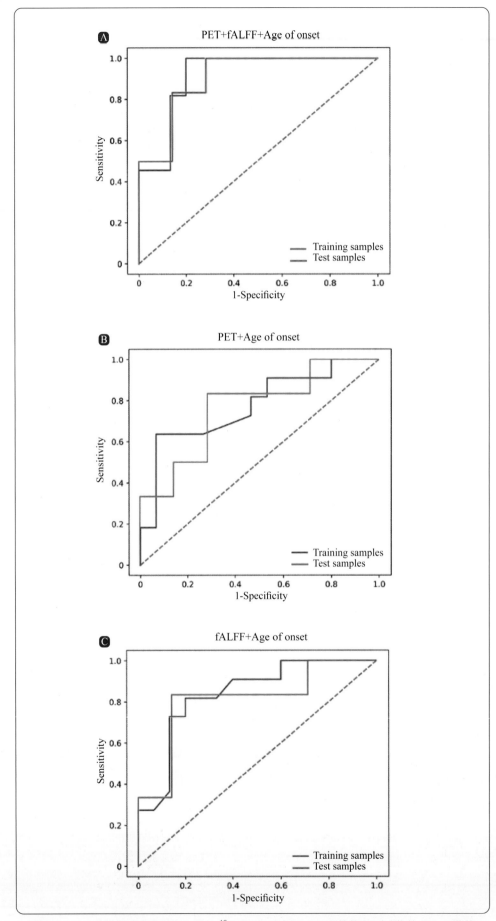

图 1-1-9　内侧颞叶癫痫患者一体化 ^{18}F-FDG PET/fMRI 训练集和测试集的 ROC 曲线

European Radiology
https://doi.org/10.1007/s00330-021-08490-9

NUCLEAR MEDICINE

Individual [18F]FDG PET and functional MRI based on simultaneous PET/MRI may predict seizure recurrence after temporal lobe epilepsy surgery

Jingjuan Wang[1] · Kun Guo[1] · Bixiao Cui[1] · Yaqin Hou[1] · Guoguang Zhao[2] · Jie Lu[1,3]

Received: 3 September 2021 / Revised: 21 October 2021 / Accepted: 28 November 2021
© The Author(s), under exclusive licence to European Society of Radiology 2021

Abstract

Objectives To investigate the individual measures of brain glucose metabolism, neural activity obtained from simultaneous [18F]FDG PET/MRI, and their association with surgical outcomes in medial temporal lobe epilepsy due to hippocampal sclerosis (mTLE-HS).

Methods Thirty-nine unilateral mTLE-HS patients who underwent anterior temporal lobectomy were classified as having completely seizure-free (Engel class IA; $n = 22$) or non-seizure-free (Engel class IB–IV; $n = 17$) outcomes at 1 year after surgery. Preoperative [18F]FDG PET and functional MRI (fMRI) were obtained from a simultaneous PET/MRI scanner, and individual glucose metabolism and fractional amplitude of low-frequency fluctuation (fALFF) were evaluated by standardizing these with respect to healthy controls. These abnormality measures and clinical data from each patient were incorporated into a machine learning framework (gradient boosting decision tree and logistic regression analysis) to estimate seizure recurrence. The predictive values of features were evaluated by the receiver operating characteristic (ROC) curve in the training and test cohorts.

Results The machine learning classification model showed [18F]FDG PET and fMRI variations in contralateral hippocampal network and age of onset identify unfavorable surgical outcomes effectively. In the validation dataset, the logistic regression model with [18F]FDG PET and fALFF obtained from simultaneous [18F]FDG PET/MRI gained the maximum area under the ROC curve of 0.905 for seizure recurrence, higher than 0.762 with 18[F]-FDG PET, and 0.810 with fALFF alone.

Conclusion Machine learning model suggests individual [18F]FDG PET and fMRI variations in contralateral hippocampal network based on 18[F]-FDG PET/MRI could serve as a potential biomarker of unfavorable surgical outcomes.

Key Points

- *Individual [18F]FDG PET and fMRI obtained from preoperative [18F]FDG PET/MR were investigated.*
- *Individual differences were further assessed based on a seizure propagation network.*
- *Machine learning can classify surgical outcomes with 90.5% accuracy.*

Keywords Temporal lobe epilepsy · Prognosis · Metabolism · Functional magnetic resonance imaging · Machine learning

Abbreviations

[18F]FDG	[18F]Fluorodeoxyglucose
ALFF	Amplitude of low-frequency fluctuation
ATL	Anterior temporal lobectomy
BOLD	Blood oxygen level–dependent
GBDT	Gradient boosting decision tree
HC	Healthy control
HS	Hippocampal sclerosis
MRI	Magnetic resonance imaging
PET	Positron emission tomography
ROC	Receiver operating characteristic
SPM	Statistical parametric mapping
TLE	Temporal lobe epilepsy

Jingjuan Wang and Kun Guo contributed equally to this work.

✉ Jie Lu
imaginglu@hotmail.com

1 Department of Radiology and Nuclear Medicine, Xuanwu Hospital Capital Medical University, Beijing 100053, China

2 Department of Neurosurgery, Xuanwu Hospital Capital Medical University, Beijing, China

3 Key Laboratory of Magnetic Resonance Imaging and Brain Informatics, Beijing, China

Published online: 13 January 2022

🙋 Springer

WANG M, CUI B, SHAN Y, et al.Non-invasive glucose metabolism quantification method based on unilateral ICA image derived input function by hybrid PET/MR in ischemic cerebrovascular disease.IEEE J Biomed Health Inform, 2022, 26(10): 5122-5129.

【研究简介】

研究背景：缺血性脑血管病（ischemic cerebrovascular disease，ICVD）是致死率较高的疾病之一，颅内 – 颅外动脉搭桥手术是缺血性脑血管病常用治疗方式之一，影像学在评价手术疗效中起着重要作用。脑葡萄糖代谢率（cerebral metabolic rate for glucose，CMRGlc）是评估脑葡萄糖代谢的有效定量指标，动态 ^{18}F-FDG PET 图像可进行非侵入性量化分析。本研究采用动态 ^{18}F-FDG PET/MR 基于图像衍生输入函数（image-derived input function，IDIF）的无创量化方法，探究缺血性脑血管病手术干预后 CMRGlc 的代谢变化。

资料与方法：本研究纳入 16 例健康者和 27 例接受搭桥手术的缺血性脑血管病患者，应用一体化 ^{18}F-FDG PET/MR 成像，包括 70 分钟的动态 PET 采集，用于分割颈动脉的磁共振血管成像（MR angiography，MRA）、勾画梗死区的结构图像和用于执行运动校正的 3D T1 成像。通过 Patlak 分析，使用具有部分体积校正的图像衍生输入函数创建体素 CMRGlc 图（图 1–1–10）；使用 50 ~ 60 分钟的 ^{18}F-FDG PET 计算 SUVR；提取 7 个感兴趣区（灰质、白质、大脑前动脉、大脑中动脉、大脑后动脉、基底动脉和小脑动脉区域）的 CMRGlc 值与 SUVR 值，比较患者术前和术后同侧和对侧差异。

研究结果：对照组 16 例健康者在双侧和单侧图像衍生输入函数测量之间的 CMRGlc 值无显著差异〔组内相关系数（intraclass correlation coefficient，ICC）：0.91 ~ 0.98〕。27 例缺血性脑血管病患者在手术干预后所有区域的 CMRGlc 值均显著增加（$P < 0.05$）（百分比变化：7.4% ~ 22.5%），相应 SUVR 值仅大脑后动脉和基底动脉区域存在显著差异（$P < 0.05$），CMRGlc 与美国国立卫生研究院卒中量表（National Institutes of Health Stroke Scale，NIHSS）评分显著相关（$r = -0.54$，$P=0.0041$）（图 1–1–11）。

研究结论：该研究表明通过图像衍生输入函数可无创实现缺血性脑血管病的脑葡萄糖代谢，对缺血性脑血管病患者的精准诊疗有重要临床意义。

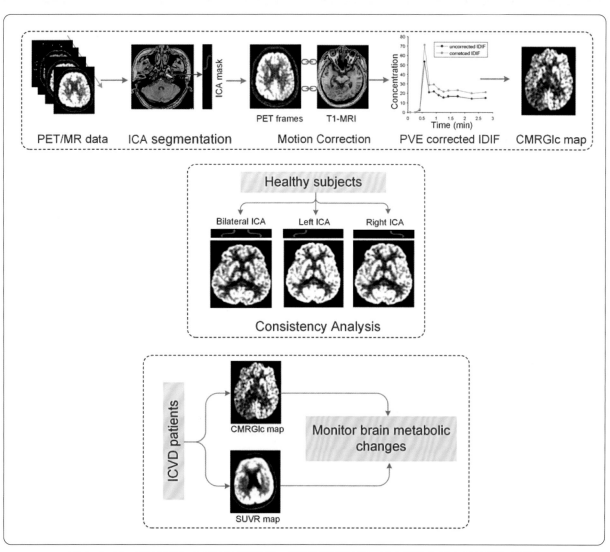

图 1-1-10　研究框架：图像后处理流程；健康对照组验证；缺血性脑血管病患者组临床测试

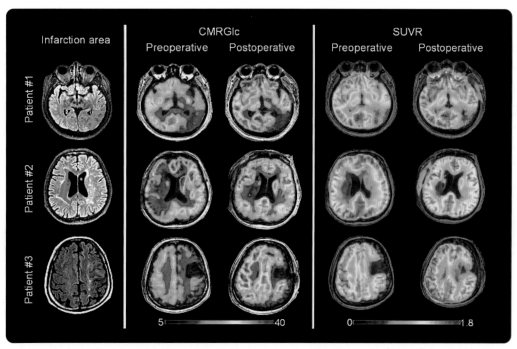

图 1-1-11　3 例缺血性脑血管病患者搭桥术前、术后的 CMRGlc 和 SUVR 比较

【附本文原文首页】

5122   IEEE JOURNAL OF BIOMEDICAL AND HEALTH INFORMATICS, VOL. 26, NO. 10, OCTOBER 2022   EMB   ComSoc   IEEE Signal Processing Society

Non-Invasive Glucose Metabolism Quantification Method Based on Unilateral ICA Image Derived Input Function by Hybrid PET/MR in Ischemic Cerebrovascular Disease

Min Wang ⓘ, Bixiao Cui, Yi Shan, Hongwei Yang, Zhuangzhi Yan ⓘ, Lalith Kumar Shiyam Sundar, Ian Alberts, Axel Rominger ⓘ, Thomas Wendler ⓘ, Kuangyu Shi, Yan Ma, Jiehui Jiang ⓘ, *Associate Member, IEEE*, and Jie Lu ⓘ

Abstract—The non-invasive quantification of the cerebral metabolic rate for glucose (CMRGlc) and the characterization of cerebral metabolism in the cerebrovascular territories are helpful in understanding ischemic cerebrovascular disease (ICVD). Firstly, we investigated a non-invasive quantification approach based on an image-derived input function (IDIF) in ICVD. Second, we studied the metabolic changes in CMRGlc after surgical intervention. We evaluated the hypothesis that the IDIF method based on the unilateral internal carotid artery could address challenges in ICVD quantification. The CMRGlc and standardized uptake value ratio (SUVR) were used to measure glucose metabolism activity. Healthy controls showed no significant differences in CMRGlc values between bilateral and unilateral IDIF measurements (intraclass correlation coefficient [ICC]: 0.91–0.98). Patients with ICVD showed significantly increased CMRGlc values after surgical intervention for all territories (percentage changes: 7.4%–22.5%). In contrast, SUVR showed minor differences between postoperative and preoperative patients, indicating that it was a poor biomarker for the diagnosis of ICVD. A significant association between CMRGlc and the National Institutes of Health Stroke Scale (NIHSS) scores was observed (r=-0.54). Our findings suggested that IDIF could be a valuable tool for CMRGlc quantification in patients with ICVD and may advance personalized precision interventions.

Index Terms—Glucose metabolism, ischemic cerebrovascular disease, noninvasive quantification, PET/MR, vascular territory.

Manuscript received 16 February 2022; revised 14 June 2022 and 11 July 2022; accepted 19 July 2022. Date of publication 22 July 2022; date of current version 5 October 2022. This work was supported in part by the National Natural Science Foundation of China under Grants 81974261, 82130058, and 82020108013, in part by the Xuanwu Hospital Science Program for Fostering Young Scholars under Grant QNPY2021037, in part by Shanghai Municipal Science and Technology Major Project under Grants 2017SHZDZX01 and 2018SHZDZX03, and in part by 111 Project under Grant D20031. *(Min Wang and Bixiao Cui contributed equally to this work.) (Corresponding author: Jiehui Jiang; Jie Lu.)*

Min Wang, Zhuangzhi Yan, and Jiehui Jiang are with the School of Life Science, Shanghai University, Shanghai 200444, China (e-mail: wmwin@shu.edu.cn; zzyan@shu.edu.cn; jiangjiehui@shu.edu.cn).

Bixiao Cui, Yi Shan, Hongwei Yang, and Jie Lu are with the Department of Radiology and Nuclear Medicine, Xuanwu Hospital, Capital Medical University, Key Laboratory of MRI and Brain Informatics, Beijing 100053, China (e-mail: bixiao1311@163.com; shanyiedu@hotmail.com; yhongw1993@163.com; imaginglu@hotmail.com).

Lalith Kumar Shiyam Sundar is with the Quantitative Imaging and Medical Physics, Center for Medical Physics and Biomedical Engineering, Medical University of Vienna, 1090 Vienna, Austria (e-mail: lalith.shiyamsundar@meduniwien.ac.at).

Ian Alberts, Axel Rominger, and Kuangyu Shi are with the Department of Nuclear Medicine Inselspital, Bern University Hospital, University of Bern, 3012 Bern, Switzerland (e-mail: ian.alberts@insel.ch; axel.rominger@insel.ch; kuangyu.shi@dbmr.unibe.ch).

Thomas Wendler is with the Chair for Computer-Aided Medical Procedures and Augmented Reality, Technical University of Munich, 85748 Munich, Germany (e-mail: wendler@tum.de).

Yan Ma is with the Department of Neurosurgery, Xuanwu Hospital, Capital Medical University, Beijing 100053, China (e-mail: leavesyan@sina.com).

This article has supplementary downloadable material available at https://doi.org/10.1109/JBHI.2022.3193190, provided by the authors.

Digital Object Identifier 10.1109/JBHI.2022.3193190

I. INTRODUCTION

ISCHEMIC cerebrovascular disease (ICVD) is a chronic, occlusive cerebrovascular disease which leads to a cascade of metabolic and molecular changes [1]. Progressive steno-occlusive in the terminal portion of the internal carotid artery (ICA) or middle cerebral artery (MCA) is one of the etiologies. The Ministry of Health China Stroke Prevention Project Committee (CSPPC) reported population screening for stroke risks is an important step in primary prevention [2]. The pathophysiological changes that lead to irreversible tissue damage and the progression of cerebral compensation based on brain-feeding arteries play a critical role in therapeutic interventions for ICVD. In recent years, superficial temporal artery-MCA (STA-MCA) bypass has been introduced as a surgical revascularization approach to potentially recover the supply of sufficient biochemical substrates and reduce stroke occurrence [3]. Previous studies focusing on brain metabolism changes showed that the post procedural asymmetry index values for cerebral blood flow and glucose metabolism were significantly lower after surgery than before surgery [4]–[7]. Therefore, quantifying these pathophysiological changes and regional metabolism is critical for monitoring clinical outcomes and recovery effects [8]–[10].

Maintaining normal brain homeostasis is an energy-consuming process that requires a continuous supply of glucose.

CUI B, SHAN Y, ZHANG T, et al.Crossed cerebellar diaschisis-related supratentorial hemodynamic and metabolic status measured by PET/MR in assessing postoperative prognosis in chronic ischemic cerebrovascular disease patients with bypass surgery.Ann Nucl Med, 2022；36(9): 812-822.

【研究简介】

研究背景： 脑缺血状态是搭桥手术的一个重要指标，血流动力学和葡萄糖代谢是评估脑缺血状态的重要因素。交叉性小脑失联络征（crossed cerebellar diaschisis，CCD）与幕上血流灌注和葡萄糖代谢减少有关，本研究探讨慢性症状性缺血性脑血管病患者在搭桥手术前 CCD 相关幕上血流和代谢状态与预后的关系。

资料与方法： 本研究纳入 24 例慢性缺血性脑血管病患者，在搭桥手术前接受一体化 PET/MR 检查。动脉自旋标记（arterial spin labelling，ASL）和 ^{18}F-FDG PET 分别可测量血流和代谢，通过 PET 图像区分 CCD 状态。搭桥手术前获得患侧血流量减低区、代谢减低区和血流代谢同步减低区（梗死区除外）的幕上不对称指数（asymmetry index，AI）和体积（图 1-1-12），使用 NIHSS 评价患者缺血状态；比较 CCD 阳性（CCD+）组和 CCD 阴性（CCD-）组之间的差异。

研究结果： 24 例慢性缺血性脑血管病患者，其中 14 例（58%）诊断为 CCD 阳性。CCD 阳性患者术前 NIHSS 和 mRS 评分显著高于 CCD 阴性［1.0（1.0）：0.0（1.0），$P=0.013$；1.0（1.5）：0.0（1.5），$P=0.048$］。术后 CCD 阳性的 NIHSS 和 mRS 评分显著下降（$P=0.011$；$P=0.008$，图 1-1-13）；幕上血流减低区脑血流量（cerebral blood flow，CBF）AI 值或体积无统计学差异（$P > 0.05$），CCD 阳性患者代谢减低区、血流代谢同步减低区代谢 AI 值更高和减低体积更大（均 $P < 0.01$）。术前 NIHSS 评分与代谢减低区代谢 AI 值（$r =0.621$，$P=0.001$）、代谢 AI 共同降低区域（$r=0.571$，$P=0.004$）显著相关（图 1-1-14）。

研究结论： 慢性缺血性脑血管病患者搭桥术后 CCD 阳性患者较 CCD 阴性患者血流和代谢改善显著，一体化 PET/MR CCD 相关幕上血流和代谢状态有助于指导个体化治疗。

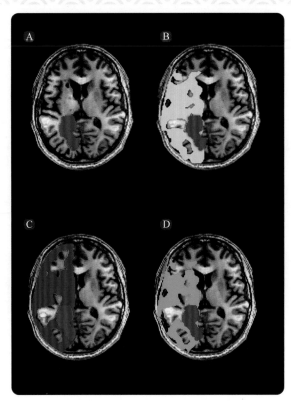

图 1-1-12　红色表示梗死区（图 A），黄色和蓝色分别表示血流减低区（图 B）和代谢减低区（图 C），绿色代表血流代谢同步减低区（图 D）

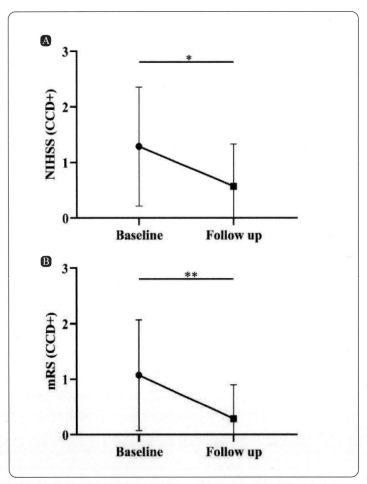

图 1-1-13　CCD 阳性组和 CCD 阴性组的基线和随访 NIHSS 和 mRS 评分比较（**$P < 0.01$，*$P < 0.05$）

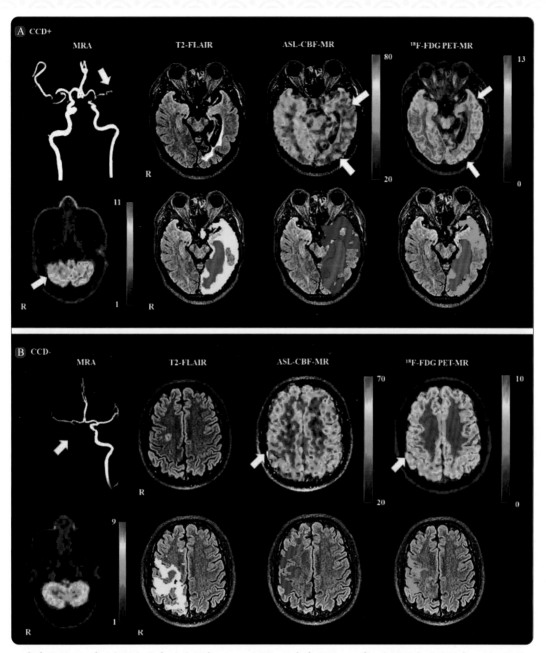

A. 患者男性, 44 岁, 左侧大脑中动脉闭塞, CCD 阳性; B. 患者男性, 62 岁, 右侧颈内动脉闭塞, CCD 阴性。
图像顺序依次为 MRA、T$_2$-FLAIR、ASL-CBF-MR、^{18}F-FDG PET-MR、小脑 ^{18}F-FDG PET、幕上感兴趣区(红色－幕上梗死区, 黄色－血流减低区, 蓝色－代谢减低区, 绿色－血流代谢同步减低区)。
图 1-1-14 CCD 阳性和 CCD 阴性患者 ^{18}F-FDG PET-MR 图像

首都医科大学宣武医院一体化 PET／MR 成果集

Annals of Nuclear Medicine
https://doi.org/10.1007/s12149-022-01766-0

ORIGINAL ARTICLE

Crossed cerebellar diaschisis-related supratentorial hemodynamic and metabolic status measured by PET/MR in assessing postoperative prognosis in chronic ischemic cerebrovascular disease patients with bypass surgery

Bixiao Cui[1,2] · Yi Shan[1,2] · Tianhao Zhang[3,4] · Yan Ma[5] · Bin Yang[5] · Hongwei Yang[1,2] · Liqun Jiao[5] · Baoci Shan[3,4,6] · Jie Lu[1,2]

Received: 10 March 2022 / Accepted: 6 June 2022
© The Author(s) 2022

Abstract

Objective Cerebral ischemic status is an indicator of bypass surgery. Both hemodynamics and glucose metabolism are significant factors for evaluating cerebral ischemic status. The occurrence of crossed cerebellar diaschisis (CCD) is influenced by the degree of supra-tentorial perfusion and glucose metabolism reduction. This study aimed to investigate the relationship between the CCD-related supra-tentorial blood flow and metabolic status before bypass surgery in patients with chronic and symptomatic ischemic cerebrovascular disease and the prognosis of surgery.

Methods Twenty-four participants with chronic ischemic cerebrovascular disease who underwent hybrid positron emission tomography (PET)/magnetic resonance (MR) before bypass surgery were included. Arterial spin labeling (ASL)-MR and FDG-PET were used to measure blood flow and metabolism, respectively. The PET images were able to distinguish CCD. The supratentorial asymmetry index (AI) and volume in the decreased blood flow region, decreased metabolism region and co-decreased region on the affected side, except for the infarct area, were respectively obtained before bypass surgery. The neurological status was determined using the National Institutes of Health Stroke Scale (NIHSS) and modified Rankin Scale (mRS) scores. Differences between CCD-positive (CCD +) and CCD-negative (CCD−) groups were investigated.

Results Fourteen (58%) of the 24 patients were diagnosed as CCD +. Before surgery, the NIHSS and mRS scores of the CCD + were significantly higher than those of the CCD− (1.0(1.0) vs. 0.0(1.0), $P = 0.013$; 1.0(1.5) vs. 0.0(1.5), $P = 0.048$). After the surgery, the NIHSS and mRS scores of the CCD + showed a significant decrease (0.0(1.0) to 0.0(0.0), $P = 0.011$; 0.0(0.5) to 0.0(0.0), $P = 0.008$). Significant differences were observed in the supra-tentorial decreased metabolism region (all $Ps \leq 0.05$) between the CCD + and CCD− groups, but no differences were observed in the preprocedural decreased supratentorial blood flow region ($P > 0.05$). The preprocedural NIHSS score was strongly correlated with the metabolism AI value in the decreased metabolism region ($r = 0.621$, $P = 0.001$) and the co-decreased region ($r = 0.571$, $P = 0.004$).

Conclusions Supratentorial blood flow and metabolism are important indicators of CCD. This study showed that CCD + patients benefited more from bypass surgery than CCD− patients. Staging based on CCD-related supra-tentorial blood flow and metabolic status by hybrid PET/MR may help to personalize treatment.

Keywords Positron emission tomography/Magnetic resonance · Glucose metabolism · Cerebral blood flow · Surgery · Crossed cerebellar diaschisis

Introduction

Data from a nationwide community-based study indicated that ischemic stroke accounts for approximately 70% of all incident stroke cases [1]. For patients with a clinical presentation of ischemic attacks and ineffective medical therapy, superficial temporal artery-middle cerebral artery

---

Bixiao Cui and Yi Shan contributed equally to this work.

✉ Jie Lu
imaginglu@hotmail.com

Extended author information available on the last page of the article

Published online: 05 July 2022

SONG S, SHAN Y, WANG L, et al.MGMT promoter methylation status shows no effect on [^{18}F] FET uptake and CBF in gliomas: a stereotactic image-based histological validation study.Eur Radiol, 2022, 32(8): 5577-5587.

【研究简介】

研究背景：脑胶质瘤的发病率为（5~8）/100万，是最常见的原发恶性脑肿瘤，治疗前的精准诊断能够指导制订个体化治疗方案，从而改善预后并进一步提高脑胶质瘤患者的生存率。6O-甲基鸟嘌呤-DNA甲基转移酶（O^6-methylguanine-DNA methyltransferase，MGMT）启动子甲基化作为胶质瘤重要分子标记物，逐渐应用于指导治疗决策。本研究利用O-（2-^{18}F-氟乙基）-L-酪氨酸{O-［2-（^{18}F）fluoroethyl］-L-tyrosine，^{18}F-FET}PET/MR探究胶质瘤MGMT启动子甲基化状态对^{18}F-FET PET代谢及ASL的CBF的影响，并采用点对点穿刺活检方式分析胶质瘤MGMT启动子状态与PET/ASL参数的联系。

资料与方法：回顾性地分析了57例经病理证实为脑胶质瘤患者，均接受了术前一体化^{18}F-FET PET/MR-ASL检查（图1-1-15）和穿刺活检。基于PET/MR图像对肿瘤区域进行体积分割，并计算PET的肿瘤-脑组织靶本比（tumor-to-brain ratio，TBR）和ASL的CBF平均值及最大值。

研究结果：基于PET/MR图像进行肿瘤分割的MGMT启动子甲基化与未甲基化胶质瘤的TBR$_{mean}$、TBR$_{max}$、CBF$_{mean}$和CBF$_{max}$均无显著差异（图1-1-16）。采取点对点穿刺活检的方法分析胶质瘤MGMT启动子甲基化状态对PET和ASL灌注的影响，发现11例穿刺活检患者中有3例肿瘤内不同穿刺部位的MGMT启动子甲基化状态不同；肿瘤MGMT启动子甲基化状态与^{18}F-FET PET摄取值及CBF值无相关，肿瘤MGMT启动子甲基化率与对应部位的TBR和CBF无相关（图1-1-17，图1-1-18）。

研究结论：研究证实基于一体化PET/MR的^{18}F-FET PET显像和ASL不能预测脑胶质瘤MGMT启动子甲基化状态，MGMT启动子甲基化状态与^{18}F-FET PET摄取和CBF无内在联系。

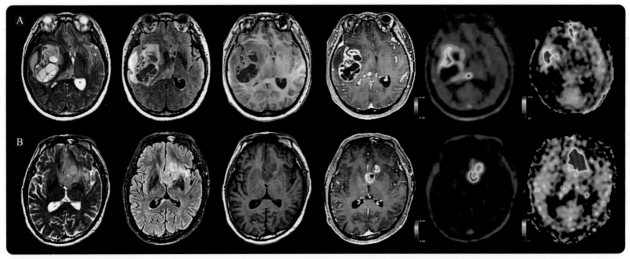

图 1-1-15　MGMT 启动子甲基化状态（A）和非甲基化状态（B）的胶质瘤患者的 T_2WI（第一列），FLAIR（第二列）、T_1WI（第三列）、T_1WI 增强（第四列）、^{18}F-FET PET（第五列）和 CBF（第六列）图像

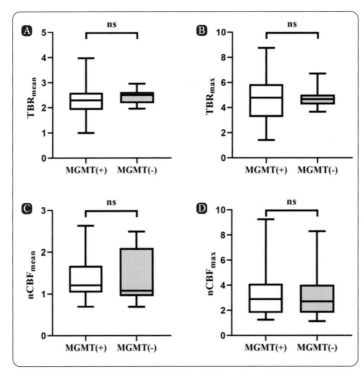

图 1-1-16　箱式图显示基于 PET/MR 图像进行肿瘤分割，MGMT 启动子甲基化组与未甲基化组胶质瘤的 TBR_{mean}、TBR_{max}、CBF_{mean} 和 CBF_{max} 均无显著差异

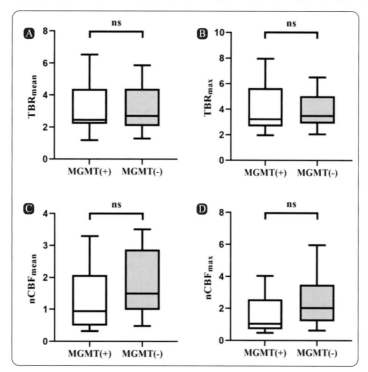

图 1-1-17　箱式图显示基于穿刺活检点对点影像 – 病理分析，MGMT 启动子甲基化与未甲基化胶质瘤的 TBR_{mean}、TBR_{max}、CBF_{mean} 和 CBF_{max} 均无显著差异

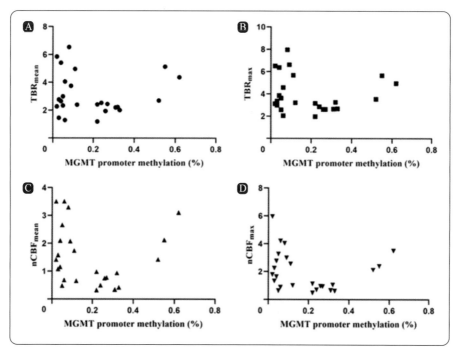

图 1-1-18　基于穿刺活检点对点影像 – 病理分析，MGMT 启动子甲基化率与其对应部位的 TBR 和 CBF 无显著相关

European Radiology
https://doi.org/10.1007/s00330-022-08606-9

MOLECULAR IMAGING

MGMT promoter methylation status shows no effect on [18F]FET uptake and CBF in gliomas: a stereotactic image-based histological validation study

Shuangshuang Song [1,2,3] · Yi Shan [1,3] · Leiming Wang [4] · Ye Cheng [5] · Hongwei Yang [1,3] · Guoguang Zhao [5] · Zhenguang Wang [2] · Jie Lu [1,3]

Received: 19 October 2021 / Revised: 17 December 2021 / Accepted: 22 January 2022
© The Author(s), under exclusive licence to European Society of Radiology 2022

Abstract

Objectives To investigate the effects of O^6-methylguanine DNA methyltransferase (MGMT) promoter methylation status of gliomas on O-(2-^{18}F-fluoroethyl)-L-tyrosine ([18F]FET) uptake and cerebral blood flow (CBF) of arterial spin labeling (ASL), evaluated by hybrid PET/MR. Stereotactic biopsy was used to validate the findings.

Methods A set of whole tumor and reference volumes of interest (VOIs) based on PET/FLAIR imaging were delineated and transferred to the corresponding [18F]FET PET and CBF maps in 57 patients with newly diagnosed gliomas. The mean and max tumor-to-brain ratio (TBR) and normalized CBF (nCBF) were calculated. The predictive efficacy of [18F]FET PET and CBF in determining MGMT promoter methylation status of glioma were evaluated by whole tumor analysis and stereotactic biopsy. The correlation between PET/MR parameters and MGMT promoter methylation were analyzed using histological specimens acquired from multiple stereotactic biopsies.

Results Based on the analysis of whole tumor volume and biopsy site, TBRmean, TBRmax, nCBFmean, and nCBFmax showed no statistically significant differences between gliomas with and without MGMT promoter methylation (all $p > 0.05$). Furthermore, stereotactic biopsy demonstrated that TBRmean, TBRmax, nCBFmean, and nCBFmax showed no correlation with MGMT promoter methylation ($r = -0.117$, $p = 0.579$; $r = -0.161$, $p = 0.443$; $r = -0.271$, $p = 0.191$; $r = -0.300$, $p = 0.145$; respectively).

Conclusions MGMT promoter methylation status shows no effect on [18F]FET uptake and CBF of ASL in gliomas. Stereotactic biopsy validates it and further reveals there is no correlation of [18F]FET PET uptake and CBF with the percentages of MGMT promoter methylation.

Key Points
• *Based on whole tumor VOI assessment, MGMT promoter methylation status shows no effect on [18F]FET uptake and CBF of ASL in gliomas.*
• *For WHO grade IV glioblastomas, [18F]FET PET and ASL parameters based on hybrid PET/MR fail to predict the MGMT promoter methylation status.*
• *Stereotactic image–based histology reveals that there is no correlation of [18F]FET PET uptake and CBF with the status and percentages of MGMT promoter methylation in gliomas.*

Keywords Glioma · MGMT promoter methylation · Positron-emission tomography · Perfusion magnetic resonance imaging · Molecular typing

---

✉ Jie Lu
  imaginglu@hotmail.com

1 Department of Radiology and Nuclear Medicine, Xuanwu Hospital, Capital Medical University, No.45 Changchun Street, Xicheng District, 100053 Beijing, People's Republic of China

2 Department of Nuclear Medicine, The Affiliated Hospital of Qingdao University, Qingdao, Shandong, China

3 Beijing Key Laboratory of Magnetic Resonance Imaging and Brain Informatics, Beijing 100053, China

4 Department of Pathology, Xuanwu Hospital, Capital Medical University, Beijing, China

5 Department of Neurosurgery, Xuanwu Hospital, Capital Medical University, Beijing, China

Published online: 22 February 2022

 Springer

LI W, ZHAO Z, LIU M, et al.Multimodal classification of Alzheimer's disease and amnestic mild cognitive impairment: integrated ^{18}F-FDG PET and DTI study.J Alzheimers Dis, 2022, 85(3): 1063-1075.

【研究简介】

研究背景：阿尔茨海默病（Alzheimer's disease，AD）是一种以进行性认知功能障碍为特征的神经退行性疾病，遗忘型轻度认知障碍（amnestic mild cognitive impairment，aMCI）是阿尔茨海默病的临床前期阶段，每年有 10% ~ 15% 的遗忘型轻度认知障碍患者进展为阿尔茨海默病。[18]F-FDG PET 反映大脑葡萄糖代谢水平，弥散张量成像（diffusion tensor imaging，DTI）评估脑白质的微观结构变化。本研究利用一体化 PET/MR，定量分析阿尔茨海默病及遗忘型轻度认知障碍患者脑代谢和脑白质结构与健康对照组之间的差异，探讨多模态影像结合能否提高阿尔茨海默病鉴别诊断的准确度。

资料与方法：本研究共纳入 140 例（30 例阿尔茨海默病患者、60 例遗忘型轻度认知障碍患者和 50 例健康对照）受试者，阿尔茨海默病根据 NINCDS-ADRDA 诊断标准、遗忘型轻度认知障碍诊断基于 Petersen 标准进行诊断。所有受试者均经过标准的临床神经心理学评估和脑部 ^{18}F-FDG PET/MR 扫描，并测量不同脑区定量参数：[18]F-FDG-SUVR、DTI-FA 和 DTI-MD，比较单模态 ^{18}F-FDG PET、DTI 和多模态（[18]F-FDG PET+DTI）对阿尔茨海默病、遗忘型轻度认知障碍和健康受试者鉴别诊断性能。

研究结果：阿尔茨海默病和遗忘型轻度认知障碍患者葡萄糖代谢较健康受试者减低（SPM 阈值设置为在体素级别未校正 $P < 0.001$; FDR 在集群级别校正 $P < 0.05$）（图 1-1-19A）。与其他两组相比，阿尔茨海默病患者的葡萄糖代谢显著降低（图 1-1-19B）。定义 9 个感兴趣区为：前扣带回皮质（anterior cingulate cortex，ACC）、后扣带回皮质（posterior cingulate cortex，PCC）、角回、缘上回、楔前叶、顶上小叶、海马、海马旁回、颞中回，选择基于 TBSS 的 FA、MD 作为观察指标。轻度认知障碍与健康受试者相比，阿尔茨海默病与轻度认知障碍、健康受试者相比，所有感兴趣区的 FA 减低，MD 增高（图 1-1-20）。联合使用 FDG-PET 和 DTI 可以更好地鉴别健康受试者、轻度认知障碍和阿尔茨海默病，鉴别阿尔茨海默病和健康人 AUC 值为 0.96，单独使用 ^{18}F-FDG PET 的 AUC 值为 0.93（图 1-1-21）。

研究结论：基于一体化 PET/MR 的 ^{18}F-FDG PET 和 DTI 能够定量测量阿尔茨海默病患者脑葡萄糖代谢和脑白质微结构变化，两种模态联合提高阿尔茨海默病鉴别诊断的准确率，有助于阿尔茨海默病病理生理学的理解。

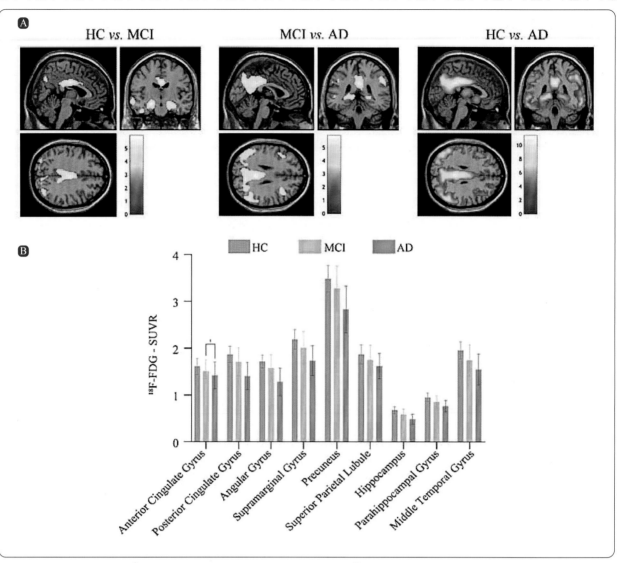

图 1-1-19　阿尔茨海默病、轻度认知障碍和健康受试者 3 组 ^{18}F-FDG-SUVR 体素及感兴趣区水平比较

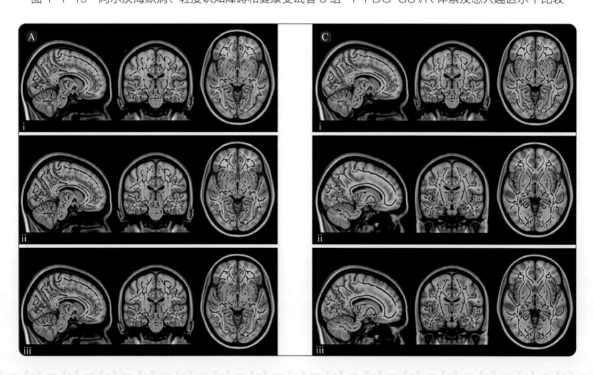

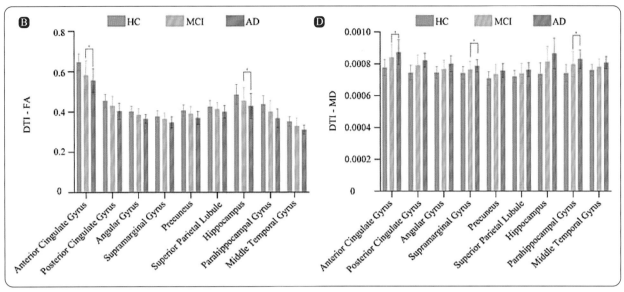

图 1-1-20 阿尔茨海默病、轻度认知障碍和健康受试者 3 组间 TBSS 的比较结果

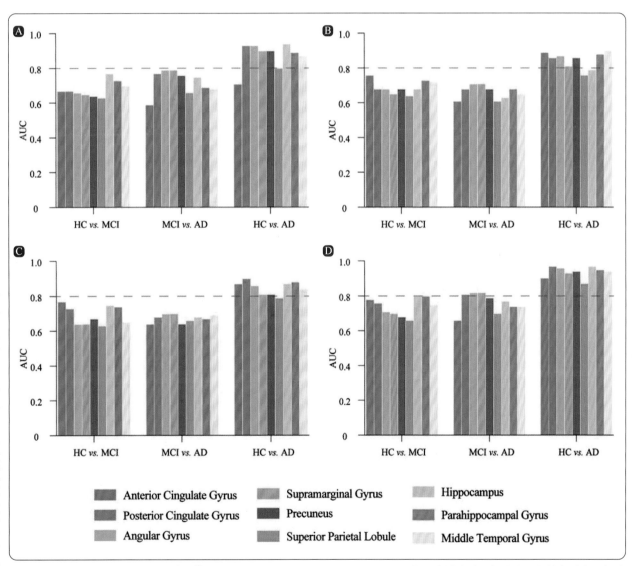

图 1-1-21 直方图显示单模态（A.^{18}F-FDG SUVR；B.DTI-FA；C.DTI-MD）和多模态（D）分类阿尔茨海默病、轻度认知障碍、健康受试者的 AUC 结果

Journal of Alzheimer's Disease 85 (2022) 1063–1075
DOI 10.3233/JAD-215338
IOS Press

1063

首都医科大学宣武医院一体化 PET/MR 成果集

Multimodal Classification of Alzheimer's Disease and Amnestic Mild Cognitive Impairment: Integrated ^{18}F-FDG PET and DTI Study

Weihua Li[a,b,1], Zhilian Zhao[a,b,1], Min Liu[a,b], Shaozhen Yan[a,b], Yanhong An[a,b], Liyan Qiao[c], Guihong Wang[d], Zhigang Qi[a,b] and Jie Lu[a,b,*]

[a]*Department of Radiology and Nuclear Medicine, Xuanwu Hospital, Capital Medical University, Beijing, China*
[b]*Beijing Key Laboratory of Magnetic Resonance Imaging and Brain Informatics, Beijing, China*
[c]*Department of Neurology, Yuquan Hospital, Clinical Neuroscience Institute, Medical Center, Tsinghua University, Beijing, China*
[d]*Department of Neurology, Tiantan Hospital, Capital Medical University, Beijing, China*

Accepted 17 October 2021
Pre-press 10 December 2021

Abstract.
Background: Alzheimer's disease (AD) is a progressive neurodegenerative disease characterized by cognitive decline and memory impairment. Amnestic mild cognitive impairment (aMCI) is the intermediate stage between normal cognitive aging and early dementia caused by AD. It can be challenging to differentiate aMCI patients from healthy controls (HC) and mild AD patients.
Objective: To validate whether the combination of ^{18}F-fluorodeoxyglucose positron emission tomography (^{18}F-FDG PET) and diffusion tensor imaging (DTI) will improve classification performance compared with that based on a single modality.
Methods: A total of thirty patients with AD, sixty patients with aMCI, and fifty healthy controls were included. AD was diagnosed according to the National Institute of Neurological and Communicative Diseases and Stroke/Alzheimer's Disease and Related Disorders Association (NINCDS-ADRDA) criteria for probable. aMCI diagnosis was based on Petersen's criteria. The ^{18}F-FDG PET and DTI measures were each used separately or in combination to evaluate sensitivity, specificity, and accuracy for differentiating HC, aMCI, and AD using receiver operating characteristic analysis together with binary logistic regression. The rate of accuracy was based on the area under the curve (AUC).
Results: For classifying AD from HC, we achieve an AUC of 0.96 when combining two modalities of biomarkers and 0.93 when using ^{18}F-FDG PET individually. For classifying aMCI from HC, we achieve an AUC of 0.79 and 0.76 using the best individual modality of biomarkers.
Conclusion: Our results show that the combination of two modalities improves classification performance, compared with that using any individual modality.

Keywords: Alzheimer's disease, diffusion tensor imaging, ^{18}F-FDG PET, mild cognitive impairment

---

[1]These authors contributed equally to this work.

*Correspondence to: Jie Lu, MD, PhD, Department of Radiology and Nuclear Medicine, Xuanwu Hospital, Capital Medical University, Beijing, China. E-mail: imaginglu@hotmail.com.

INTRODUCTION

Alzheimer's disease (AD) is a progressive neurodegenerative disease characterized by cognitive decline and memory impairment, and it is the most

ZANG Z, SONG T, LI J, et al.Modulation effect of substantia nigra iron deposition and functional connectivity on putamen glucose metabolism in Parkinson's disease.Hum Brain Mapp, 2022, 43(12): 3735-3744.

【研究简介】

研究背景： 帕金森病（Parkinson's disease，PD）是老年人群中第二位常见的神经退行性疾病，主要临床表现为静止性震颤、肌肉僵直、运动迟缓等运动功能障碍。黑质－纹状体通路的神经衰退是帕金森病最显著的特征之一。研究表明帕金森病患者黑质铁沉积增多，且与多巴胺减少密切相关。本研究从影像学角度探讨帕金森病患者黑质铁沉积与纹状体代谢的关系。

资料与方法： 本研究纳入 34 例帕金森病患者与 25 例性别、年龄匹配的健康志愿者，同步获取 PET 与 MRI 图像。获取 PET 图像的 SUVR、磁敏感成像的 R2* 值及 fMRI 数据的黑质－壳核功能连接。进一步通过基于线性回归的调制分析（modulation analysis）探讨黑质铁沉积与壳核代谢之间的关联。

研究结果： 帕金森病患者黑质铁沉积增加（图 1-1-22A）、壳核葡萄糖代谢增加（图 1-1-22B）及黑质－壳核功能连接降低（图 1-1-22C）。黑质铁沉积与壳核代谢无显著相关，而黑质铁沉积与黑质－壳核功能连接的交互作用与壳核代谢显著相关（图 1-1-23）。

研究结论： 本研究通过 PET/MR 同步扫描，发现帕金森病患者黑质铁沉积、壳核代谢增加而黑质－壳核功能连接降低。研究通过调制分析进一步发现，黑质铁沉积与壳核代谢无显著相关，而黑质铁沉积与黑质－壳核功能连接的交互作用与壳核代谢有显著关系，表明黑质铁沉积与黑质－壳核功能连接共同调控壳核活动，揭示了帕金森病黑质铁沉积对壳核代谢的调控机制。

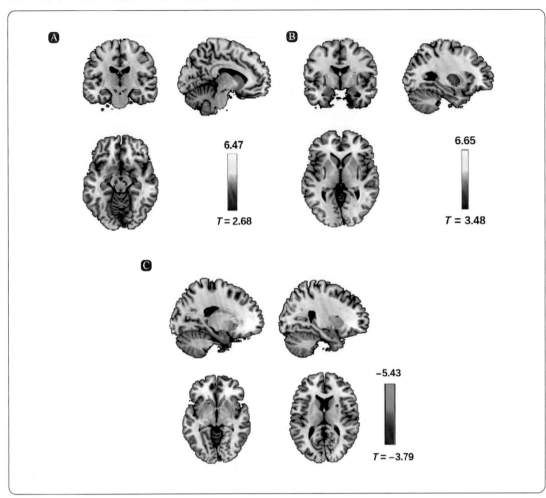

A. 黑质铁沉积；B. 壳核代谢；C. 黑质－壳核功能连接。

图 1-1-22　帕金森病患者黑质铁沉积、壳核代谢及黑质－壳核功能连接异常示意

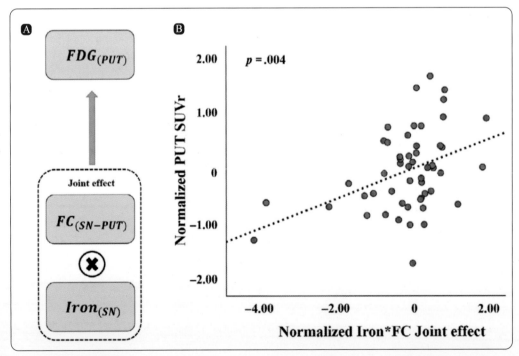

图 1-1-23　A. 黑质铁沉积与黑质－壳核功能连接对壳核葡萄糖代谢调控机制示意；B. 黑质铁沉积与黑质－壳核功能连接的交互作用与壳核代谢显著相关

Received: 26 October 2021 | Revised: 4 March 2022 | Accepted: 5 April 2022

DOI: 10.1002/hbm.25880

RESEARCH ARTICLE

WILEY

Modulation effect of substantia nigra iron deposition and functional connectivity on putamen glucose metabolism in Parkinson's disease

Zhenxiang Zang[1,2] | Tianbin Song[1,2] | Jiping Li[3] | Shaozhen Yan[1,2] | Binbin Nie[4] | Shanshan Mei[5] | Jie Ma[1,2] | Yu Yang[1,2] | Baoci Shan[4] | Yuqing Zhang[3] | Jie Lu[1,2]

[1]Department of Radiology and Nuclear Medicine, Xuanwu Hospital, Capital Medical University, Beijing, China

[2]Beijing Key Laboratory of Magnetic Resonance Imaging and Brain Informatics, Beijing, China

[3]Beijing Institute of Functional Neurosurgery, Xuanwu Hospital, Capital Medical University, Beijing, China

[4]Beijing Engineering Research Center of Radiographic Techniques and Equipment, Institute of High Energy Physics, Chinese Academy of Sciences, China

[5]Department of Neurology, Xuanwu Hospital, Capital Medical University, Beijing, China

Correspondence

Jie Lu, Department of Radiology and Nuclear Medicine, Xuanwu Hospital, Capital Medical University, Changchun Road, No. 45, Beijing 100053, China.
Email: imaginglu@hotmail.com

Funding information

Beijing Municipal Administration of Hospitals' Ascent Plan, Grant/Award Number: DFL20180802; Huizhi Ascent Project of Xuanwu Hospital, Grant/Award Number: HZ2021ZCLJ005

Abstract

Neurodegeneration of the substantia nigra affects putamen activity in Parkinson's disease (PD), yet in vivo evidence of how the substantia nigra modulates putamen glucose metabolism in humans is missing. We aimed to investigate how substantia nigra modulates the putamen glucose metabolism using a cross-sectional design. Resting-state fMRI, susceptibility-weighted imaging, and [^{18}F]-fluorodeoxyglucose-PET (FDG-PET) data were acquired. Forty-two PD patients and 25 healthy controls (HCs) were recruited for simultaneous PET/MRI scanning. The main measurements of the current study were R_2^* images representing iron deposition (28 PD and 25 HCs), standardized uptake value ratio (SUVr) images representing FDG-uptake (33 PD and 25 HCs), and resting state functional connectivity maps from resting state fMRI (34 PD and 25 HCs). An interaction term based on the general linear model was used to investigate the joint modulation effect of nigral iron deposition and nigral-putamen functional connectivity on putamen FDG-uptake. Compared with HCs, we found increased iron deposition in the substantia nigra ($p = .007$), increased FDG-uptake in the putamen (left: $P_{FWE} < 0.001$; right: $P_{FWE} < 0.001$), and decreased functional connectivity between the substantia nigra and the anterior putamen (left $P_{FWE} < 0.001$, right: $P_{FWE} = 0.007$). We then identified significant interaction effect of nigral iron deposition and nigral-putamen connectivity on FDG-uptake in the putamen ($p = .004$). The current study demonstrated joint modulation effect of the substantia nigra iron deposition and nigral-putamen functional connectivity on putamen glucose metabolic distribution, thereby revealing in vivo pathological mechanism of nigrostriatal neurodegeneration of PD.

KEYWORDS

nigral iron deposition, nigrostriatal functional connectivity, Parkinson's disease, putamen metabolism distribution

第一章 一体化 PET/MR 科研成果

ZANG Z, SONG T, LI J, et al.Simultaneous PET/fMRI revealed increased motor area input to subthalamic nucleus in Parkinson's disease.Cereb Cortex, 2022, 33(1): 167-175.

【研究简介】

研究背景： 帕金森病是老年人群中常见的神经退行性疾病，主要临床表现为静止性震颤、肌肉僵直等运动障碍。丘脑底核是帕金森病患者的异常运动环路中最重要的节点。针对丘脑底核的侵入性电生理研究，如深部脑刺激，虽然能够揭示丘脑底核的致病及治疗机制，但是很难在术前实施。因此，寻求一种无创的方法用于识别运动区与丘脑底核之间的信息流动对于评估帕金森病的治疗策略至关重要。本研究旨在使用 ^{18}F-FDG-PET/fMRI 研究帕金森病患者皮质 - 丘脑底核连接通路的有向连接。

资料与方法： 本研究纳入 34 例帕金森病患者与 25 例健康志愿者，同步获取 PET 与 fMRI 图像。获取 PET 图像的 SUVR 和 fMRI 数据的丘脑底核功能连接。采用代谢连接映射（Metabolic Connectivity Mapping，MCM）评估丘脑底核的有向连接，计算两个脑区 FDG 与功能连接的空间一致性，判断两个脑区之间的信息流动方向。

研究结果： 帕金森病患者在感觉运动区的 FDG SUVR 和丘脑底核功能连接均异常增加（P FDR < 0.05），且空间上高度重叠（图 1-1-24）。MCM 分析显示，健康对照与帕金森病组丘脑底核的 MCM 值均显著高于感觉运动皮层（$P < 0.05$），表明信息从感觉运动皮层向丘脑底核流动。其中，帕金森病患者左侧中央前回的皮质与丘脑底核的 MCM 差值显著升高（$P=0.013$；图 1-1-25），表明帕金森病患者左侧中央前回到丘脑底核的有向连接异常增加。

研究结论： 通过 PET/fMRI 同步扫描，发现帕金森病患者感觉运动区域的葡萄糖代谢增加与丘脑底核功能连接增加高度重叠，其中，左侧中央前回到丘脑底核的信息流入异常增高。本研究不仅从能量代谢的角度揭示帕金森病患者运动皮层到丘脑底核的有向连接，更为非侵入性的脑刺激（如经颅磁刺激等）治疗提供了精准靶点。

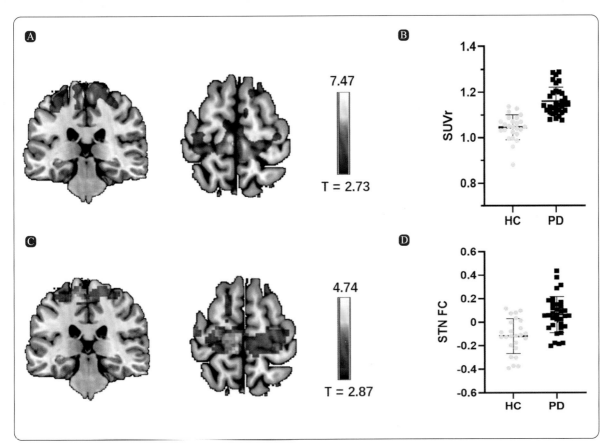

图 1-1-24　帕金森病患者感觉运动区葡萄糖代谢（图 A、图 B）及丘脑底核 - 感觉运动区功能连接（图 C、图 D）增高

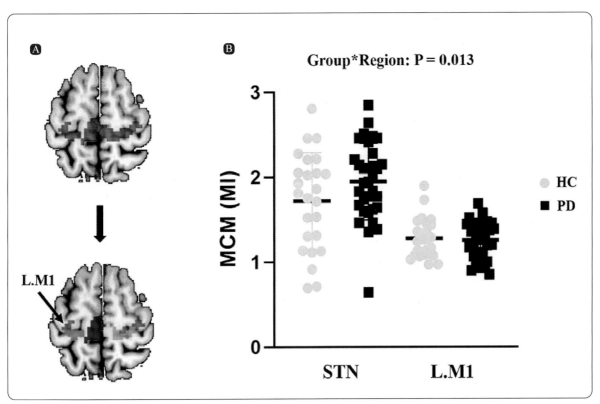

A. 帕金森病患者葡萄糖代谢、丘脑底核功能连接升高重叠区域；B.MCM 方法显示，帕金森病患者左侧中央前回与丘脑底核的 MCM 值显著升高，提示左侧中央前回到丘脑底核的有向连接升高。

图 1-1-25　帕金森病患者 MCM 示意

首
都
医
科
大
学
宣
武
医
院
一
体
化
PET/MR
成
果
集

Cerebral Cortex, 2022, 00, 1–9

https://doi.org/10.1093/cercor/bhac059
Original Article

Simultaneous PET/fMRI revealed increased motor area input to subthalamic nucleus in Parkinson's disease

Zhenxiang Zang ⓘ PhD[1,2], Tianbin Song MD[1,2], Jiping Li MD[3], Binbin Nie PhD[4], Shanshan Mei MD[5], Chun Zhang MD[1,2], Tao Wu MD[6], Yuqing Zhang MD[3], Jie Lu MD[1,2,*]

[1] Department of Radiology and Nuclear Medicine, Xuanwu Hospital, Capital Medical University, Changchun Rd. 45, Xicheng district, Beijing 100053, China,
[2] Beijing Key Laboratory of Magnetic Resonance Imaging and Brain Informatics, Changchun Rd. 45, Xicheng district, Beijing 100053, China,
[3] Beijing Institute of Functional Neurosurgery, Xuanwu Hospital, Capital Medical University, Changchun Rd. 45, Xicheng district, Beijing 100053, China,
[4] Beijing Engineering Research Center of Radiographic Techniques and Equipment, Institute of High Energy Physics, Chinese Academy of Sciences, Yuquan Rd. 19, Shijingshan district, Beijing 100049, China,
[5] Department of Neurology, Xuanwu Hospital, Capital Medical University, Changchun Rd. 45, Xicheng district, Beijing 100053, China,
[6] Department of Neurobiology, Neurology and Geriatrics, Xuanwu Hospital of Capital Medical University, National Clinical Research Center for Geriatric Disorders, Changchun Rd. 45, Xicheng district, Beijing 100053, China
*Corresponding author: Xuanwu Hospital, Changchun Rd No. 45, Beijing 100053, China. Email: imaginglu@hotmail.com

Abstract

Invasive electrophysiological recordings in patients with Parkinson's disease (PD) are extremely difficult for cross-sectional comparisons with healthy controls. Noninvasive approaches for identifying information flow between the motor area and the subthalamic nucleus (STN) are critical for evaluation of treatment strategy. We aimed to investigate the direction of the cortical-STN hyperdirect pathway using simultaneous ^{18}F-FDG-PET/functional magnetic resonance imaging (fMRI). Data were acquired during resting state on 34 PD patients and 25 controls. The ratio of standard uptake value for PET images and the STN functional connectivity (FC) maps for fMRI data were generated. The metabolic connectivity mapping (MCM) approach that combines PET and fMRI data was used to evaluate the direction of the connectivity. Results showed that PD patients exhibited both increased FDG uptake and STN-FC in the sensorimotor area ($P_{FDR} < 0.05$). MCM analysis showed higher cortical-STN MCM value in the PD group ($F = 6.63$, $P = 0.013$) in the left precentral gyrus. There was a high spatial overlap between the increased glucose metabolism and increased STN-FC in the sensorimotor area in PD. The MCM approach further revealed an exaggerated cortical input to the STN in PD, supporting the precentral gyrus as a target for treatment such as the repetitive transcranial magnetic stimulation.

Key words: Parkinson's disease; subthalamic nucleus; causal effect.

Introduction

Parkinson's disease (PD) is a common neurodegenerative disease in aged population, which is characterized by resting tremor, akinesia, or postural instability (Maiti et al. 2017). In addition to the dopaminergic neurodegeneration of the substantia nigra as well as the nigrostriatal pathway, the subthalamic nucleus (STN) is also one of the core subcortical regions that plays a critical pathological role in the motor loop (Rodriguez-Oroz et al. 2001; Calabresi et al. 2014). The cortical-STN hyperdirect pathway has been described as a monosynaptic axonal connection (Nambu et al. 2002), which is strongly associated with motor inhibition (Chen et al. 2020). By using deep brain stimulation (DBS), Oswal et al. (2021) have found that exaggerated high beta activity is generated in the cortex and can spread to STN and provoke the generation of pathological activity. These observations in PD patients have been largely based on invasive electrophysiological recordings (Litvak et al. 2011; Kahan et al. 2014, 2019; Oswal et al. 2016).

Although the invasive studies have established ground truth of electrophysiological pathological characteristics of the cortical-STN hyperdirect pathway in PD patients, they were on other hand extremely difficult if not impossible for presurgery PD patients, not mentioning cross-sectional comparisons with healthy controls (HCs). Noninvasive evaluation of causal effect of the cortical-STN hyperdirect pathway may not only help revealing the pathology of PD but also significantly benefit presurgery evaluations. Resting-state functional magnetic resonance imaging (rsfMRI) is a widely used approach to uncover the neural basis of pathophysiology in human (Greicius 2008). Consistent increased functional connectivity (FC) between STN and the primary sensorimotor motor cortex has been found in a variety of rsfMRI studies (Baudrexel et al. 2011; Shen et al. 2017) and was proved to predict behavioral improvement of post-surgery DBS (Horn et al. 2017). In addition, ^{18}F-fluorodeoxyglucose -positron emission tomography (FDG-PET) is a golden-standard imaging

Received: October 28, 2021. **Revised:** January 23, 2022. **Accepted:** January 25, 2022

SHAN Y, WANG Z, SONG S, et al.Integrated positron emission tomography/ magnetic resonance imaging for resting-state functional and metabolic imaging in human brain: what is correlated and what is impacted.Front Neurosci, 2022, 16: 824152.

【研究简介】

研究背景：一体化 PET/MR 利用 ^{18}F-FDG PET 及 fMRI 数据同步获得脑代谢及脑功能信息，但静息态 ^{18}F-FDG PET 的采集过程需患者保持视听封闭状态，以免外界因素影响脑组织摄取示踪剂的过程，而 fMRI 扫描会对人体产生以噪声为主的多因素效应，因此二者同步扫描，可能影响人脑 PET 的精准定量。本研究应用一体化 PET/MR 从体素及网络水平探讨 fMRI 扫描对静息态 PET 参数的影响。

资料与方法：本研究纳入 24 例健康志愿者（女性 10 例，男性 14 例，31～66 岁），采用随机自身对照方案，将 22 分钟的静息态 ^{18}F-FDG PET 头部扫描分为无 fMRI 扫描（MRI-off）与有 fMRI 扫描（MRI-on）两种模式，每个模式持续 11 分钟。计算基于体素水平的 fMRI 指标［包括局部一致性（regional homogeneity, ReHo）、ALFF、fALFF 和度中心性（degree centrality, DC）］及 PET 定量指标［包括 SUV、SUVR 斜率、局部脑葡萄糖代谢率（rCMRGlu）］。采用配对双样本 t 检验评估 SUV、SUVR 斜率及脑功能 – 代谢偶联参数分别在 MRI-off 和 MRI-on 两种模式下的统计学差异。采用独立成分分析（independent-component analysis，ICA）比较在 MRI-off 和 MRI-on 模式下静息态 PET 脑代谢网络的空间分布差异。

研究结果：MRI-off 和 MRI-on 两种模式的全脑 SUVR 无统计学差异（$P > 0.05$），但 MRI-on 模式全脑 SUVR 的斜率显著高于 MRI-off 模式（$P < 0.001$，图 1–1–26）。ICA 结果显示 MRI-off 和 MRI-on 模式分别获得的 PET 脑代谢网络，视觉观察的空间分布无显著差异；MRI-on 模式较 MRI-off 模式脑代谢活跃的脑区主要位于额极、额上回、颞中回和枕极（图 1–1–27）。脑功能 – 代谢偶联参数（fMRI 各指标与 rCMRGlu 的相关系数）在 MRI-off 和 MRI-on 模式下均显著相关（$P < 0.05$），其中 ReHo 与 rCMRGlu 的相关系数最高。在视觉网络（平均相关系数 0.523 ± 0.057）及 DMN（平均相关系数 0.461 ± 0.099），rCMRGlu 与 fMRI 各指标的相关系数最高（图 1–1–28）。

研究结论：同步扫描 fMRI 会影响脑的瞬时能量代谢改变，但不影响静息态 PET 体素水平及脑代谢网络的定量研究，因此一体化 PET/fMR 扫描适用于同步测定脑功能及代谢水平的研究。

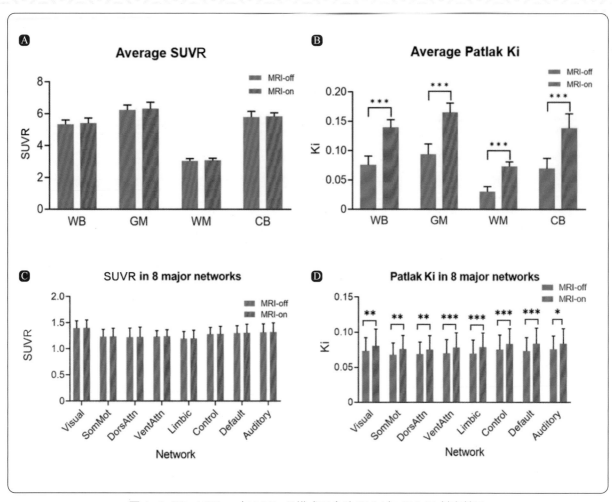

图 1-1-26　MRI-on 与 MRI-off 模式下全脑 SUV 与 SUVR 斜率差异

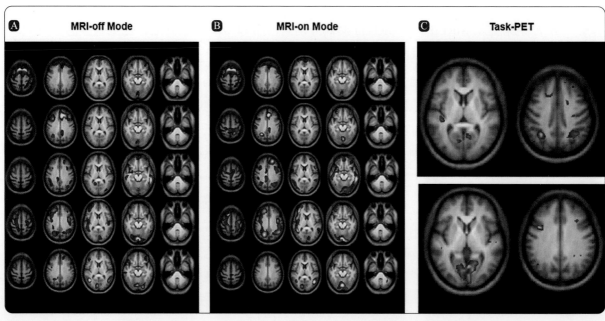

图 1-1-27　MRI-on 与 MRI-off 模式下全脑代谢网络的空间分布差异

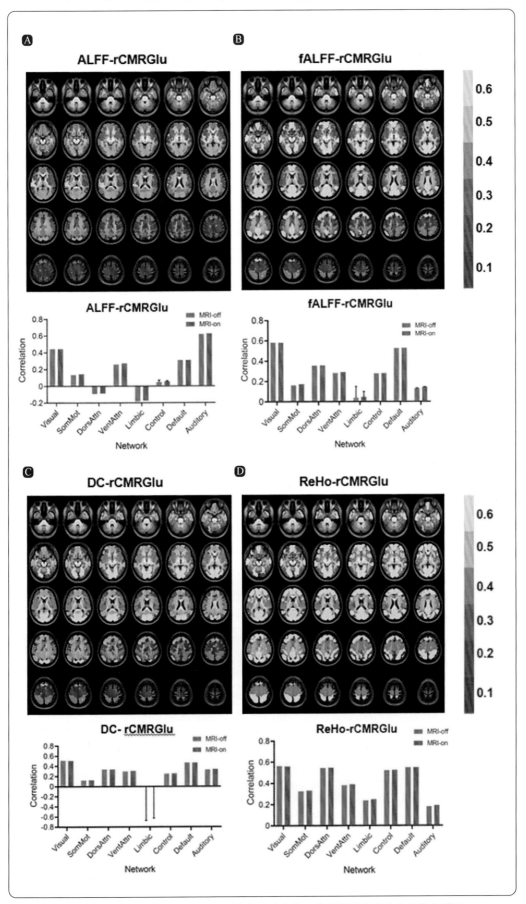

图 1-1-28　MRI-on 与 MRI-off 模式下脑功能 – 代谢偶联参数的空间分布差异

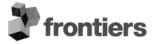

Author's Proof

Before checking your proof, please see the instructions below.

- Carefully read the entire proof and mark all corrections in the appropriate place, using the Adobe Reader commenting tools (**Adobe Help**).
- Provide your corrections in a single PDF file or post your comments in the Production Forum making sure to reference the relevant query/line number. Upload or post all your corrections directly in the Production Forum to avoid any comments being missed.
- We do not accept corrections in the form of edited manuscripts nor via email.
- Do not provide scanned, handwritten corrections.
- Before you submit your corrections, please make sure that you have checked your proof carefully as once you approve it, you won't be able to make any further corrections.
- To ensure the timely publication of your article, please submit the corrections within 48 hours. After submitting, do not email or query asking for confirmation of receipt.

Do you need help? Visit our **Production Help Center** for more information. If you can't find an answer to your question, contact your Production team directly by posting in the Production Forum.

Quick Check-List

- ☐ **Author names** - Complete, accurate and consistent with your previous publications.
- ☐ **Affiliations** - Complete and accurate. Follow this style when applicable: Department, Institute, University, City, Country.
- ☐ **Tables** - Make sure our formatting style did not change the meaning/alignment of your Tables.
- ☐ **Figures** - Make sure we are using the latest versions.
- ☐ **Funding and Acknowledgments** - List all relevant funders and acknowledgments.
- ☐ **Conflict of Interest** - Ensure any relevant conflicts are declared.
- ☐ **Supplementary files** - Ensure the latest files are published and that no line numbers and tracked changes are visible.
  Also, the supplementary files should be cited in the article body text.
- ☐ **Queries** - Reply to all typesetters queries below.
- ☐ **Content** - Read all content carefully and ensure any necessary corrections are made.

Author Queries Form

Query No.	Details Required	Author's Response
Q1	Your article has been copyedited to ensure that we publish the highest quality work possible. Please check it carefully to make sure that it is correct and that the meaning was not lost during the process.	
Q2	The citation and surnames of all of the authors have been highlighted. Check that they are correct and consistent with the authors' previous publications, and correct if need be. Please note that this may affect the indexing of your article in repositories such as PubMed.	
Q3	There is a discrepancy between the styling of the author names in the submission system and the manuscript. We have used [Bixiao Cui] instead of [Xiao Bi Cui]. Please confirm that it is correct.	

TIAN D, YANG H, LI Y, et al.The effect of Q. Clear reconstruction on quantification and spatial resolution of ^{18}F-FDG PET in simultaneous PET/MR.EJNMMI Phys, 2022, 9(1): 1.

【研究简介】

研究背景：Q. Clear 是 PET 基于贝叶斯概率统计的正则化最大期望值（block sequence regularization expectation-maximization，BSREM）重建算法，对提高 PET/CT 图像质量和定量精度具有重要价值，目前有关 PET/MR 图像的研究较少。本研究评估 Q. Clear 对 ^{18}F-FDG PET/MR 系统的影响，并确定最佳惩罚因子 β 值。

资料与方法：根据 NEMA NU 2-2012 标准，在 GE SIGNA PET/MR 扫描美国国家电气制造商协会 / 国际电工委员会（National Electrical Manufacturers Association/International Electrotechnical Commission，NEMA/IEC）图像质量模型。评估对比度恢复（CR）、背景变异性（BV，图 1-1-29）、信噪比（SNR，图 1-1-30）和空间分辨率等指标，临床资料采用病变 SNR、信号背景比（SBR）、噪声水平（图 1-1-31）和视觉评分进行评估。对 OSEM+TOF 和 Q. Clear 重建的 PET 图像进行可视化比较和统计分析，其中 OSEM+TOF 采用点扩展函数作为默认程序，Q. Clear 采用 β 值分别为 100、200、300、400、500、800、1100 和 1400。

研究结果：体模数据随 β 值增加，内部球体的 CR 和 BV 降低；β 值为 400 时，Q. Clear 重建的图像 SNR 达到峰值，较 OSEM+TOF 重建图像分辨率更好。临床数据与 OSEM+TOF 相比，β 值为 400 的 Q. Clear 的 SNR 中位数（从 58.8 到 166.0）增加了 138%，SBR 的中位数增加了 59%（从 4.2 到 6.8），噪声水平中位数减少了 38%（从 0.14 到 0.09）。两名医师的视觉评估，β 值在 200 到 400 之间的 Q. Clear 优于 OSEM+TOF，其中 β 值为 400 最佳。

研究结论：Q. Clear 超级迭代技术与传统 OSEM+TOF 重建方法相比，可有效提高 ^{18}F-FDG 的图像质量及定量精度，且使用惩罚因子 β 值 400 最佳。

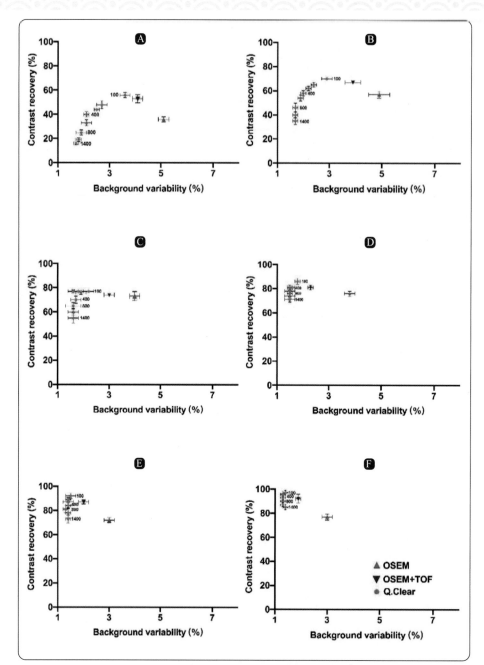

图 1-1-29　体模各尺寸直径球体 CR 值和 BV 值的比较

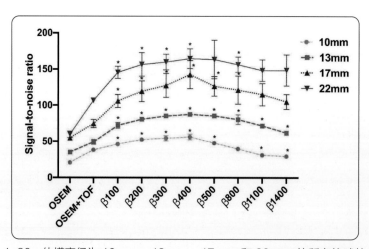

图 1-1-30　体模直径为 10 mm、13 mm、17 mm 和 22 mm 的所有热球的 SNR

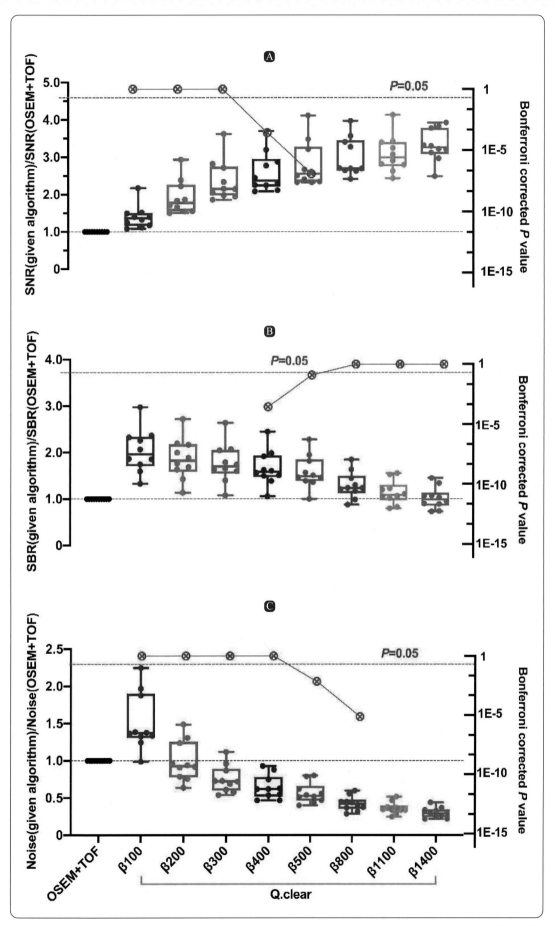

图 1-1-31　箱线图显示不同重建算法对体部肿瘤患者 SNR（图 A）、SBR（图 B）和噪声水平值（图 C）影响

首都医科大学宣武医院一体化 PET/MR 成果集

Tian *et al. EJNMMI Physics* (2022) 9:1
https://doi.org/10.1186/s40658-021-00428-w

EJNMMI Physics

ORIGINAL RESEARCH

Open Access

The effect of Q.Clear reconstruction on quantification and spatial resolution of 18F-FDG PET in simultaneous PET/MR

Defeng Tian[1], Hongwei Yang[1], Yan Li[1], Bixiao Cui[1] and Jie Lu[1,2]*

*Correspondence:
imaginglu@hotmail.com
[1] Department of Radiology and Nuclear Medicine, Xuanwu Hospital, Capital Medical University, 45# Changchun Street, Xicheng District, Beijing, China
Full list of author information is available at the end of the article

Disclaimer This study was supported by the Beijing Municipal Administration of Hospitals' Ascent Plan (No. DFL20180802) and National Natural Science Foundation of China (No. 81974261). All authors read and approved the final manuscript.

Abstract

Background: Q.Clear is a block sequential regularized expectation maximization penalized-likelihood reconstruction algorithm for Positron Emission Tomography (PET). It has shown high potential in improving image reconstruction quality and quantification accuracy in PET/CT system. However, the evaluation of Q.Clear in PET/MR system, especially for clinical applications, is still rare. This study aimed to evaluate the impact of Q.Clear on the ^{18}F-fluorodeoxyglucose (FDG) PET/MR system and to determine the optimal penalization factor β for clinical use.

Methods: A PET National Electrical Manufacturers Association/ International Electrotechnical Commission (NEMA/IEC) phantom was scanned on GE SIGNA PET/MR, based on NEMA NU 2-2012 standard. Metrics including contrast recovery (CR), background variability (BV), signal-to-noise ratio (SNR) and spatial resolution were evaluated for phantom data. For clinical data, lesion SNR, signal to background ratio (SBR), noise level and visual scores were evaluated. PET images reconstructed from OSEM + TOF and Q.Clear were visually compared and statistically analyzed, where OSEM + TOF adopted point spread function as default procedure, and Q.Clear used different β values of 100, 200, 300, 400, 500, 800, 1100 and 1400.

Results: For phantom data, as β value increased, CR and BV of all sizes of spheres decreased in general; images reconstructed from Q.Clear reached the peak SNR with β value of 400 and generally had better resolution than those from OSEM + TOF. For clinical data, compared with OSEM + TOF, Q.Clear with β value of 400 achieved 138% increment in median SNR (from 58.8 to 166.0), 59% increment in median SBR (from 4.2 to 6.8) and 38% decrement in median noise level (from 0.14 to 0.09). Based on visual assessment from two physicians, Q.Clear with β values ranging from 200 to 400 consistently achieved higher scores than OSEM + TOF, where β value of 400 was considered optimal.

Conclusions: The present study indicated that, on ^{18}F-FDG PET/MR, Q.Clear reconstruction improved the image quality compared to OSEM + TOF. β value of 400 was optimal for Q.Clear reconstruction.

Keywords: PET/MR, Q.Clear, Penalization factor β, OSEM

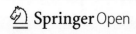
Springer Open

DONG QY, LI TR, JIANG XY, et al.Glucose metabolism in the right middle temporal gyrus could be a potential biomarker for subjective cognitive decline: a study of a Han population.Alzheimers Res Ther, 2021, 13(1): 74.

【研究简介】

研究背景：主观认知下降（subjective cognitive decline，SCD）是认知功能正常但阿尔茨海默病患病风险增加的一种状态，识别主观认知下降的葡萄糖代谢特征有助于超早期定位代谢变化脑区。本研究旨在通过主观认知下降患者脑内感兴趣区分析，探讨其葡萄糖代谢改变模式。

资料与方法：本研究队列来自两个三级医疗中心，属于 SILCODE 研究项目（NCT03370744）。队列 1 包括 26 例健康对照（normal control，NC）和 32 例主观认知下降患者；队列 2 包括 36 例健康对照、23 例主观认知下降、32 例遗忘型轻度认知障碍、32 例阿尔茨海默病痴呆（AD dementia，ADDs）和 22 例路易体痴呆（dementia with Lewy bodies，DLB）患者。受试者均进行 ^{18}F-FDG PET 和 MRI 检查，队列 1 的受试者进行了淀粉样蛋白 PET 显像。感兴趣区分析基于解剖自动标记（anatomical automatic labeling，AAL）模板。采用多重置换检验和重复交叉验证分析健康对照组和主观认知下降组间代谢差异；采用受试者工作特征曲线评价葡萄糖代谢对各组的区分能力；采用 Pearson 相关分析探讨葡萄糖代谢与神经心理量表、皮层淀粉样蛋白沉积的相关性。

研究结果：主观认知下降患者右侧颞中回葡萄糖代谢水平与主观记忆抱怨评分（r =-0.239，P=0.009）、抑郁评分（r =-0.200，P=0.030）和长期延迟记忆水平（r =0.207，P=0.025）呈正相关，与皮层淀粉样蛋白沉积呈轻度正相关（r =-0.246，P=0.066）（图 1-1-32）。右侧颞中回葡萄糖代谢水平在健康对照组、主观认知下降组、遗忘型轻度认知障碍组、阿尔茨海默病痴呆组、路易体痴呆组逐渐降低（图 1-1-33），诊断效能与传统后扣带皮层或楔前叶葡萄糖代谢相当（健康对照 *vs.* 阿尔茨海默病痴呆、遗忘型轻度认知障碍或路易体痴呆），优于传统模型（健康对照 *vs.* 主观认知下降）。

研究结论：右侧颞中回葡萄糖代谢减低是主观认知下降的典型特征，随疾病进展代谢逐渐减低，与传统依赖于主观症状判断的方法相比，可以提高主观认知下降诊断特异度。

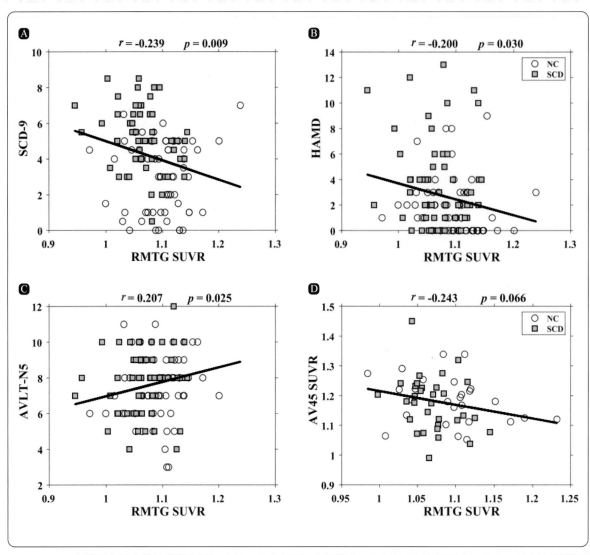

图 1-1-32　A. 右侧颞中回葡萄糖代谢水平与 SCD-9 主观记忆抱怨评分；B.HAMD 抑郁评分；C.AVLT-N5 听觉词语学习测验 - 长期延迟记忆评分；D.AV45SUVR 皮层淀粉样蛋白沉积相关性

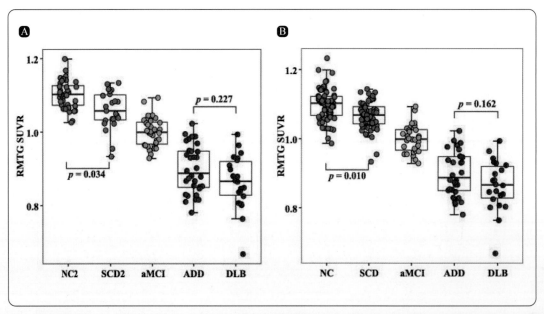

图 1-1-33　健康对照组、主观认知下降组、遗忘型轻度认知障碍组、阿尔茨海默病痴呆组、路易体痴呆组右侧颞中回葡萄糖代谢水平组间比较

Dong *et al. Alzheimer's Research & Therapy*   (2021) 13:74
https://doi.org/10.1186/s13195-021-00811-w

Alzheimer's
Research & Therapy

RESEARCH   **Open Access**

Glucose metabolism in the right middle temporal gyrus could be a potential biomarker for subjective cognitive decline: a study of a Han population

Check for updates

Qiu-Yue Dong[1†], Tao-Ran Li[2†], Xue-Yan Jiang[2,3], Xiao-Ni Wang[2], Ying Han[2,4,5,6*] and Jie-Hui Jiang[1*]

第一章 一体化 PET/MR 科研成果

Abstract

Introduction: Subjective cognitive decline (SCD) represents a cognitively normal state but at an increased risk for developing Alzheimer's disease (AD). Recognizing the glucose metabolic biomarkers of SCD could facilitate the location of areas with metabolic changes at an ultra-early stage. The objective of this study was to explore glucose metabolic biomarkers of SCD at the region of interest (ROI) level.

Methods: This study was based on cohorts from two tertiary medical centers, and it was part of the SILCODE project (NCT03370744). Twenty-six normal control (NC) cases and 32 SCD cases were in cohort 1; 36 NCs, 23 cases of SCD, 32 cases of amnestic mild cognitive impairment (aMCIs), 32 cases of AD dementia (ADDs), and 22 cases of dementia with Lewy bodies (DLBs) were in cohort 2. Each subject underwent [18F]fluoro-2-deoxyglucose positron emission tomography (PET) imaging and magnetic resonance imaging (MRI), and subjects from cohort 1 additionally underwent amyloid-PET scanning. The ROI analysis was based on the Anatomical Automatic Labeling (AAL) template; multiple permutation tests and repeated cross-validations were conducted to determine the metabolic differences between NC and SCD cases. In addition, receiver operating characteristic curves were used to evaluate the capabilities of potential glucose metabolic biomarkers in distinguishing different groups. Pearson correlation analysis was also performed to explore the correlation between glucose metabolic biomarkers and neuropsychological scales or amyloid deposition.

(Continued on next page)

* Correspondence: hanying@xwh.ccmu.edu.cn; jiangjiehui@shu.edu.cn
†Qiu-Yue Dong and Tao-Ran Li authors contribute equally to this work, as first co-authors of equal status.
²Department of Neurology, Xuanwu Hospital of Capital Medical University, Beijing, China
¹Key laboratory of Specialty Fiber Optics and Optical Access Networks, Joint International Research Laboratory of Specialty Fiber Optics and Advanced Communication, School of Information and Communication Engineering, Shanghai University, Shanghai, China
Full list of author information is available at the end of the article

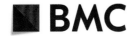

CHEN Y, WANG J, CUI C, et al.Evaluating the association between brain atrophy, hypometabolism, and cognitive decline in Alzheimer's disease: a PET/MRI study.Aging (Albany NY), 2021, 13(5): 7228-7246.

【研究简介】

研究背景： 研究表明阿尔茨海默病患者大脑受损最严重的区域为海马和默认网络（default-mode network，DMN）相关脑区，但同时探讨这两个关键部位的功能及结构损伤与认知关系的研究较少。一体化 PET/MR 可同步获得脑代谢及脑结构信息，是研究阿尔茨海默病多模态神经影像特征与认知表现之间关系的理想工具。本研究应用一体化 PET/MR，联合分析海马和 DMN 的结构与代谢的多模态影像特征，探索其与认知功能的相关性，以期进一步理解阿尔茨海默病认知损害的潜在神经机制，为治疗方案的研究提供新思路。

资料与方法： 本研究招募 23 例阿尔茨海默病患者和 24 例年龄、性别和教育水平相匹配的认知正常老年人作为健康对照组，所有受试者进行临床病史采集、神经心理学量表评估、一体化 PET/MR ^{18}F-FDG PET 及 MRI 高分辨 T_1WI 图像。定义海马和 DMN 为感兴趣区，利用 SPM12 对进行分析，提取感兴趣代谢及结构信息，采用多元线性回归模型研究脑区损伤与认知的关系。

研究结果： 阿尔茨海默病组的 DMN 脑代谢显著低于健康对照组（$P < 0.001$）（图 1-1-34 B1-1），控制灰质体积萎缩后依然存在（$P < 0.001$）（图 1-1-34 B2-1）。^{18}F-FDG-PET 数据的全脑分析结果显示阿尔茨海默病组 DMN 脑代谢降低最显著（图 1-1-35）；基于感兴趣区的灰质体积及 VBM 结果均显示，阿尔茨海默病组双侧海马及 DMN 的灰质萎缩最显著（$P < 0.001$，FWE 校正）（图 1-1-34C，图 1-1-36）；多元线性回归结果显示，多种认知任务的受损与 DMN 的低代谢及海马和 DMN 区域灰质萎缩呈显著相关。

研究结论： 海马和 DMN 相关脑区的代谢和结构联合受损，能够预测阿尔茨海默病患者的认知功能下降，有助于理解阿尔茨海默病患者认知下降的神经机制。

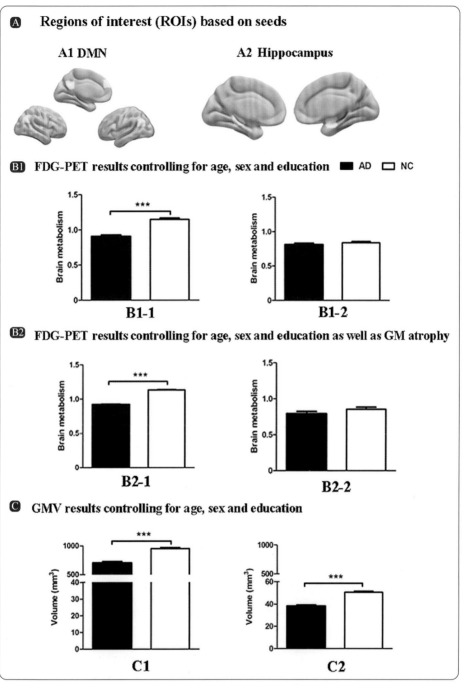

图 1-1-34　基于感兴趣区分析阿尔茨海默病组与健康对照组在 ^{18}F-FDG SUVR 和灰质体积的组间差异

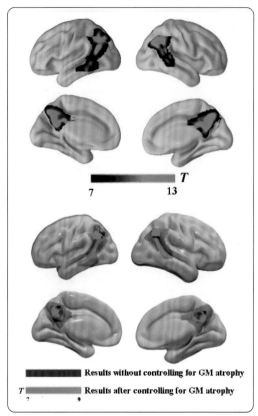

图 1-1-35　控制灰质萎缩前后全脑验证性分析阿尔茨海默病组与健康对照组的 ^{18}F-FDG SUVR 组间差异

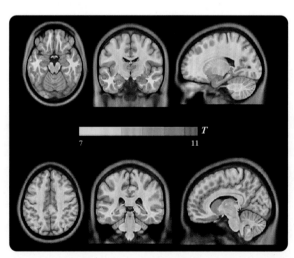

图 1-1-36　VBM 分析阿尔茨海默病组与健康对照组脑灰质体积组间差异

www.aging-us.com   AGING 2021, Vol. 13, No. 5

Research Paper

Evaluating the association between brain atrophy, hypometabolism, and cognitive decline in Alzheimer's disease: a PET/MRI study

Yifan Chen[1,*], Junkai Wang[2,3,4,*], Chunlei Cui[1], Yusheng Su[1], Donglai Jing[5], LiYong Wu[5], Peipeng Liang[3,4], Zhigang Liang[1]

[1]Department of Nuclear Medicine, Xuanwu Hospital, Capital Medical University, Beijing, China
[2]Department of Psychology, Tsinghua University, Beijing, China
[3]School of Psychology, Capital Normal University, Beijing, China
[4]Beijing Key Laboratory of Learning and Cognition, Beijing, China
[5]Department of Neurology, Xuanwu Hospital, Capital Medical University, Beijing, China
*Equal contribution

Correspondence to: Zhigang Liang, Peipeng Liang; email: zhgliang@ccmu.edu.cn, ppliang@cnu.edu.cn
Keywords: hybrid PET/MR, Alzheimer's disease, hippocampus, default mode network, gray matter volume
Received: September 13, 2020   Accepted: January 14, 2021   Published: February 26, 2021

ABSTRACT

Glucose metabolism reduction and brain volume losses are widely reported in Alzheimer's disease (AD). Considering that neuroimaging changes in the hippocampus and default mode network (DMN) are promising important candidate biomarkers and have been included in the research criteria for the diagnosis of AD, it is hypothesized that atrophy and metabolic changes of the abovementioned regions could be evaluated concurrently to fully explore the neural mechanisms underlying cognitive impairment in AD. Twenty-three AD patients and Twenty-four age-, sex- and education level-matched normal controls underwent a clinical interview, a detailed neuropsychological assessment and a simultaneous 18F-fluoro-2-deoxy-D-glucose positron emission tomography (18F-FDG PET)/high-resolution T1-weighted magnetic resonance imaging (MRI) scan on a hybrid GE SIGNA PET/MR scanner. Brain volume and glucose metabolism were examined in patients and controls to reveal group differences. Multiple linear regression models were employed to explore the relationship between multiple imaging features and cognitive performance in AD. The AD group had significantly reduced volume in the hippocampus and DMN regions (P < 0.001) relative to that of normal controls determined by using ROI analysis. Compared to normal controls, significantly decreased metabolism in the DMN (P < 0.001) was also found in AD patients, which still survived after controlling for gray matter atrophy (P < 0.001). These findings from ROI analysis were further confirmed by whole-brain confirmatory analysis (P < 0.001, FWE-corrected). Finally, multiple linear regression results showed that impairment of multiple cognitive tasks was significantly correlated with the combination of DMN hypometabolism and atrophy in the hippocampus and DMN regions. This study demonstrated that combining functional and structural features can better explain the cognitive decline of AD patients than unimodal FDG or brain volume changes alone. These findings may have important implications for understanding the neural mechanisms of cognitive decline in AD.

INTRODUCTION

Alzheimer's disease (AD) is a progressive neuro-degenerative disorder with insidious onset followed by cognitive decline [1]. Prior studies have revealed that individuals with mild cognitive impairment (MCI), which represents a transitional stage between normal aging and a very early phase of AD, will face many

文章 15

DU W, DING C, JIANG J, et al.Women exhibit lower global left frontal cortex connectivity among cognitively unimpaired elderly individuals: a pilot study from SILCODE.J Alzheimers Dis, 2021, 83(2): 653-663.

【研究简介】

研究背景： 研究表明认知正常老年人的认知储备存在性别差异，左侧额叶全脑功能连接（global left frontal cortex connectivity，gLFC-connectivity）是认知储备的神经生理基础，本研究旨在探讨认知正常老年人 gLFC 的性别差异。

资料与方法： 本研究纳入中国认知下降纵向研究（Sino Longitudinal Study on Cognitive Decline，SILCODE）招募的 113 例健康对照和 132 例主观认知下降患者，其中女性受试者分别为 66 例、92 例（数据 1）。88 例受试者进行了 β- 淀粉样蛋白（amyloid β-protein，Aβ）PET 显像，其中 32 例为 Aβ 阳性、56 例为 Aβ 阴性。46 例受试者进行了静息态 fMRI（数据 2），采用基于种子点的脑功能连接分析方法计算全脑各体素与左侧额叶间的功能连接强度，验证 gLFC 的可重复性；采用独立样本 t 检验分析健康对照组与主观认知下降组、Aβ 阳性组与 Aβ 阴性组间 gLFC 的性别差异；采用偏相关分析计算 gLFC 与认知评分的相关性。

研究结果： 健康对照组、主观认知下降组、Aβ 阴性组、Aβ 阳性组女性 gLFC 均显著低于男性（$P=0.001$，$P=0.020$，$P=0.006$，$P=0.025$）（图 1-1-37，图 1-1-38）。将年龄、教育程度、颅内总体积和 APOE 4 携带状态作为协变量分析，Aβ 阳性组女性与男性受试者间 gLFC 未见显著差异；主观认知下降组 gLFC 与老年抑郁量表得分呈负相关（$r=-0.176$，$P=0.047$）。

研究结论： 认知正常老年人的认知储备存在性别差异，女性显著低于男性，gLFC-connectivity 可能是认知储备的神经生理基础。

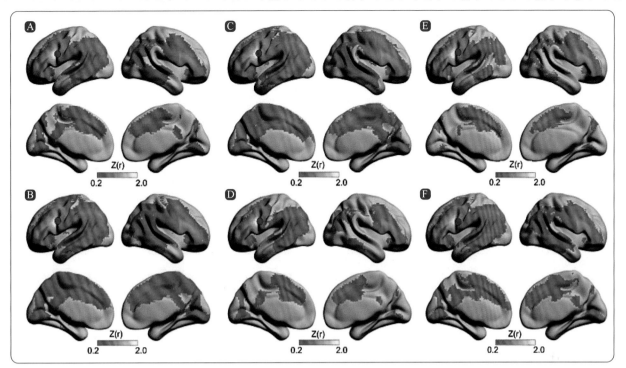

图 1-1-37　数据 1（图 A）、数据 2（图 B）、数据 1 男性（图 C）、数据 1 女性（图 D）、数据 1 健康对照组（图 E）、数据 1 主观认知下降组（图 F）基于种子点的 gLFC-connectivity 图

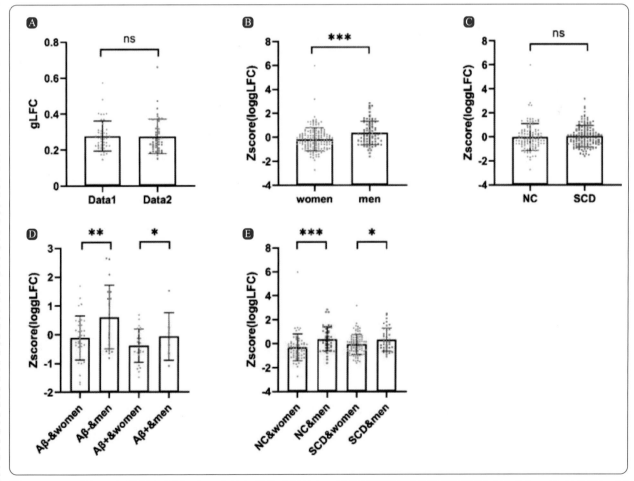

图 1-1-38　数据 1 与数据 2（图 A）、女性与男性（图 B）、健康对照组与主观认知下降组（图 C）、Aβ 阳性组与 Aβ 阴性组（图 D）及其他亚组间（图 E）gLFC 差异

Journal of Alzheimer's Disease 83 (2021) 653–663
DOI 10.3233/JAD-210376
IOS Press

Women Exhibit Lower Global Left Frontal Cortex Connectivity Among Cognitively Unimpaired Elderly Individuals: A Pilot Study from SILCODE

Wenying Du[a], Changchang Ding[b], Jiehui Jiang[b,*] and Ying Han[a,c,d,e,*]
[a]*Department of Neurology, Xuanwu Hospital of Capital Medical University, Beijing, China*
[b]*Institute of Biomedical Engineering, School of Communication and Information Engineering, Shanghai University, Shanghai, China*
[c]*School of Biomedical Engineering, Hainan University, Haikou, China*
[d]*Center of Alzheimer's Disease, Beijing Institute for Brain Disorders, Beijing, China*
[e]*National Clinical Research Center for Geriatric Disorders, Beijing, China*

Accepted 23 June 2021
Pre-press 27 July 2021

Abstract.
Background: Mounting evidence suggests that sex differences exist in cognitive reserve (CR) for cognitively unimpaired (CU) elderly individuals. Global left frontal connectivity (gLFC connectivity) is a reliable neural substrate of CR.
Objective: The purpose of this study was to explore sex differences in gLFC connectivity among CU elderly individuals.
Methods: One hundred thirteen normal controls (NCs) (women = 66) and 132 individuals with subjective cognitive decline (SCD) (women = 92) were recruited from the Sino Longitudinal Study on Cognitive Decline (SILCODE) (data 1). Among them, 88 subjects underwent amyloid-β (Aβ) imaging, including 32 Aβ+ and 56 Aβ– subjects. Forty-six subjects underwent another rs-fMRI examination (data 2) to validate the repeatability of the calculation of gLFC connectivity, which was determined through seed-based functional connectivity between the LFC and voxels throughout the whole brain. Independent-sample t-tests were used to evaluate the sex differences in gLFC connectivity across different subgroups (NC versus SCD, Aβ+ versus Aβ–). Partial correlation analysis was used to calculate the correlations between gLFC connectivity and cognitive assessments.
Results: Women exhibited lower gLFC connectivity in both the NC ($p = 0.001$) and SCD ($p = 0.020$) subgroups than men. Women also exhibited lower gLFC connectivity in both the Aβ– ($p = 0.006$) and Aβ+ ($p = 0.025$) groups. However, the significant difference disappeared in the Aβ+ group when considering the covariates of age, education, total intracranial volume, and *APOE4*-carrying status. In addition, gLFC connectivity values were negatively correlated with Geriatric Depression Scale scores in the SCD group ($r = –0.176$, $p = 0.047$).
Conclusion: Women showed lower gLFC connectivity among CU elderly individuals.

Keywords: Amyloid deposition, cognitive reserve, global left frontal cortex connectivity, sex differences, subjective cognitive decline

INTRODUCTION

Alzheimer's disease (AD), with a long progressive course, is the main cause of dementia. Cascade theory

---

*Correspondence to: Ying Han, Department of Neurology, XuanWu Hospital of Capital Medical University, No.45 Changchun Street, Xicheng District, Beijing 100053, China. Tel.: +86 13621011941; E-mail: hanying@xwh.ccmu.edu.cn. and Jiehui Jiang, Institute of Biomedical Engineering, School of Communication and Information Engineering, Shanghai University, 99 Shangda Road, Shanghai 200444, China. Tel.: +86 021 66135299; E-mail: jiangjiehui@shu.edu.cn.

CHU M, LIU L, WANG J, et al.Investigating the roles of anterior cingulate in behavioral variant frontotemporal dementia: a PET/MRI study.J Alzheimers Dis, 2021, 84(4): 1771-1779.

【研究简介】

研究背景：ACC 在行为变异型额颞叶痴呆（behavioral variant of frontotemporal dementia，bvFTD）患者的行为缺陷和执行功能障碍中起重要作用，但其机制尚不明确。本研究旨在通过一体化 PET/MR 同步采集 T_1WI 与 ^{18}F-FDG PET 数据，分析行为变异型额颞叶痴呆患者 ACC 灰质体积和 SUVR 改变与疾病严重程度的关系。

资料与方法：本研究纳入 21 例行为变异型额颞叶痴呆患者和 21 例健康对照。受试者均接受一体化 PET/MR 检查和标准化神经心理评估。基于体素水平计算灰质体积及 SUVR 并进行组间比较，采用 Pearson 偏相关分析探讨 ACC 灰质体积、SUVR 与行为缺陷和执行功能障碍严重程度的相关性。

研究结果：与健康对照相比，行为变异型额颞叶痴呆患者 ACC 灰质体积减少、葡萄糖代谢减低（图 1-1-39）。Pearson's 偏相关分析显示 ACC SUVR 与额叶行为量表总分（左侧 ACC $r = -0.85$，右侧 ACC $r = -0.85$，$P < 0.0001$）、脱抑制得分（左侧 ACC $r = -0.72$，$P = 0.002$，右侧 ACC $r = -0.75$，$P < 0.0001$）和淡漠得分（左侧 ACC $r = -0.87$，右侧 ACC $r = -0.85$，$P < 0.0001$）显著相关（图 1-1-40）。

研究结论：行为变异型额颞叶痴呆患者行为缺陷与 ACC 葡萄糖代谢减低有关，^{18}F-FDG PET 是评估患者 ACC 损伤的重要方法。

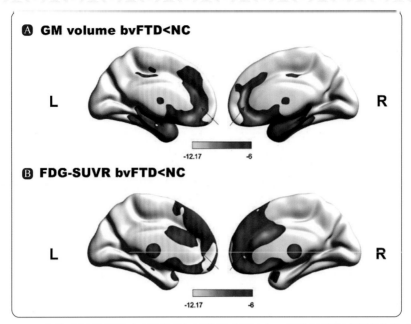

图 1-1-39　行为变异型额颞叶痴呆患者灰质体积（图 A）、葡萄糖代谢（图 B）改变模式

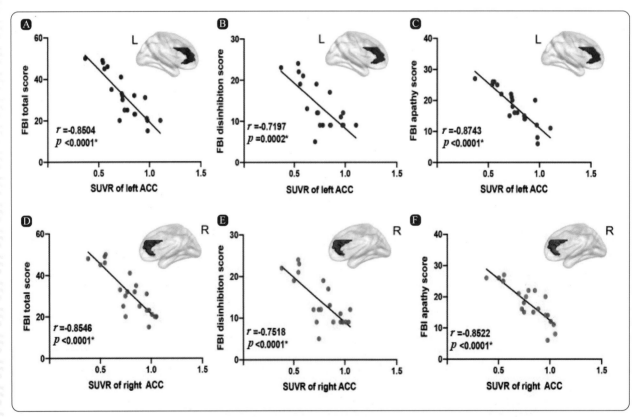

图 1-1-40　行为变异型额颞叶痴呆患者额叶行为量表得分与双侧 ACC SUVR 相关分析
（蓝色：左侧 ACC，红色：右侧 ACC）

Journal of Alzheimer's Disease 84 (2021) 1771–1779
DOI 10.3233/JAD-215127
IOS Press

1771

第一章 一体化 PET/MR 科研成果

Investigating the Roles of Anterior Cingulate in Behavioral Variant Frontotemporal Dementia: A PET/MRI Study

Min Chu[a,1], Li Liu[a,b,1], Jingjuan Wang[c], Lin Liu[a,d], Yu Kong[a], Donglai Jing[a,e], Kexin Xie[a], Yue Cui[a], Bo Cui[a], Jing Zhang[a], Hong Ye[a], Junjie Li[a], Lin Wang[a], Pedro Rosa-Neto[f], Serge Gauthier[f] and Liyong Wu[a,*]

[a]*Department of Neurology, Xuanwu Hospital, Capital Medical University, Beijing, China*
[b]*Department of Neurology, Shenyang Fifth People Hospital, Shenyang, China*
[c]*Department of Nuclear Medicine, Xuanwu Hospital, Capital Medical University, Beijing, China*
[d]*Department of Neurology, Second Hospital of ShanXi Medical University, Taiyuan, China*
[e]*Department of Neurology, Rongcheng People's Hospital, Hebei, China*
[f]*McGill Centre for Studies in Aging, Alzheimer's Disease Research Unit, Montreal, Canada*

Accepted 28 September 2021
Pre-press 25 October 2021

Abstract.
Background: The anterior cingulate cortex (ACC) seems to play an important role in behavioral deficits and executive dysfunctions in patients with behavioral variant frontotemporal dementia (bvFTD), while its specific and independent contribution requires clarification.
Objective: To identify whether ACC abnormalities in gray matter (GM) volume and standardized uptake value ratio (SUVR) images are associated with disease severity of bvFTD, by analyzing hybrid T1 and ^{18}F-fluorodeoxyglucose positron emission tomography (^{18}F-FDG PET).
Methods: We enrolled 21 bvFTD patients and 21 healthy controls in the study. Each subject underwent a hybrid PET/MRI study and a standardized neuropsychologic assessment battery. GM volume and SUVR are voxel-wise calculated and compared. Then we estimate the mean value inside ACC for further partial Pearson's correlation to explore the association between GM volume/SUVR of the ACC and severity of behavioral deficit as well as executive dysfunction.
Results: ACC was shown to be involved in both atrophy and hypometabolism patterns. The partial Pearson's correlation analysis showed that the SUVR of the ACC was strongly correlated with frontal behavior inventory total score (left $r = -0.85$, right $r = -0.85$, $p < 0.0001$), disinhibition subscale score (left $r = -0.72$, $p = 0.002$; right $= -0.75$, $p < 0.0001$), and apathy subscale score (left $= -0.87$, right $= -0.85$, $p < 0.0001$).
Conclusion: These findings demonstrated decreased ACC activity contributes to behavioral disturbances of both apathetic and disinhibition syndromes of bvFTD, which can be sensitively detected using ^{18}F-FDG PET.

Keywords: Anterior cingulate cortex, atrophy, ^{18}F-fluorodeoxyglucose positron emission tomography, frontotemporal dementia, hypometabolism, magnetic resonance imaging

---

[1]These authors contributed equally to this work.
*Correspondence to: Li-yong Wu, MD, PhD, Department of Neurology, Xuanwu Hospital, Capital Medical University, Beijing 100053, China. Tel.: +86 10 83923051; Fax: +86 10 83157841; E-mail: wmywly@hotmail.com.

DING C, DU W, ZHANG Q, et al.Coupling relationship between glucose and oxygen metabolisms to differentiate preclinical Alzheimer's disease and normal individuals.Hum Brain Mapp, 2021, 42(15): 5051-5062.

【研究简介】

研究背景： 临床前阿尔茨海默病的发现为阿尔茨海默病早期干预提供了重要的时间窗，一体化 PET/MR 葡萄糖和氧代谢之间的耦合关系可以早期显示临床前阿尔茨海默病的脑生理信息。

资料与方法： 本研究纳入 27 例健康对照组、20 例临床前阿尔茨海默病患者和 15 例认知障碍患者。每个受试者进行基于 ^{18}F-FDG PET 计算葡萄糖 SUVR、fMRI 计算异常 ReHo 和 fALFF 分析，并计算全脑和 DMN SUVR 与 ReHo、fALFF 的偏 Spearaman 相关值，使用受试者工作特征曲线评估其诊断性能。

研究结果： 35 例患者中 98% 的受试者 SUVR 和 fALFF/ReHo 存在显著相关；与健康对照组相比，临床前阿尔茨海默病组和认知障碍组 DMN 的 SUVR/fALFF、SUVR/ReHo 偏 Spearman 相关值显著减低；而与对照组相比，临床前阿尔茨海默病组的全脑偏 Spearman 相关值无显著差异（图 1-1-41）；DMN 的 SUVR/ReHo 相关值分类临床前阿尔茨海默病组 AUC 最高（0.787）（图 1-1-42）。

研究结论： 临床前阿尔茨海默病阶段 DMN 区域的葡萄糖和氧代谢之间的耦合关系发生了变化，有助于指导临床进行早期诊断。

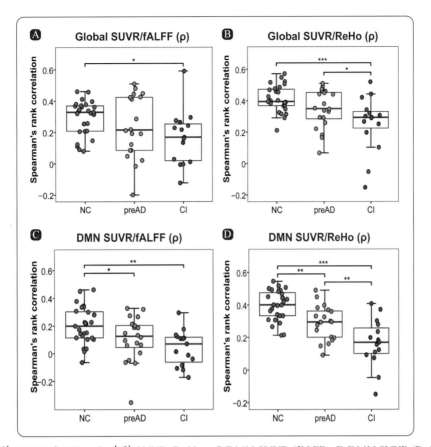

A. 全脑 SUVR/fALFF ; B. 全脑 SUVR/ReHo; C.DMN SUVR/fALFF; D.DMN SUVR/ReHo。

图 1-1-41 健康对照组、临床前阿尔茨海默病组、认知障碍组个体水平灰质体素的 FDG SUVR 和不同 fMRI 相关性比较

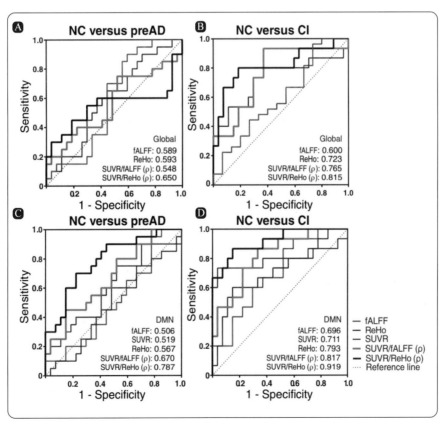

图 1-1-42 全脑（图 A、图 B）及 DMN（图 C、图 D）健康对照组和临床前阿尔茨海默病组、健康对照组和认知障碍组 fALFF、ReHo、DMN SUVR/fALFF、DMN SUVR/ReHo 的受试者工作特征曲线

Received: 10 March 2021 | Revised: 10 June 2021 | Accepted: 12 July 2021

DOI: 10.1002/hbm.25599

RESEARCH ARTICLE

WILEY

Coupling relationship between glucose and oxygen metabolisms to differentiate preclinical Alzheimer's disease and normal individuals

Changchang Ding[1] | Wenying Du[2] | Qi Zhang[1] | Luyao Wang[3] |
Ying Han[2,4,5,6] | Jiehui Jiang[1]

[1]Key Laboratory of Specialty Fiber Optics and Optical Access Networks, Joint International Research Laboratory of Specialty Fiber Optics and Advanced Communication, School of Communication and Information Engineering, Shanghai University, Shanghai, China

[2]Department of Neurology, Xuanwu Hospital of Capital Medical University, Beijing, China

[3]School of Mechatronical Engineering, Beijing Institute of Technology, Beijing, China

[4]Center of Alzheimer's Disease, Beijing Institute for Brain Disorders, Beijing, China

[5]National Clinical Research Center for Geriatric Disorders, Beijing, China

[6]Biomedical Engineering Institute, Hainan University, Haikou, China

Correspondence
Jiehui Jiang, School of Communication and Information Engineering, Shanghai University, 99 Shangda Road, Shanghai 200444, China.
Email: jiangjiehui@shu.edu.cn

Funding information
Higher Education Discipline Innovation Project, Grant/Award Number: D20031; National Natural Science Foundation of China, Grant/Award Numbers: 61603236, 61633018, 82001773, 82020108013

Abstract

The discovery of preclinical Alzheimer's disease (preAD) provides a wide time window for the early intervention of AD. The coupling relationships between glucose and oxygen metabolisms from hybrid PET/MRI can provide complementary information on the brain's physiological state for preAD. In this study, we purpose to explore the change of coupling relationship among 27 normal controls (NCs), 20 preADs, and 15 cognitive impairments (CIs). For each subject, we calculated the Spearman partial correlation between the fractional amplitude of low-frequency fluctuations (fALFF) and the regional homogeneity (ReHo) from functional image (fMRI), and the standard uptake value ratio (SUVR) from [18F] fluorodeoxyglucose positron emission tomography (^{18}F-FDG PET), in the whole-brain and default mode network (DMN) as a novel potential biomarker. The diagnostic performance of this biomarker was evaluated by the receiver operating characteristic analysis. Significant Spearman correlations between the FDG SUVR and the fALFF/ReHo were found in 98% of subjects. For the DMN-based biomarker, there was a significant decreasing trend for the preAD and CI groups compared to the NC group, whereas no significant difference in preAD based on whole-brain. The correlation ρ value for the FDG SUVR/ReHo showed the highest area under curve of the preAD classification (0.787). The results imply the coupling relationship changed during the preAD stage in the DMN area.

KEYWORDS
default mode network, functional magnetic resonance imaging, position emission tomography, preclinical Alzheimer's disease

1 | INTRODUCTION

Alzheimer's disease (AD) is a neurodegenerative disease characterized by progressive cognitive decline. Amyloid-β (Aβ) and tau

Changchang Ding and Wenying Du should be considered joint first author.

CHENG Y, SONG S, WEI Y, et al.Glioma imaging by O-(2-^{18}F-Fluoroethyl)-L-tyrosine PET and diffusion-weighted MRI and correlation with molecular phenotypes, validated by PET/MR-guided biopsies.Front Oncol, 2021, 11: 743655.

【研究简介】

研究背景： 脑胶质瘤分子病理的预测是临床诊治的热点问题，对放化疗及综合治疗方案具有决策意义。胶质瘤存在较高的组织学和分子异质性，本研究基于一体化 ^{18}F-FET PET/MR 同步多模态显像对肿瘤进行立体定向穿刺活检，以探索 ^{18}F-FET PET 联合 DWI 预测肿瘤分子基因型的价值。

资料与方法： 11 例患者在 PET/MR 检查后一周内进行穿刺活检，根据 ^{18}F-FET PET 显像和 MRI 增强图像，每例患者选取 1 ~ 7 个活检部位，共获得 36 个穿刺活检样本。穿刺结束后患者行 3D T_1WI 及 3D FLAIR 扫描，采用 3D Slicer 软件的"通用配准模块"将术前及术中 MRI 图像配准，确认穿刺部位，测量穿刺取材区域术前 PET 的平均及最大 TBR（TBR$_{mean}$、TBR$_{max}$）、DWI 的平均及最小 ADC 和 eADC 值。穿刺活检样本均由病理科两位主治以上级别医师，依据 2016 年 WHO 脑肿瘤分类标准进行组织病理和基因型分析。

研究结果： 具有人端粒酶逆转录酶（*hTERT*）突变的肿瘤区域 TBR 较高、ADC 较低，肿瘤蛋白 *P53* 突变与较低的 TBR 和较高的 ADC 值相关，a- 地中海贫血 / 智力迟钝综合征 X 连锁基因（*ATRX*）突变与较高的 ADC 值相关，1p/19q 联合缺失和表皮生长因子受体（EGFR）突变与较低的 ADC 值相关，异枸橼酸脱氢酶 1（isocitrate dehydrogenase-1，IDH-1）突变与较高的 TBR$_{mean}$ 值相关，TBR$_{max}$/TBR$_{mean}$/ADC/eADC 值与磷酸酶和张力素同源突变（*PTEN*）或 MGMT 启动子甲基化之间无显著相关（图 1-1-43）。PET 的 TBR、DWI 的 ADC 和 eADC 在不同胶质瘤级别和基因型存在显著差异（图 1-1-44 ~ 图 1-1-46）。

研究结论： 一体化 PET/MR 可预测胶质瘤级别，以及 *IDH1*、*hTERT*、*TP53*、*EGFR* 等突变，^{18}F-FET PET 联合 DWI-ADC 能够提高预测胶质瘤分级及相关基因突变的准确度及特异度，有助于实现影像参数和分子突变的精准"点对点"对应。

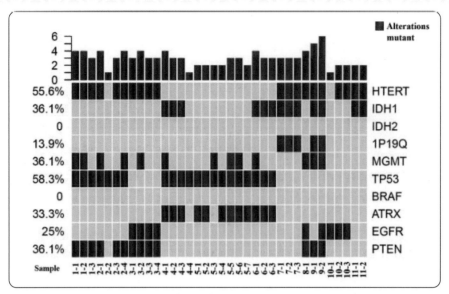

图 1-1-43　脑胶质瘤患者肿瘤穿刺点的级别及分子亚型分布情况

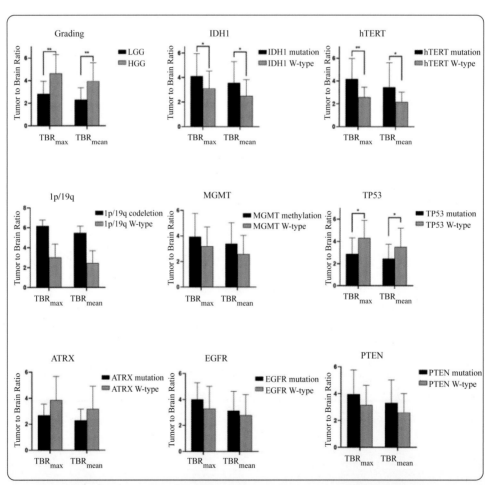

图 1-1-44　不同级别和基因型胶质瘤的 ^{18}F-FET PET 的 TBR 比较

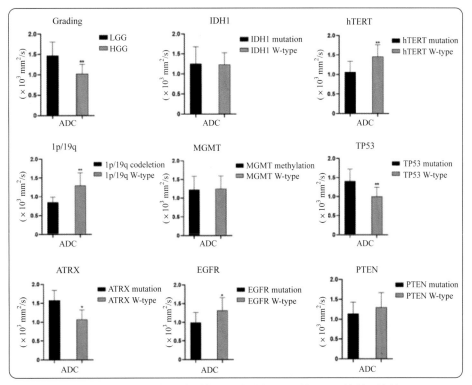

图 1-1-45　不同级别和基因型胶质瘤 DWI 的 ADC 的差异比较

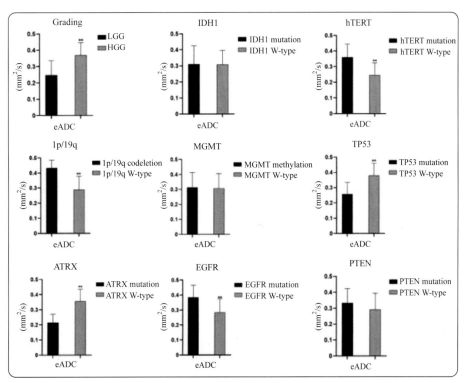

图 1-1-46　不同级别和基因型胶质瘤 DWI 的 eADC 差异比较

首都医科大学宣武医院一体化 PET/MR 成果集

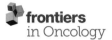

ORIGINAL RESEARCH
published: 29 November 2021
doi: 10.3389/fonc.2021.743655

Glioma Imaging by O-(2-18F-Fluoroethyl)-L-Tyrosine PET and Diffusion-Weighted MRI and Correlation With Molecular Phenotypes, Validated by PET/MR-Guided Biopsies

Ye Cheng[1,2,3†], Shuangshuang Song[4,5,6†], Yukui Wei[1,2], Geng Xu[1,2], Yang An[1,2], Jie Ma[5], Hongwei Yang[5], Zhigang Qi[4], Xinru Xiao[1,2], Jie Bai[1,2], Lixin Xu[1,2], Zeliang Hu[7], Tingting Sun[8], Leiming Wang[7*], Jie Lu[4,5*] and Qingtang Lin[1,2*]

[1] Department of Neurosurgery, Xuanwu Hospital, Capital Medical University, Beijing, China, [2] Department of Neurosurgery, China International Neuroscience Institute, Beijing, China, [3] Department of Neurosurgery, National Clinical Research Center for Geriatric Diseases, Beijing, China, [4] Department of Radiology and Nuclear Medicine, Xuanwu Hospital, Capital Medical University, Beijing, China, [5] Beijing Key Laboratory of Magnetic Resonance Imaging and Brain Informatics, Beijing, China, [6] Department of Nuclear Medicine, The Affiliated Hospital of Qingdao University, Qingdao, China, [7] Department of Pathology, Xuanwu Hospital, Capital Medical University, Beijing, China, [8] Department of Medicine, Nanjing Geneseeq Technology Inc., Nanjing, China

OPEN ACCESS

Edited by:
Khan Iftekharuddin,
Old Dominion University, United States

Reviewed by:
Jens Gempt,
Technical University of Munich,
Germany
Marco Riva,
University of Milan, Italy

*Correspondence:
Leiming Wang
wangleiming0918@163.com
Jie Lu
imaginglu@hotmail.com
Qingtang Lin
linqingtang@126.com

†These authors have contributed
equally to this work

Specialty section:
This article was submitted to
Neuro-Oncology and
Neurosurgical Oncology,
a section of the journal
Frontiers in Oncology

Received: 21 July 2021
Accepted: 11 November 2021
Published: 29 November 2021

Citation:
Cheng Y, Song S, Wei Y, Xu G, An Y,
Ma J, Yang H, Qi Z, Xiao X, Bai J, Xu L,
Hu Z, Sun T, Wang L, Lu J and Lin Q
(2021) Glioma Imaging by O-(2-18F-
Fluoroethyl)-L-Tyrosine PET and
Diffusion-Weighted MRI and
Correlation With Molecular
Phenotypes, Validated
by PET/MR-Guided Biopsies.
Front. Oncol. 11:743655.
doi: 10.3389/fonc.2021.743655

Gliomas exhibit high intra-tumoral histological and molecular heterogeneity. Introducing stereotactic biopsy, we achieved a superior molecular analysis of glioma using O-(2-18F-fluoroethyl)-L-tyrosine (FET)-positron emission tomography (PET) and diffusion-weighted magnetic resonance imaging (DWI). Patients underwent simultaneous DWI and FET-PET scans. Correlations between biopsy-derived tumor tissue values, such as the tumor-to-background ratio (TBR) and apparent diffusion coefficient (ADC)/exponential ADC (eADC) and histopathological diagnoses and those between relevant genes and TBR and ADC values were determined. Tumor regions with human telomerase reverse transcriptase (hTERT) mutation had higher TBR and lower ADC values. Tumor protein P53 mutation correlated with lower TBR and higher ADC values. α-thalassemia/mental-retardation-syndrome-X-linked gene (ATRX) correlated with higher ADC values. 1p/19q codeletion and epidermal growth factor receptor (EGFR) mutations correlated with lower ADC values. Isocitrate dehydrogenase 1 (IDH1) mutations correlated with higher TBRmean values. No correlation existed between TBRmax/TBRmean/ADC/eADC values and phosphatase and tensin homolog mutations (PTEN) or O6-methylguanine-DNA methyltransferase (MGMT) promoter methylation. Furthermore, TBR/ADC combination had a higher diagnostic accuracy than each single imaging method for high-grade and IDH1-, hTERT-, and EGFR-mutated gliomas. This is the first study establishing the accurate diagnostic criteria for glioma based on FET-PET and DWI.

Keywords: hybrid PET/MR, 18F-FET, DWI, glioma phenotyping, biopsy

SONG S, WANG L, YANG H, et al.Static ^{18}F-FET PET and DSC-PWI based on hybrid PET/MR for the prediction of gliomas defined by IDH and 1p/19q status.Eur Radiol, 2021, 31(6): 4087-4096.

【研究简介】

研究背景：异枸橼酸脱氢酶（isocitrate dehydrogenase，IDH）突变和 1p/19q 编码缺失是脑胶质瘤分类的重要分子生物标志物之一。研究表明 IDH 突变状态与胶质瘤的诊断、治疗及预后密切相关，本研究旨在利用一体化 PET/MR 探索 ^{18}F-FET PET 的胶质瘤氨基酸代谢信息联合灌注加权成像（DSC-PWI）的脑血容量（cerebral blood volume，CBV）信息，预测胶质瘤分级、IDH 突变及 1p/19q 突变。

资料与方法：本研究纳入 52 例经病理证实的胶质瘤患者，术前均进行了一体化 ^{18}F-FET PET/MR DSC-PWI 检查。基于 PET/MR 图像对肿瘤病灶进行体积分割（图 1-1-47），计算 TBR 的均值和最大值、标准 CBV（normalized CBV，nCBV）的均值和最大值，综合评估二者在胶质瘤分级、IDH 突变及 1p/19q 突变的预测效能，采用 ROC 曲线和 AUC 进行对比统计分析。

研究结果：高低级别胶质瘤的 TBR_{mean}、TBR_{max}、$rCBV_{mean}$ 及 $rCBV_{max}$ 均有显著差异（P 均小于 0.05），其中 nCBVmean 鉴别高低级别胶质瘤的 AUC 高达 0.920，敏感度与特异度分别为 91.67%、90.00%（图 1-1-48）。TBR_{mean}、TBR_{max}、及 $rCBV_{mean}$ 均可鉴别 IDH- 野生型胶质母细胞瘤和 IDH- 突变不伴 1p/19q 联合缺失型星形细胞瘤（P 分别为 0.049、0.034 和 0.029）；IDH- 野生型胶质母细胞瘤组和 IDH- 突变伴 1p/19q 联合缺失型少突胶质细胞瘤组的 $rCBV_{mean}$ 存在统计学差异（$P < 0.001$）。IDH- 突变型星形细胞瘤和 IDH 突变伴 1P/19q 联合缺失型少突胶质细胞瘤（图 1-1-49）的所有参数均无统计学差异。TBR_{max} 和 $rCBV_{mean}$ 在 IDH- 突变型与 IDH- 野生型胶质瘤间的分布有显著差异，其预测胶质瘤 IDH 亚型的 AUC 分别为 0.678 和 0.815。

研究结论：^{18}F-FET PET 和 DSC-PWI 同步信息是脑胶质瘤分级和 IDH 突变的无创影像学标志物，^{18}F-FET PET 联合 CBV 可以进一步提高 IDH 突变型星形细胞瘤和 IDH 野生型胶质母细胞瘤的鉴别效能，然而二者鉴别少突胶质细胞瘤的效能有限。

第一章 一体化 PET/MR 科研成果

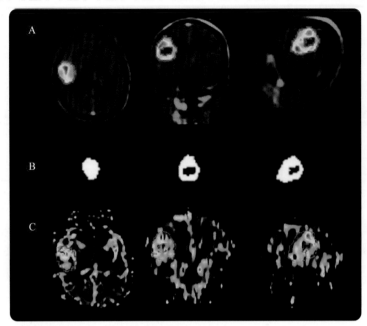

图 1-1-47　IDH-野生型胶质母细胞瘤患者（53 岁，男性）的 ^{18}F-FET PET 图像（图 A），3D 肿瘤病灶区域体积分割（图 B）和 CBV 图（图 C）

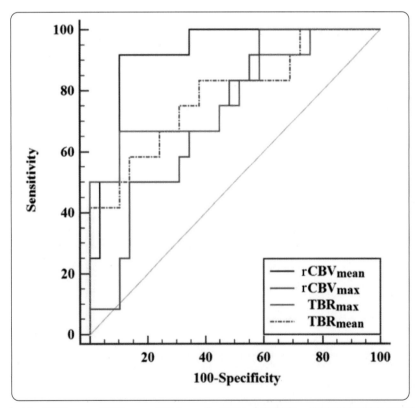

图 1-1-48　TBR_{mean}、TBR_{max}、$rCBV_{mean}$ 或 $rCBV_{max}$ 鉴别高、低级别胶质瘤的 ROC 曲线

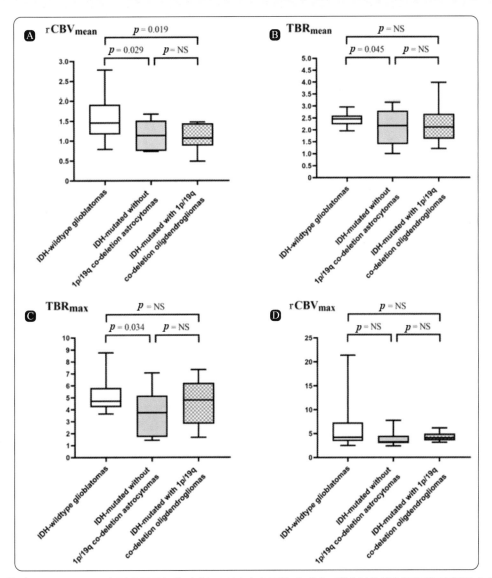

图 1-1-49　箱式图显示 IDH 野生型胶质母细胞瘤组、IDH 突变不伴 1p/19q 联合缺失型星形细胞瘤组及少突胶质细胞瘤组的 TBR$_{mean}$、TBR$_{max}$、rCBV$_{mean}$ 和 rCBV$_{max}$ 比较

European Radiology (2021) 31:4087–4096
https://doi.org/10.1007/s00330-020-07470-9

NEURO

Static ^{18}F-FET PET and DSC-PWI based on hybrid PET/MR for the prediction of gliomas defined by IDH and 1p/19q status

Shuangshuang Song[1,2] · Leiming Wang[3] · Hongwei Yang[4] · Yongzhi Shan[5] · Ye Cheng[5] · Lixin Xu[5] ·
Chengyan Dong[6] · Guoguang Zhao[5] · Jie Lu[1,2]

Received: 3 June 2020 / Revised: 26 August 2020 / Accepted: 4 November 2020 / Published online: 19 November 2020
© European Society of Radiology 2020

Abstract

Objectives To investigate the predictive value of static O-(2-^{18}F-fluoroethyl)-L-tyrosine positron emission tomography (^{18}F-FET PET) and cerebral blood volume (CBV) for glioma grading and determining isocitrate dehydrogenase (IDH) mutation and 1p/19q codeletion status.

Methods Fifty-two patients with newly diagnosed gliomas who underwent simultaneous ^{18}F-FET PET and dynamic susceptibility contrast perfusion-weighted imaging (DSC-PWI) examinations on hybrid PET/MR were retrospectively enrolled. The mean and max tumor-to-brain ratio (TBR) and normalized CBV (nCBV) were calculated based on whole tumor volume segmentations with reference to PET/MR images. The predictive efficacy of FET PET and CBV in glioma according to the 2016 World Health Organization (WHO) classification was evaluated by receiver operating characteristic curve analyses with the area under the curve (AUC).

Results TBRmean, TBRmax, nCBVmean, and nCBVmax differed between low- and high-grade gliomas, with the highest AUC of nCBVmean (0.920). TBRmax and nCBVmean showed significant differences between gliomas with and without IDH mutation ($p = 0.032$ and 0.010, respectively). Furthermore, TBRmean, TBRmax, and nCBVmean discriminated between IDH-wildtype glioblastomas and IDH-mutated astrocytomas ($p = 0.049$, 0.034 and 0.029, respectively). The combination of TBRmax and nCBVmean showed the best predictive performance (AUC, 0.903). Only nCBVmean differentiated IDH-mutated with 1p/19q codeletion oligodendrogliomas from IDH-wildtype glioblastomas ($p < 0.001$) (AUC, 0.829), but none of the parameters discriminated between oligodendrogliomas and astrocytomas.

Conclusions Both FET PET and DSC-PWI might be non-invasive predictors for glioma grades and IDH mutation status. FET PET combined with CBV could improve the differentiation of IDH-mutated astrocytomas and IDH-wildtype glioblastomas. However, FET PET and CBV might be limited for identifying oligodendrogliomas.

Key Points

• *Static ^{18}F-FET PET and DSC-PWI parameters differed between low- and high-grade gliomas, with the highest AUC of the mean value of normalized CBV.*

• *Static ^{18}F-FET PET and DSC-PWI parameters based on hybrid PET/MR showed predictive value in identifying glioma IDH mutation subtypes, which have gained importance for both determining the diagnosis and prognosis of gliomas according to the 2016 WHO classification.*

• *Static ^{18}F-FET PET and DSC-PWI parameters have limited potential in differentiating IDH-mutated with 1p/19q codeletion oligodendrogliomas from IDH-wildtype glioblastomas or IDH-mutated astrocytomas.*

Shuangshuang Song and Leiming Wang contribute equally to this work as
co-first author.

✉ Jie Lu
  imaginglu@hotmail.com

1 Department of Radiology, Xuanwu Hospital, Capital Medical
   University, No. 45 Changchun Street, Xicheng District,
   Beijing 100053, China

2 Beijing Key Laboratory of Magnetic Resonance Imaging and Brain
   Informatics, Beijing, China

3 Department of Pathology, Xuanwu Hospital, Capital Medical
   University, Beijing, China

4 Department of Nuclear Medicine, Xuanwu Hospital, Capital Medical
   University, Beijing, China

5 Department of Neurosurgery, Xuanwu Hospital, Capital Medical
   University, Beijing, China

6 GE Healthcare, Beijing, China

 Springer

GUO K, CUI B, SHANG K, et al.Assessment of localization accuracy and postsurgical prediction of simultaneous ¹⁸F-FDG PET/MRI in refractory epilepsy patients. Eur Radiol, 2021, 31(9): 6974-6982.

【研究简介】

研究背景：癫痫临床特征是反复性、自发性癫痫发作，全世界人群的发生率为 1%～2%，其中 1/3 患者用药控制效果并不理想，因此外科手术是癫痫治疗的常用方案，手术治疗的前提及治疗效果取决于致痫区的精准定位。

资料与方法：本研究纳入 98 例经病理证实为难治性癫痫的患者，行外科手术前进行 PET/MR 检查，术后追踪随访 1 年。两名放射科 – 核医学科医师对患者的 PET/MR 图像进行视觉分析定位致痫区，以病理和手术后 1 年随访结果为定位准确的"金标准"，计算 ¹⁸F-FDG PET/MR 定位致痫区的灵敏性、特异度、准确度，分析 PET/MR 定位结果与手术切除部位一致时，与预后的相关性（图 1-1-50～图 1-1-53）。

研究结果：¹⁸F-FDG PET/MR 成像对难治性癫痫致痫区的定位灵敏性、特异度和准确度分别为 95.3%、8.8%、65.3%，多因素 Logistic 回归分析显示 PET/MR 结果与手术部位一致（OR=14.741，95% CI 3.934～55.033，$P < 0.001$）是影响手术预后的独立危险因素。

研究结论：¹⁸F-FDG PET/MR 提供的综合影像信息，能够提高难治性癫痫的致痫区定位灵敏性，有助于进一步改善外科手术预后。

第一章 一体化 PET/MR 科研成果

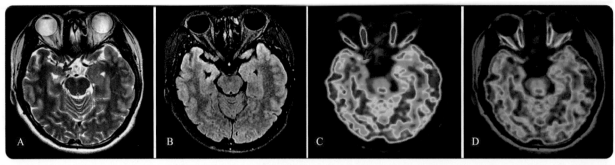

图 1-1-50　患者女性，21 岁，癫痫反复发作伴有意识障碍 13 年，横轴位 T$_2$WI（图 A）和 T$_2$-FLAIR（图 B）显示右侧海马体体积减小和信号增高（箭头）。^{18}F-FDG PET（图 C）和 PET/MR（图 D）显示局灶性代谢减低。术后病理诊断为海马硬化（箭头）

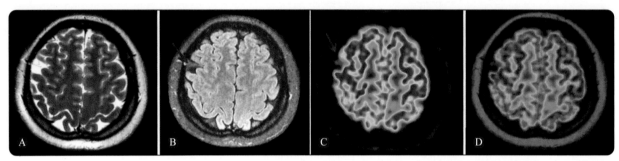

图 1-1-51　患者女性，35 岁，癫痫发作 28 年，横轴位 T$_2$WI（图 A）、T$_2$-FLAIR（图 B）显示脑沟增宽，右侧额叶条状高信号（箭头）。^{18}F-FDG PET（图 C）和 PET/MR（图 D）显示 MRI 异常部位病灶局灶性代谢减低。术后病理诊断为结节性硬化（箭头）

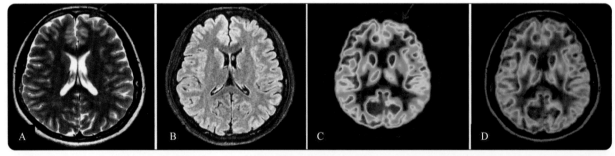

图 1-1-52　患者女性，22 岁，癫痫发作 17 年，横轴位 T$_2$WI（图 A）和 T$_2$-FLAIR（图 B）显示左上额叶皮质可疑皮质增厚（箭头）。^{18}F-FDG PET（图 C）和 PET/MR（图 D）显示左上额叶局灶性代谢减低。术后病理诊断为局灶性皮质发育不良（箭头）

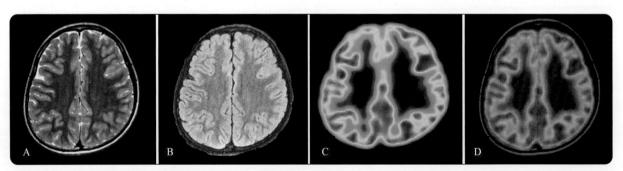

图 1-1-53　患者男性，6 岁，癫痫发作 4 年余，横轴位 T$_2$WI（图 A）和 T$_2$-FLAIR（图 B）未见异常信号。^{18}F-FDG PET（图 C）和 PET/MR（图 D）显示双侧额叶皮层局灶性代谢减低

European Radiology
https://doi.org/10.1007/s00330-021-07738-8

NUCLEAR MEDICINE

Assessment of localization accuracy and postsurgical prediction of simultaneous ^{18}F-FDG PET/MRI in refractory epilepsy patients

Kun Guo[1] · Bixiao Cui[1] · Kun Shang[1] · Yaqin Hou[1] · Xiaotong Fan[2] · Hongwei Yang[1] · Guoguang Zhao[2] · Jie Lu[1,3,4]

Received: 7 April 2020 / Revised: 16 December 2020 / Accepted: 2 February 2021
© European Society of Radiology 2021

Abstract
Objectives To evaluate the accuracies of simultaneous ^{18}F-fluorodeoxyglucose positron emission tomography/magnetic resonance imaging ([^{18}F]-FDG PET/MRI) in preoperative localization and the postsurgical prediction.
Methods This retrospective study was performed on ninety-eight patients diagnosed with refractory epilepsy whose presurgical evaluation included [^{18}F]-FDG PET/MRI, with 1-year post-surgery follow-up between August 2016 and December 2018. PET/MRI images were interpreted by two radiologists and a nuclear medicine physician to localize the EOZ using standard visual analysis and asymmetry index based on standard uptake value (SUV). The localization accuracy and predictive performance of simultaneous ^{18}F-FDG PET/MRI based on the surgial pathology and postsurgical outcome were evaluated.
Results A total of 41.8% (41/98) patients were found to have a definitely structural abnormality on the MR portion of PET/MRI; 93.9% (92/98) were shown hypometabolism on the PET portion of the hybrid PET/MRI. PET/MRI identified 18 cases with subtle structural abnormalities on MRI re-read. Six percent (6/98) of patients PET/MRI were negative. A total of 65.3% (64/98) patients showed seizure-free at 1-year follow-up after epilepsy surgery. The sensitivity, specificity, and accuracy of [^{18}F]-FDG PET/MRI was 95.3%, 8.8%, and 65.3% for seizure onset localization based on surgical pathology and postsurgical outcome, respectively. Multivariate regression analysis indicated that concordant of EOZ localization between PET/MRI and surgical resection range, which was a good positive predictor of seizure freedom (Engel I) (OR = 14.741, 95% CI 3.934–55.033, $p < 0.001$).
Conclusions [^{18}F]-FDG PET/MRI used as two combined modalities providing additional sensitivity when detecting possible epileptic foci and will probably improve the surgical outcome.
Key Points
• *Sensitivity, specificity, and accuracy of [^{18}F]-FDG PET/MRI were 95.3%, 8.8%, and 65.3% for seizure onset localization based on surgical pathology and postsurgical outcome, respectively.*
• *Concordance of EOZ localization between PET/MRI and surgical resection range was a good positive predictor of seizure freedom; presurgical [^{18}F]-FDG PET/MRI will probably improve the surgical outcome.*

Keywords Epilepsy · Positron emission tomography · Magnetic resonance imaging · Surgery · Prognosis

✉ Jie Lu
imaginglu@hotmail.com

[1] Department of Nuclear Medicine, Xuanwu Hospital, Capital Medical University, Beijing, China

[2] Department of Neurosurgery, China INI, Xuanwu Hospital, Capital Medical University, Beijing, China

[3] Department of Radiology, Xuanwu Hospital, Capital Medical University, Beijing, China

[4] Beijing Key Laboratory of Magnetic Resonance Imaging and Brain Informatics, Beijing, China

Abbreviations

[^{18}F]-FDG PET/MRI	^{18}F-fluorodeoxyglucose positron emission tomography/magnetic resonance imaging
AI	Asymmetry index
CD	Cortical dysplasia
CI	Confidence interval
EOZ	Epileptogenic onset zone
FCD	Focal cortical dysplasia
HS	Hippocampus sclerosis
OR	Odds ratio
SVA	Standard visual analysis
TSC	Tuberous sclerosis complex

Published online: 27 February 2021

 Springer

LI X, YU T, REN Z, et al.Localization of the epileptogenic zone by multimodal neuroimaging and high-frequency oscillation.Front Hum Neurosci, 2021, 15: 677840.

【研究简介】

研究背景：准确定位致痫区是难治性癫痫患者获得良好手术效果的关键因素，然而目前缺乏可以精确定位致痫区的影像技术，本研究旨在综合应用多种影像技术提高致痫区定位精度。

资料与方法：回顾性分析 15 例手术的难治性癫痫患者 PET/MR、液体 – 白质抑制序列（FLAWS）及高频震荡（high frequency oscillation，HFO）自动分析脑电信息（图 1–1–54），检测患者的异常脑区。比较 PET-MRI、FLAWS 和 HFO 与传统方法的结果，以评估其诊断价值。使用每种模态标记每例患者的致痫区，以确定三种模态之间定位的相关性。

研究结果：与传统方法相比，PET/MR、FLAWS 和 HFOs 可以提供更多潜在致癫痫灶的信息（图 1–1–55）。PET/MR、FLAWS 和 HFOs 检测致痫区的敏感度分别为 68.75%、53.85% 和 87.50%，特异度分别为 80.00%、33.33% 和 100.00%。术后良好患者 HFO 标记的电极触点切除率显著高于术后不良的患者（$P < 0.05$）。颅内电极覆盖神经影像学显示的所有异常区域，依据 HFO 分析结果，完全去除重叠的致痫区，患者术后癫痫发作（$P < 0.01$）。

研究结论：多模态方法可以更准确检测致痫区，HFO 分析有助于定义真正的致痫区，无创 PET/MR 和 FLAWS 结果联合 HFO 分析指导植入颅内电极是定位致痫区优化分析方法。

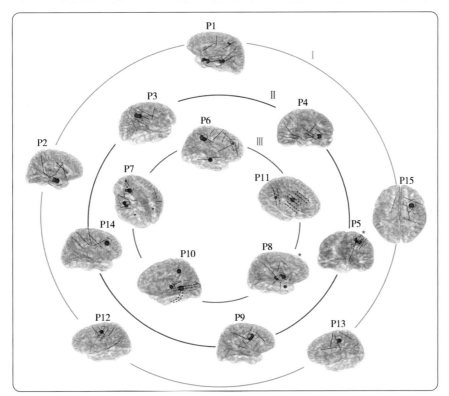

15例患者的硬膜下电极（P10和P11）或SEEG位置。大多数电极显示为黑色，白色表示大脑模型无法显示的对侧电极。蓝色、红色和绿色球体分别表示使用PET/MR、FLAWS和HFO检测的可疑异常，不同的体积表明不同的显著性水平。红色虚线标记切除病灶的体积。患者根据病理结果分为3组（Engel Ⅰ、Ⅱ和Ⅲ），*表示患者进行了射频消融术。

图 1-1-54　癫痫患者可疑致病区颅内电极放置部位

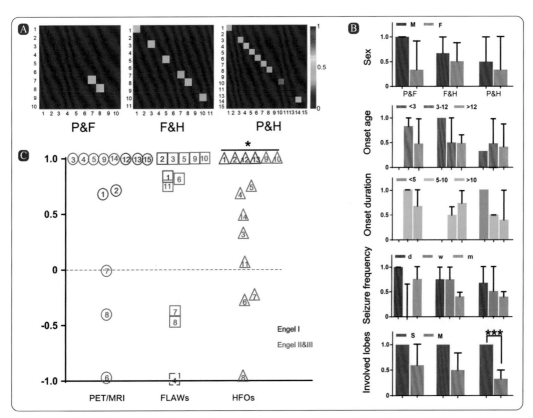

A.PET/MR和FLAWS（P&F）、FLAWS和HFOs（F&H）、PET/MR和HFOs（P&H）的一致性；B.不同性别、发作年龄、发作持续时间、发作频率和病变脑叶检测一致性；C.使用3种方法得到每个患者的病灶手术切除/未切除比值。

图 1-1-55　PET/MR、FLAWS和HFOs 3种技术定位致病区的一致性分析

首都医科大学宣武医院一体化 PET/MR 成果集

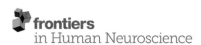

ORIGINAL RESEARCH
published: 08 June 2021
doi: 10.3389/fnhum.2021.677840

Localization of the Epileptogenic Zone by Multimodal Neuroimaging and High-Frequency Oscillation

Xiaonan Li[1,2,3], Tao Yu[2], Zhiwei Ren[2], Xueyuan Wang[2], Jiaqing Yan[4], Xin Chen[2], Xiaoming Yan[2], Wei Wang[1,2,3], Yue Xing[1,2,3], Xianchang Zhang[5], Herui Zhang[3], Horace H. Loh[3], Guojun Zhang[2]* and Xiaofeng Yang[1,2,3]*

[1] Laboratory of Brain Disorders, Collaborative Innovation Center for Brain Disorders, Ministry of Science and Technology, Beijing Institute of Brain Disorders, Capital Medical University, Beijing, China, [2] Xuanwu Hospital, Capital Medical University, Beijing, China, [3] Bioland Laboratory, Guangzhou, China, [4] College of Electrical and Control Engineering, North China University of Technology, Beijing, China, [5] MR Collaboration, Siemens Healthcare Ltd., Beijing, China

OPEN ACCESS

Edited by:
Felix Scholkmann,
University Hospital Zürich, Switzerland

Reviewed by:
Ahmet Ademoglu,
Boğaziçi University, Turkey
James Ward Antony,
Princeton University, United States

*Correspondence:
Xiaofeng Yang
xiaofengyang@yahoo.com
Guojun Zhang
zgj62051@163.com

Specialty section:
This article was submitted to
Brain Imaging and Stimulation,
a section of the journal
Frontiers in Human Neuroscience

Received: 08 March 2021
Accepted: 23 April 2021
Published: 08 June 2021

Citation:
Li X, Yu T, Ren Z, Wang X, Yan J,
Chen X, Yan X, Wang W, Xing Y,
Zhang X, Zhang H, Loh HH, Zhang G
and Yang X (2021) Localization of the
Epileptogenic Zone by Multimodal
Neuroimaging and High-Frequency
Oscillation.
Front. Hum. Neurosci. 15:677840.
doi: 10.3389/fnhum.2021.677840

Accurate localization of the epileptogenic zone (EZ) is a key factor to obtain good surgical outcome for refractory epilepsy patients. However, no technique, so far, can precisely locate the EZ, and there are barely any reports on the combined application of multiple technologies to improve the localization accuracy of the EZ. In this study, we aimed to explore the use of a multimodal method combining PET-MRI, fluid and white matter suppression (FLAWS)—a novel MRI sequence, and high-frequency oscillation (HFO) automated analysis to delineate EZ. We retrospectively collected 15 patients with refractory epilepsy who underwent surgery and used the above three methods to detect abnormal brain areas of all patients. We compared the PET-MRI, FLAWS, and HFO results with traditional methods to evaluate their diagnostic value. The sensitivities, specificities of locating the EZ, and marking extent removed versus not removed [RatioChann(ev)] of each method were compared with surgical outcome. We also tested the possibility of using different combinations to locate the EZ. The marked areas in every patient established using each method were also compared to determine the correlations among the three methods. The results showed that PET-MRI, FLAWS, and HFOs can provide more information about potential epileptic areas than traditional methods. When detecting the EZs, the sensitivities of PET-MRI, FLAWS, and HFOs were 68.75, 53.85, and 87.50%, and the specificities were 80.00, 33.33, and 100.00%. The RatioChann(ev) of HFO-marked contacts was significantly higher in patients with good outcome than those with poor outcome ($p < 0.05$). When intracranial electrodes covered all the abnormal areas indicated by neuroimaging with the overlapping EZs being completely removed referred to HFO analysis, patients could reach seizure-free ($p < 0.01$). The periphery of the lesion marked by neuroimaging may be epileptic, but not every lesion contributes to seizures. Therefore, approaches in multimodality can detect EZ more accurately, and HFO analysis may help in defining real epileptic areas that may be missed in the neuroimaging results. The implantation of intracranial electrodes guided by non-invasive PET-MRI and FLAWS findings as well as HFO analysis would be an optimized multimodal approach for locating EZ.

Keywords: epileptogenic zone, neuroimaging, high-frequency oscillations, PET-MRI, FLAWS, multimodal method

WANG J, SUN H, CUI B, et al.The relationship among glucose metabolism, cerebral blood flow, and functional activity: a hybrid PET/fMRI study.Mol Neurobiol, 2021, 58(6): 2862-2873.

【研究简介】

研究背景： ^{18}F-FDG PET 和 fMRI 可从不同方面评估大脑活动，包括 ^{18}FDG-PET 的区域葡萄糖摄取（rGU）、ASL 的区域脑血流（rCBF）及血氧水平依赖（blood oxygenation level dependent，BOLD）fMRI 的脱氧血红蛋白动态变化，然而 3 者之间的关联尚不清楚。

资料与方法： 本研究纳入 24 例健康受试者，基于一体化 PET/MR 同步获得 ^{18}F-FDG PET 代谢、ASL 血流和 fMRI 图像。为获得模态间共同像素模板 intersection mask，将所有受试者的视野模板 FOV mask 与 50% 的灰质模板相乘，在 intersection mask 内分别计算脑区 SUVR、CBF 和低频振荡 ALFF、Reho、DC。单样本方差检验获得每个模态数据的空间分布，配对 t 检验获得模态间的空间敏感度，像素水平和脑区水平跨像素间和跨被试间的相关性。

研究结果： 健康受试者 ASL-rCBF、rGU、fALFF、ReHo 和 DC 空间分布大致相似（图 1-1-56），在内侧前额叶、颞上回、颞中回、后扣带回、楔前叶和距状裂有较高活动。配对检验显示仅在基底节有较高代谢，双侧海马区 ASL-rCBF 高于 rGU、fALFF、ReHo，岛叶的 ASL-rCBF 和 rGU 高于其他静息态参数（图 1-1-57）。基于像素和基于脑区的跨像素相关性分析显示 rGU 和 ReHo 有最高的相关性，rGU 和静息态 fMRI 参数的相关性高于 ASL-rCBF 和静息态 fMRI 参数（图 1-1-58）。

研究结论： 一体化 PET/MR 同步获得脑区葡萄糖代谢、血流和脑活动信息，可以为大脑活动的潜在机制提供新视角。

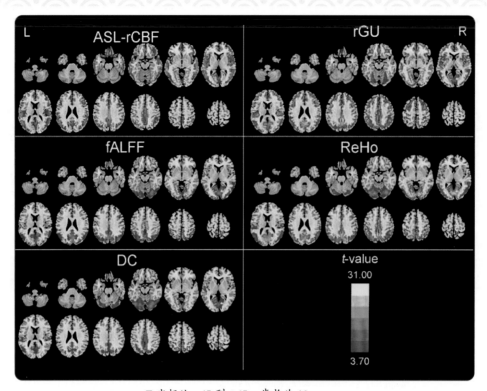

Z 坐标从 −45 到 +65，步长为 10 mm。

图 1-1-56　ASL-rCBF、rGU、fALFF、ReHo 和 DC 的单样本 t 检验结果（p < 0.05，FDR 校正）

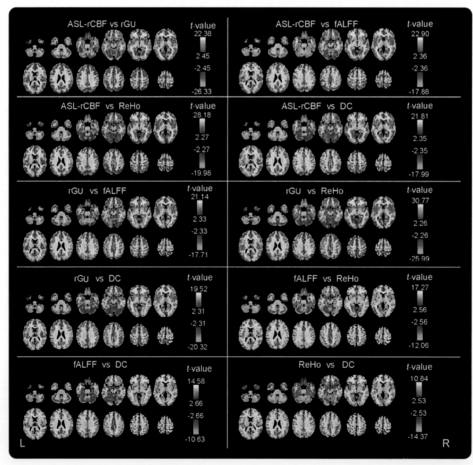

Z 坐标从 −45 到 +65，步长为 10 mm。ASL：动脉自旋标记；rCBF：局部脑血流；rGU：局部葡萄糖代谢；fALFF：低频波动振幅分数；ReHo：局部一致性；DC：度中心。

图 1-1-57　ASL-rCBF、rGU、fALFF、ReHo 和 DC 的配对 t 检验结果（P < 0.05，FDR 校正）

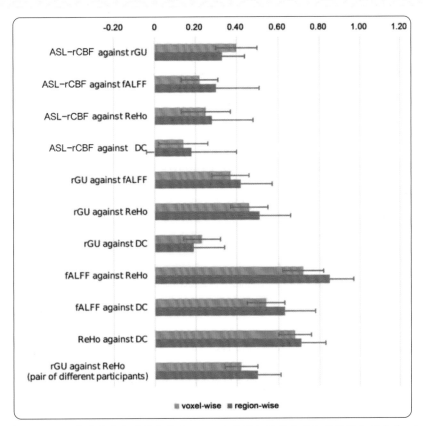

跨空间体素水平［$n=(19722\pm866)$体素］和脑区水平（$n=90$）两两相关的平均相关系数和标准差。红色是基于像素水平，紫色是基于脑区水平。

图 1-1-58　基于跨空间的相关性结果

Molecular Neurobiology (2021) 58:2862–2873
https://doi.org/10.1007/s12035-021-02305-0

The Relationship Among Glucose Metabolism, Cerebral Blood Flow, and Functional Activity: a Hybrid PET/fMRI Study

Jingjuan Wang[1] · Haiyang Sun[2,3,4] · Bixiao Cui[1] · Hongwei Yang[1] · Yi Shan[5] · Chengyan Dong[6] · Yufeng Zang[2,3,4] · Jie Lu[1,5]

Received: 15 July 2020 / Accepted: 20 December 2020 / Published online: 1 February 2021
Ⓒ The Author(s), under exclusive licence to Springer Science+Business Media, LLC part of Springer Nature 2021

Abstract

^{18}F-fluorodeoxyglucose (FDG) positron emission tomography (PET) and functional magnetic resonance imaging (fMRI) estimate brain activities from different aspects, including regional glucose uptake (rGU) by ^{18}FDG-PET, regional cerebral blood flow (rCBF) by arterial spin labeling, and dynamic changes of deoxyhemoglobin by blood oxygenation level-dependent (BOLD) functional magnetic resonance imaging (fMRI). However, the relationships between them remain incompletely understood. In the current study, twenty-four subjects (14 males, 10 females) were recruited and investigated the correlation among rGU, rCBF, and BOLD fMRI-derived metrics reflecting the neural activity, including amplitude of low-frequency fluctuation (ALFF), regional homogeneity (ReHo), and degree centrality (DC) by hybrid PET/fMRI. Correlation analyses were performed across subject and across space at both voxel level and region level, considering partial volume effects by adjusting for gray matter volume. Each pair of metrics showed significant across-space correlations. rGU against ReHo showed the highest mean correlation coefficients. rGU had higher correlations with three resting-state (RS) fMRI metrics than did ASL-rCBF. However, the across-subject correlations were not significant among functional modalities (rGU, rCBF, and RS-fMRI BOLD data) at either voxel level or region level even with a liberal threshold, except for significant across-subject correlation between RS-fMRI metrics (ALFF, ReHo, and DC). These comprehensive findings from hybrid PET/MR might provide complementary information to reveal the underlying mechanisms of the brain activity and open new perspective to interpret pathologic conditions.

Keywords Regional glucose metabolism · Cerebral blood flow · Resting-state fMRI · Correlation analysis · Hybrid PET/fMRI

Introduction

Hybrid scans of positron emission tomography (PET) and magnetic resonance imaging (MRI) are becoming increasingly popular for clinical diagnosis. PET and functional MRI (fMRI) are two of the most frequently used imaging techniques for non-invasively mapping the human brain function. Both ^{18}F-fluorodeoxyglucose (FDG)-PET and fMRI estimate brain activities from different aspects, such as energy consumption, low-frequency fluctuation, and regional cerebral blood flow (rCBF). However, the complex relationships among energy consumption, rCBF, and other fMRI metrics remain unknown.

FDG-PET is the most commonly used technique to assess regional glucose uptake (rGU), which reflects cellular activity by measuring glucose uptake. One method used in fMRI is referred to as blood oxygenation level-dependent (BOLD) imaging, which reflects the oxygen absorption by measuring the ratio changes of oxygenated to deoxygenated hemoglobin [1]. Resting-state functional MRI (RS-fMRI; i.e., without

✉ Yufeng Zang
zangyf@hznu.edu.cn

✉ Jie Lu
imaginglu@hotmail.com

1   Department of Nuclear Medicine, Xuanwu Hospital Capital Medical University, Beijing 100053, China

2   Center for Cognition and Brain Disorders, Affiliated Hospital, Hangzhou Normal University, Hangzhou 311121, China

3   Institutes of Psychological Sciences, Hangzhou Normal University, Hangzhou 311121, China

4   Zhejiang Key Laboratory for Research in Assessment of Cognitive Impairments, Hangzhou 311121, China

5   Department of Radiology, Xuanwu Hospital Capital Medical University, Beijing 100053, China

6   GE Healthcare, Beijing 100176, China

Ⓐ Springer

CUI B, ZHANG T, MA Y, et al.Simultaneous PET-MRI imaging of cerebral blood flow and glucose metabolism in the symptomatic unilateral internal carotid artery/middle cerebral artery steno-occlusive disease.Eur J Nucl Med Mol Imaging, 2020, 47(7): 1668-1677.

【研究简介】

研究背景： 缺血性脑血管病（ischemic cerebrovascular disease，ICVD）是脑血流动力学障碍导致相应供血区脑组织缺血、缺氧而出现脑组织坏死或软化，并引起短暂或持久的、局部或弥散的脑损害。CBF 是临床评价的重要指标之一，葡萄糖作为大脑的能量来源，也是反映缺血性脑血管病患者脑缺血状态的重要参数。本研究利用一体化 PET/MRI 获得相同生理状态下葡萄糖代谢和 CBF 值，评价缺血性脑血管病患者治疗前后的改变。

资料与方法： 本研究纳入 15 例慢性单侧颈内动脉 / 大脑中动脉狭窄或闭塞患者［女 2 例，男 13 例，年龄（47.33 ± 12.65）岁］，应用一体化 PET/MR 在颅内搭桥术前及术后进行检查。采用 ASL 测量 CBF 值，^{18}F-FDG PET 测量 SUVR。心脏搭桥手术前后，除梗死区及其对侧相应区域外，根据同侧和对侧大脑半球的 CBF 和 SUVR 分别计算 AI，计算术前和术后 CBF 和 SUVR 的百分比变化 ΔCBF 和 ΔSUVR，使用配对 t 检验行术前术后比较，Spearman's 检验同区域内血流和代谢参数的相关性。

研究结果： 术前慢性单侧颈内动脉 / 大脑中动脉狭窄或闭塞同侧的 CBF 和 SUVR 显著低于对侧（$P < 0.01$），术后 CBF 明显高于术前（$P < 0.05$），但术后 SUVR 并未显著提高（$P > 0.05$，图 1-1-59）。15 例患者术前患侧区域 CBF AI 与术前 SUVR AI 值之间存在显著相关（$r = 0.729$，$P < 0.01$，图 1-1-60），但 CBF 与 SUVR 之间无显著相关（$P > 0.05$）；术后 CBF 和 SUVR 的 AI 值较术前显著减低（$P < 0.05$）（图 1-1-61，图 1-1-62）。

研究结论： 一体化 PET/MR 联合血流和葡萄糖代谢信息，同时分析心脏搭桥手术患者术前、术后大脑血流动力学模式和代谢的变化，是评估慢性脑缺血患者血流动力学和代谢状态的重要手段。

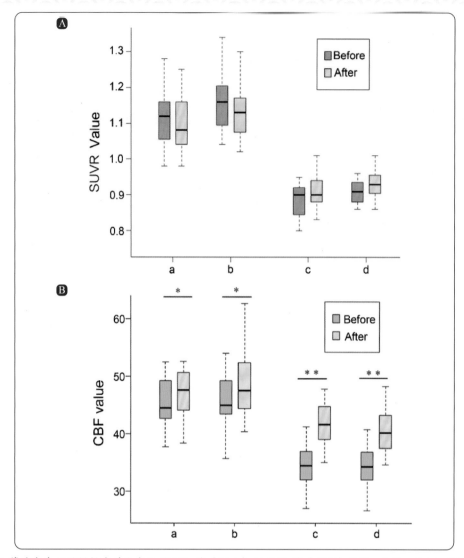

缺血性脑血管病患者心脏搭桥术前和术后 SUVR 值（图 A）与 CBF 值（图 B）比较。* $P < 0.05$，** $P < 0.01$。

图 1-1-59

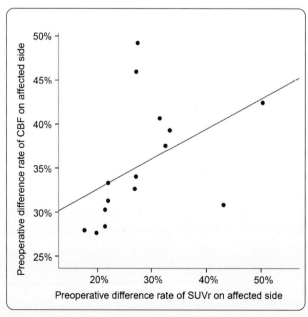

图 1-1-60　15 例缺血性脑血管病患者心脏搭桥术前血流和代谢相关性分析

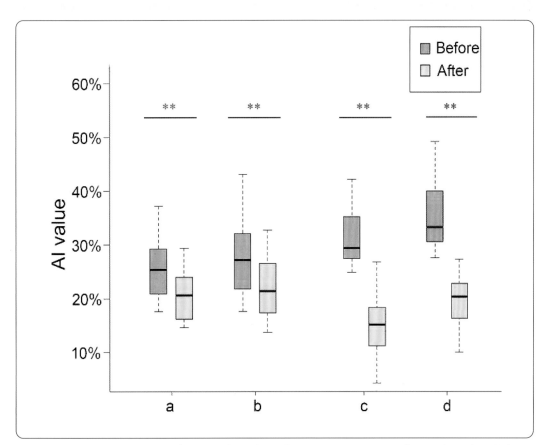

术后代谢减低区（图A）和代谢与血流同步减低区（图B）的 SUVR AI 值，以及血流减低区（图B）和代谢与血流同步减低区（图D）的 CBF AI 值比较，**$P < 0.01$。

图 1-1-61　缺血性脑血管病患者心脏搭桥术前和术后 AI 值的比较

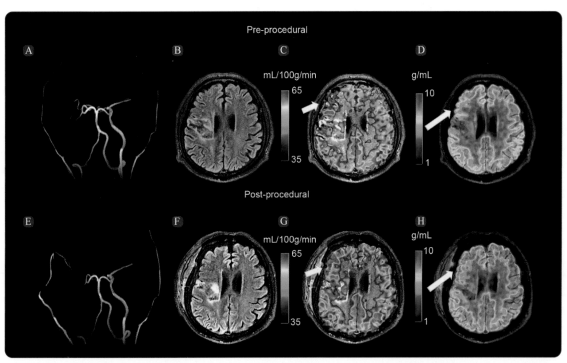

术前 MRA（图A）显示严重的 ICA 闭塞，术后 MRA（图E）显示 STA 和 MCA 之间的端侧吻合；T$_2$-FLAIR 图像（图B，图F）显示左额顶叶和胼胝体梗死；术后 CBF/MR 图像（图G）与术前图像（图C）相比，患侧血流明显提高（短箭头）；术后 ^{18}F-FDG PET/MRI 图像（图H）与术前（图D）相比代谢改善（长箭头）。

图 1-1-62　51 岁男性，右颈内动脉闭塞，搭桥手术前后血流、代谢改变

European Journal of Nuclear Medicine and Molecular Imaging
https://doi.org/10.1007/s00259-019-04551-w

ORIGINAL ARTICLE

Simultaneous PET-MRI imaging of cerebral blood flow and glucose metabolism in the symptomatic unilateral internal carotid artery/middle cerebral artery steno-occlusive disease

Bixiao Cui[1] · Tianhao Zhang[2,3] · Yan Ma[4] · Zhongwei Chen[5] · Jie Ma[1] · Lei Ma[1] · Liqun Jiao[4] · Yun Zhou[6] · Baoci Shan[2,3,7] · Jie Lu[1,8]

Received: 28 May 2019 / Accepted: 24 September 2019
© The Author(s) 2019

Abstract

Purpose Cerebral blood flow (CBF) and glucose metabolism are important and significant factors in ischaemic cerebrovascular disease. The objective of this study was to use quantitative hybrid PET/MR to evaluate the effects of surgery treatment on the symptomatic unilateral internal carotid artery/middle cerebral artery steno-occlusive disease.

Methods Fifteen patients diagnosed with ischaemic cerebrovascular disease were evaluated using a hybrid TOF PET/MR system (Signa, GE Healthcare). The CBF value measured by arterial spin labelling (ASL) and the standardized uptake value ratio (SUVR) measured by ^{18}F-FDG PET were obtained, except for the infarct area and its contralateral side, before and after bypass surgery. The asymmetry index (AI) was calculated from the CBF and SUVR of the ipsilateral and contralateral cerebral hemispheres, respectively. The ΔCBF and ΔSUVR were calculated as the percent changes of CBF and SUVR between before and after surgery, and paired t tests were used to determine whether a significant change occurred. Spearman's rank correlation was also used to compare CBF with glucose metabolism in the same region.

Results The analysis primarily revealed that after bypass surgery, a statistically significant increase occurred in the CBF on the affected side ($P < 0.01$). The postprocedural SUVR was not significantly higher than the preprocedural SUVR ($P > 0.05$). However, the postprocedural AI values for CBF and SUVR were significantly lower after surgery than before surgery ($P < 0.01$). A significant correlation was found between the AI values for preoperative CBF and SUVR on the ipsilateral hemisphere ($P < 0.01$).

Conclusions The present study demonstrates that a combination of ASL and ^{18}F-FDG PET could be used to simultaneously analyse changes in patients' cerebral haemodynamic patterns and metabolism between before and after superficial temporal artery-middle cerebral artery (STA-MCA) bypass surgery. This therefore represents an essential tool for the evaluation of critical haemodynamic and metabolic status in patients with symptomatic unilateral ischaemic cerebrovascular disease.

Bixiao Cui and Tianhao Zhang contributed equally to this study.

This article is part of the Topical Collection on Neurology.

✉ Baoci Shan
   shanbc@ihep.ac.cn

✉ Jie Lu
   imaginglu@hotmail.com

1   Department of Nuclear Medicine, Xuanwu Hospital Capital Medical University, Beijing, China

2   Beijing Engineering Research Center of Radiographic Techniques and Equipment, Institute of High Energy Physics, Chinese Academy of Sciences, Beijing, China

3   School of Nuclear Science and Technology, University of Chinese Academy of Sciences, Beijing, China

4   Department of Neurosurgery, Xuanwu Hospital Capital Medical University, Beijing, China

5   GE Healthcare, Beijing, China

6   Mallinckrodt Institute of Radiology, Washington University in St. Louis School of Medicine, St. Louis, MO, USA

7   CAS Center for Excellence in Brain Science and Intelligence Technology, Shanghai, China

8   Department of Radiology, Xuanwu Hospital Capital Medical University, Beijing, China

Published online: 06 November 2019

⌖ Springer

YAN S, ZHENG C, CUI B, et al.Multiparametric imaging hippocampal neurodegeneration and functional connectivity with simultaneous PET/MRI in Alzheimer's disease.Eur J Nucl Med Mol Imaging, 2020, 47(10): 2440-2452.

【研究简介】

研究背景：阿尔茨海默病（alzheimer's disease，AD）是最常见的神经退行性疾病，主要表现为认知功能减退、神经精神症状和日常生活能力丧失。海马是阿尔茨海默病最早受损的脑区之一，与记忆和空间定位关系密切。海马不同亚区具有不同的功能，本研究采用一体化 PET/MR 同时评估阿尔茨海默病患者海马亚区内在神经活动、葡萄糖代谢和结构信息，为阐明海马亚区神经功能受损的潜在机制提供影像学依据。

资料与方法：本研究纳入 102 例受试者，其中认知正常对照组 42 例、轻度认知障碍 38 例和阿尔茨海默病 22 例。所有受试者均进行一体化 PET/MR（GE Signa）检查，采集 ^{18}F-FDG、fMRI 和高分辨 3D T_1WI 图像。采用 Van Cittert 迭代法对 ^{18}F-FDG PET 图像行部分容积校正（partial volume correction，PVC），计算海马 3 个亚区（CA1、CA2/3/DG 和下托）的全脑功能连接、SUVR 和体积（图 1-1-63）。

研究结果：阿尔茨海默病和轻度认知障碍患者 CA1、CA2/3/DG 和下托的功能连接、^{18}F-FDG SUVR 和体积显著降低（阿尔茨海默病＜轻度认知障碍＜健康对照，图 1-1-64）。阿尔茨海默病患者左侧 CA2/3/DG-内侧额上回功能连接与左侧 CA2/3/DG 的 ^{18}F-FDG SUVR 和体积呈显著负相关，阿尔茨海默病患者左侧 CA2/3/DG 体积与 ^{18}F-FDG SUVR 呈正相关，提示海马失连接的主要亚区是左侧 CA2/3/DG（图 1-1-65）。

研究结论：一体化 PET/MR 同步获得阿尔茨海默病患者脑代谢、功能和结构信息，有助于了解海马失连接的神经机制，为阿尔茨海默病的干预治疗提供了潜在靶点。

第一章　一体化 PET/MR 科研成果

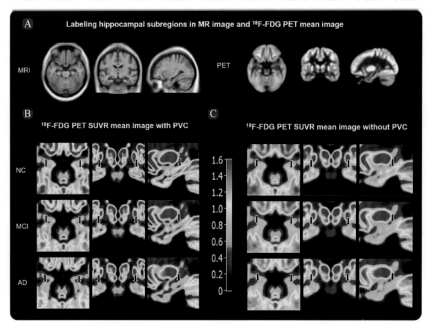

海马亚区模板（图 A）；PVC 校正后 PET 图像（图 B）较未经 PVC 校正图像（图 C）的对比度和空间分辨率更高。蓝色：CA1；红色：CA2/3/DG；绿色：下托；黑箭头：海马。

图 1-1-63　PVC 校正提高 ¹⁸F-FDG PET 图像空间分辨率

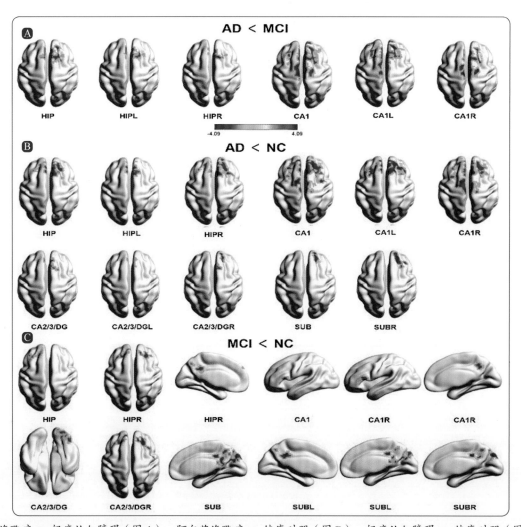

阿尔茨海默病 vs. 轻度认知障碍（图 A），阿尔茨海默病 vs. 健康对照（图 B），轻度认知障碍 vs. 健康对照（图 C）。

图 1-1-64　阿尔茨海默病和轻度认知障碍患者海马亚区全脑功能连接降低脑区

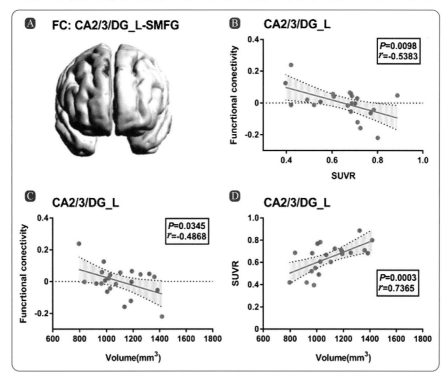

图 1-1-65 阿尔茨海默病患者左侧 CA2/3/DG-内侧前额叶功能连接强度（图 A）与 ^{18}F-FDG SUVR（图 B）和体积（图 C）均呈负相关，^{18}F-FDG SUVR 与左侧 CA2/3/DG 体积（图 D）呈正相关。

首都医科大学宣武医院一体化 PET/MR 成果集

European Journal of Nuclear Medicine and Molecular Imaging
https://doi.org/10.1007/s00259-020-04752-8

ORIGINAL ARTICLE

Multiparametric imaging hippocampal neurodegeneration and functional connectivity with simultaneous PET/MRI in Alzheimer's disease

Shaozhen Yan[1,2,3] · Chaojie Zheng[2] · Bixiao Cui[4] · Zhigang Qi[1,3] · Zhilian Zhao[1,3] · Yanhong An[1,3] · Liyan Qiao[5] · Ying Han[6] · Yun Zhou[2] · Jie Lu[1,3,4]

Received: 20 December 2019 / Accepted: 3 March 2020
© The Author(s) 2020

Abstract

Purpose The objective of this study is to investigate the hippocampal neurodegeneration and its associated aberrant functions in mild cognitive impairment (MCI) and Alzheimer's disease (AD) patients using simultaneous PET/MRI.

Methods Forty-two cognitively normal controls (NC), 38 MCI, and 22 AD patients were enrolled in this study. All subjects underwent ^{18}F-FDG PET/functional MRI (fMRI) and high-resolution T1-weighted MRI scans on a hybrid GE Signa PET/MRI scanner. Neurodegeneration in hippocampus and its subregions was quantified by regional gray matter volume and ^{18}F-FDG standardized uptake value ratio (SUVR) relative to cerebellum. An iterative reblurred Van Cittert iteration method was used for voxelwise partial volume correction on ^{18}F-FDG PET images. Regional gray matter volume was estimated from voxel-based morphometric analysis with MRI. fMRI data were analyzed after slice time correction and head motion correction using statistical parametric mapping (SPM12) with DPARSF toolbox. The regions of interest including hippocampus, cornu ammonis (CA1), CA2/3/dentate gyrus (DG), and subiculum were defined in the standard MNI space.

Results Patient groups had reduced SUVR, gray matter volume, and functional connectivity compared to NC in CA1, CA2/3/DG, and subiculum (AD < MCI < NC). There was a linear correlation between the left CA2/3DG gray matter volume and ^{18}F-FDG SUVR in AD patients ($P < 0.001$, $r = 0.737$). Significant correlation was also found between left CA2/3/DG-superior medial frontal gyrus functional connectivity and left CA2/3/DG hypometabolism in patients with AD. The functional connectivity of right CA1-precuneus in patients with MCI and right subiculum-superior frontal gyrus in patients with AD was positively correlated with mini mental status examination scores ($P < 0.05$).

Conclusion Our findings demonstrate that the associations existed at subregional hippocampal level between the functional connectivity measured by fMRI and neurodegeneration measured by structural MRI and ^{18}F-FDG PET. Our results may provide a basis for precision neuroimaging of hippocampus in AD.

Keywords Alzheimer's disease · Hippocampal subregions · Neurodegeneration · Hybrid PET/MRI · Voxel-based morphometric analysis

This article is part of the Topical Collection on Neurology

✉ Yun Zhou
    yunzhou@wustl.edu

✉ Jie Lu
    imaginglu@hotmail.com

1   Department of Radiology, Xuanwu Hospital, Capital Medical University, Beijing, China

2   Mallinckrodt Institute of Radiology, Washington University School of Medicine, 510 Kingshighway Blvd., St. Louis, MO, USA

3   Beijing Key Laboratory of Magnetic Resonance Imaging and Brain Informatics, Beijing, China

4   Department of Nuclear Medicine, Xuanwu Hospital, Capital Medical University, Beijing, China

5   Department of Neurology, Yuquan Hospital, Clinical Neuroscience Institute, Medical Center, Tsinghua University, Beijing, China

6   Department of Neurology, Xuanwu Hospital, Capital Medical University, Beijing, China

Published online: 10 March 2020

 Springer

LI TR, WU Y, JIANG JJ, et al.Radiomics analysis of magnetic resonance imaging facilitates the identification of preclinical Alzheimer's disease: an exploratory study.Front Cell Dev Biol, 2020, 8: 605734.

【研究简介】

研究背景：临床前阶段诊断阿尔茨海默病为早期干预提供了机会，目前缺乏简便的早期诊断生物标志物，本研究利用影像组学探讨多参数 MRI 提取的特征是否可作为潜在的诊断标志物。

资料与方法：本研究是中国认知衰退前瞻队列研究（NCT03370744）的一部分，所有参与者在基线时认知水平均正常。依据 PET 结果将队列 1（$n=183$）分为临床前阿尔茨海默病患者（$n=78$）和正常对照（$n=105$），80% 的受试者 MRI 数据被用作训练数据集，20% 的受试者用作测试集。队列 2（$n=51$）数据为回顾性，根据后来的认知状态分为阿尔茨海默病"转化者"和"非转化者"，该队列为单独测试数据集；队列 3 包括 37 个阿尔茨海默病转化者（13 个来自阿尔茨海默病神经成像计划），作为独立纵向的数据测试集。使用 t 检验、自相关检验和三种独立的选择算法，从每个受试者的多参数 MR 图像中提取放射组学特征，使用两个分类模型〔支持向量机（SVM）和随机森林（RF）〕来验证所保留特征的分类效能。对上述过程进行了 5 倍交叉验证并重复 100 次，将获得的稳定高频特征在队列 3 中通过配对双样本 t 检验和生存分析进行验证（图 1-1-66）。

研究结果：SVM 和 RF 模型都表现出良好的分类效率，测试集的平均准确率分别为 89.7%～95.9% 和 87.1%～90.8%，验证集的平均准确率为 81.9%～89.1% 和 83.2%～83.7%（图 1-1-67）。基于 MRI 结构像，识别出三个稳定的高频特征：右后扣带回的区域高灰度强调特征、左后扣带回的方差特征和左后扣带回的粗糙度特征，且与 β 淀粉样蛋白的沉积相关，并能预测未来的认知减退（AUC 为 0.649～0.761），此外基线变异特征水平随认知能力的下降而降低，并影响转化时间（$P < 0.05$，图 1-1-68）。

研究结论：多参数 MRI 扫描的放射组学特征可作为临床前阿尔茨海默病的潜在影像标志物，有助于临床的早期诊断。

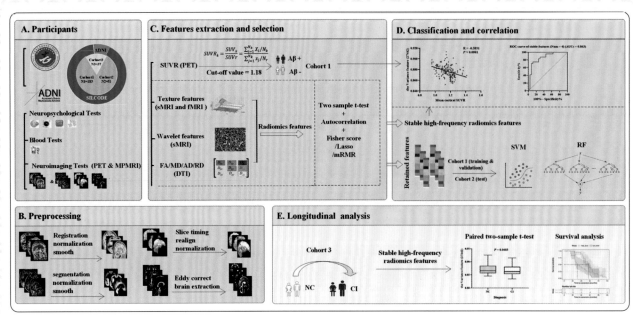

图 1-1-66 研究流程示意

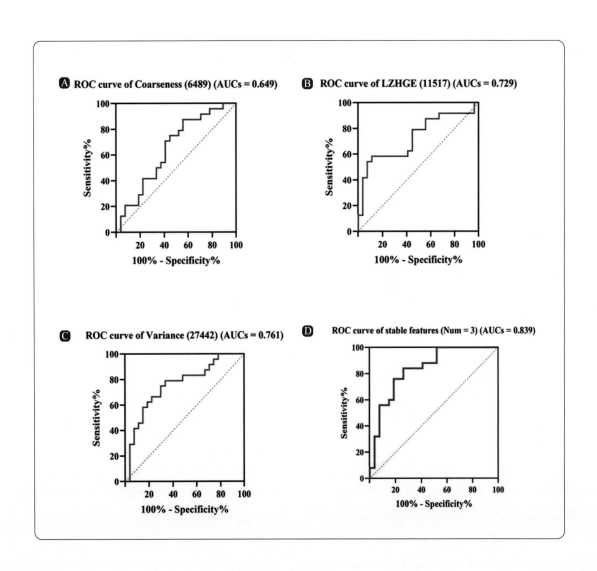

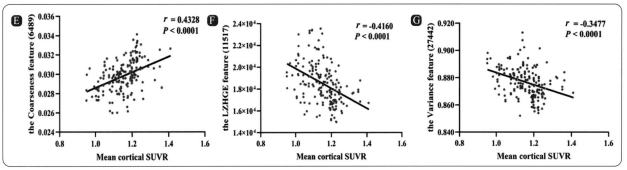

图 1-1-67　高频特征受试者特征曲线及相关性分析

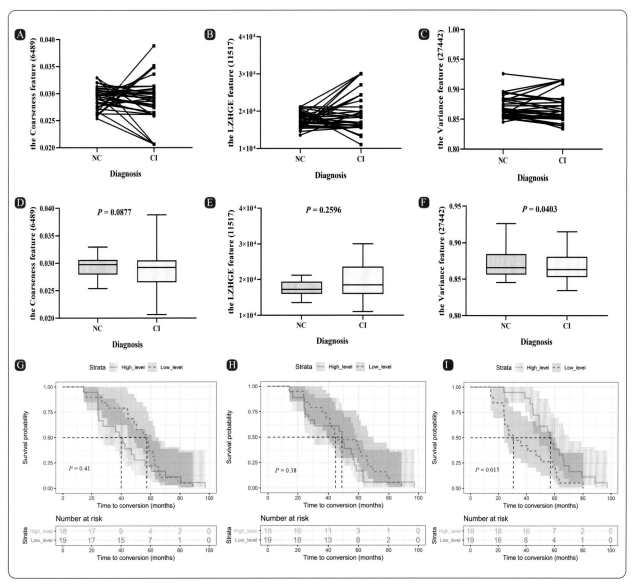

图 1-1-68　稳定高频特征的纵向变化及生存分析

第一章　一体化 PET/MR 科研成果

PET/MR

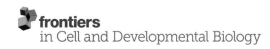

in Cell and Developmental Biology

ORIGINAL RESEARCH
published: 03 December 2020
doi: 10.3389/fcell.2020.605734

Check for updates

Radiomics Analysis of Magnetic Resonance Imaging Facilitates the Identification of Preclinical Alzheimer's Disease: An Exploratory Study

Tao-Ran Li[1†], Yue Wu[4†], Juan-Juan Jiang[4], Hua Lin[1], Chun-Lei Han[5], Jie-Hui Jiang[4]* and Ying Han[1,2,3]*

[1] Department of Neurology, Xuanwu Hospital of Capital Medical University, Beijing, China, [2] Center of Alzheimer's Disease, Beijing Institute for Brain Disorders, Beijing, China, [3] National Clinical Research Center for Geriatric Disorders, Beijing, China, [4] Key Laboratory of Specialty Fiber Optics and Optical Access Networks, Joint International Research Laboratory of Specialty Fiber Optics and Advanced Communication, School of Information and Communication Engineering, Shanghai University, Shanghai, China, [5] Turku PET Centre and Turku University Hospital, Turku, Finland

OPEN ACCESS

Edited by:
Chencheng Zhang,
Shanghai Jiao Tong University, China

Reviewed by:
Feng Bai,
Nanjing Drum Tower Hospital, China
I-Shiang Tzeng,
Chinese Culture University, Taiwan

*Correspondence:
Jie-Hui Jiang
jiangjiehui@shu.edu.cn
Ying Han
hanying@xwh.ccmu.edu.cn

†These authors have contributed equally to this work

Specialty section:
This article was submitted to
Molecular Medicine,
a section of the journal
Frontiers in Cell and Developmental
Biology

Received: *13 September 2020*
Accepted: *09 November 2020*
Published: *03 December 2020*

Citation:
Li T-R, Wu Y, Jiang J-J, Lin H,
Han C-L, Jiang J-H and Han Y (2020)
Radiomics Analysis of Magnetic
Resonance Imaging Facilitates
the Identification of Preclinical
Alzheimer's Disease: An Exploratory
Study.
Front. Cell Dev. Biol. 8:605734.
doi: 10.3389/fcell.2020.605734

Diagnosing Alzheimer's disease (AD) in the preclinical stage offers opportunities for early intervention; however, there is currently a lack of convenient biomarkers to facilitate the diagnosis. Using radiomics analysis, we aimed to determine whether the features extracted from multiparametric magnetic resonance imaging (MRI) can be used as potential biomarkers. This study was part of the Sino Longitudinal Study on Cognitive Decline project (NCT03370744), a prospective cohort study. All participants were cognitively healthy at baseline. Cohort 1 ($n = 183$) was divided into individuals with preclinical AD ($n = 78$) and controls ($n = 105$) using amyloid-positron emission tomography, and this cohort was used as the training dataset (80%) and validation dataset (the remaining 20%); cohort 2 ($n = 51$) was selected retrospectively and divided into "converters" and "nonconverters" according to individuals' future cognitive status, and this cohort was used as a separate test dataset; cohort three included 37 converters (13 from the Alzheimer's Disease Neuroimaging Initiative) and was used as another test set for independent longitudinal research. We extracted radiomics features from multiparametric MRI scans from each participant, using t-tests, autocorrelation tests, and three independent selection algorithms. We then established two classification models (support vector machine [SVM] and random forest [RF]) to verify the efficiency of the retained features. Five-fold cross-validation and 100 repetitions were carried out for the above process. Furthermore, the acquired stable high-frequency features were tested in cohort three by paired two-sample t-tests and survival analyses to identify whether their levels changed with cognitive decline and impact conversion time. The SVM and RF models both showed excellent classification efficiency, with an average accuracy of 89.7–95.9% and 87.1–90.8% in the validation set and 81.9–89.1% and 83.2–83.7% in the test set, respectively. Three stable high-frequency features were identified, all based on the structural MRI modality: the large zone high-gray-level emphasis feature of the right posterior cingulate gyrus, the variance feature of the left

LU H, JING D, CHEN Y, et al.Metabolic changes detected by 18F-FDG PET in the preclinical stage of familial Creutzfeldt-Jakob disease.J Alzheimers Dis, 2020, 77(4): 1513-1521.

【研究简介】

研究背景： 克 – 雅脑病（Creutzfeldt-Jakob disease，CJD）的病理发展过程目前尚不清楚，本研究采用 ^{18}F-FDG PET 探究克 – 雅脑病临床前阶段的脑葡萄糖代谢改变模式。

资料与方法： 本研究纳入 7 例无症状的 *G114V* 突变携带者和来自同一家族性克–雅脑病的 6 例无 *PRNP* 突变的家族成员，随访 2 年。同时招募了 10 例有症状的克–雅脑病患者。所有受试者均进行了标准化的临床检查和 ^{18}F-FDG PET 扫描。结果分 3 组进行比较：基线携带者与非携带者比较（基线分析），携带者基线与 2 年后的变化比较（随访分析），以及有症状的克 – 雅脑病患者与健康对照组的差异（克 – 雅脑病患者分析）。

研究结果： 2 年的随访中突变携带者未出现任何神经系统症状。基线分析相较于无携带者，突变携带者左侧和右侧中央后叶、左侧梭状回、左侧颞上回、左侧舌回、左侧顶上叶和左侧颞横回的代谢减低（$P < 0.001$）。随访分析发现 2 年后突变携带者右颞下回、左颞上回和左中央后回的代谢减低（$P < 0.001$），而左梭状回、左角回、左丘脑、左颞横回、右 Rolandic 区和左顶上回的代谢增加（$P < 0.001$）。克 - 雅脑病患者相较于正常人表现为右额下回三角部、右枕中回、右壳核、右丘脑和右颞中回的代谢减低（图 1–1–69 ~ 图 1–1–71）。

研究结论： 克–雅脑病的临床前阶段 ^{18}F-FDG PET 检测出顶叶和颞叶低代谢，皮层下区域出现代偿，而症状期则失代偿，有助于揭示患者发病的病理生理机制。

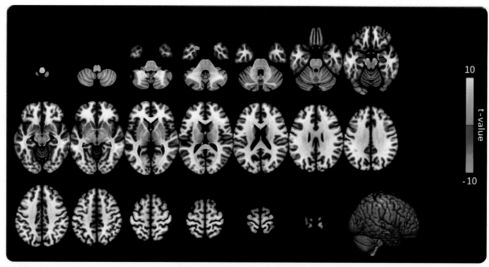

图 1-1-69　*G114V* 突变携带者与非携带者基线期 ^{18}F-FDG PET 比较

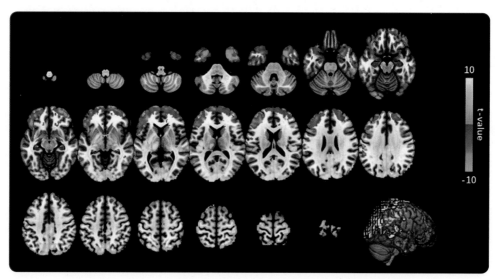

图 1-1-70　*G114V* 突变携带者 ^{18}F-FDG PET 纵向随访比较

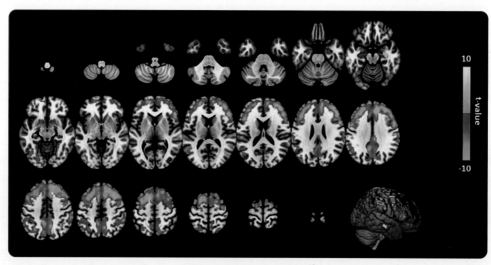

图 1-1-71　克 - 雅脑病患者与正常对照组 ^{18}F-FDG PET 比较

Journal of Alzheimer's Disease 77 (2020) 1513–1521
DOI 10.3233/JAD-200576
IOS Press

1513

Metabolic Changes Detected by ^{18}F-FDG PET in the Preclinical Stage of Familial Creutzfeldt-Jakob Disease

Hui Lu[a], Donglai Jing[a], Yaojing Chen[b], Chunlei Cui[c], Ran Gao[a], Lin Wang[a], Zhigang Liang[c], Kewei Chen[d] and Liyong Wu[a,*]

[a]*Department of Neurology, Xuanwu Hospital, Capital Medical University, Beijing, China*
[b]*State Key Laboratory of Cognitive Neuroscience and Learning, Beijing Normal University, Beijing, China*
[c]*Department of Nuclear Medicine, Xuanwu Hospital, Capital Medical University, Beijing, China*
[d]*Banner Alzheimer's Institute, Phoenix, AZ, USA*

Accepted 17 July 2020

Abstract.
Background: Pathologic processes in Creutzfeldt-Jakob disease (CJD) are not fully understood. Familial CJD (fCJD) gives opportunities to discover pathologic changes in the preclinical stage.
Objective: To investigate cerebral glucose metabolism in the preclinical stage via ^{18}F-fluorodeoxyglucose positron emission tomography (^{18}F-FDG PET) in fCJD.
Methods: Seven asymptomatic carriers of G114V mutation and six family members without *PRNP* mutation from the same fCJD kindred were included, and were followed for 2 years. Ten symptomatic CJD patients were also recruited. All subjects underwent standardized clinical examinations and ^{18}F-FDG PET scans. Results were compared in three groups: baseline carriers against non-carriers (baseline analysis), changes after 2 years in carriers (follow-up analysis), and differences between symptomatic CJD patients and healthy controls (CJD patients analysis).
Results: No carriers developed any neurological symptoms during 2-year follow-up. Baseline analysis: carriers demonstrates decreased metabolism ($p < 0.001$) in left and right postcentral, left fusiform, left superior temporal, left lingual, left superior parietal, and left Heschl gyrus. Follow-up analysis shows metabolic decline ($p < 0.001$) in right inferior temporal, left supra-marginal and left postcentral lobe, and increased metabolism ($p < 0.001$) in left fusiform, left angular, left thalamus, left Heschl's, right Rolandic operculum, and left superior parietal gyrus. CJD patients demonstrates decreased metabolism in right inferior triangularis frontal gyrus, right middle occipital gyrus, right putamen, right thalamus, and right middle temporal gyrus.
Conclusion: Hypo-metabolism of parietal and temporal lobe can be detected by ^{18}F-FDG PET in the preclinical stage of CJD. Subcortical area might compensate in the preclinical stage and decompensate in the symptomatic stage.

Keywords: Familial Creutzfeldt-Jakob disease, ^{18}F-fluorodeoxyglucose positron emission tomography, metabolism, preclinical stage

INTRODUCTION

Creutzfeldt-Jakob disease (CJD) is a transmissible spongiform encephalopathy caused by aggregation of pathologic prion protein. CJD is characterized by rapidly progressive dementia, a variety of neurological symptoms, and fatal outcome. The disease

*Correspondence to: Liyong Wu, 45 Changchun Street, Xicheng district, Beijing 100053, China. Tel.: +86 00861083198420; E-mail: wmywly@hotmail.com.

SONG S, CHENG Y, MA J, et al.Simultaneous FET-PET and contrast-enhanced MRI based on hybrid PET/MR improves delineation of tumor spatial biodistribution in gliomas: a biopsy validation study.Eur J Nucl Med Mol Imaging, 2020, 47(6): 1458-1467.

【研究简介】

研究背景： 评估胶质瘤手术范围和放化疗靶区是国内外研究的热点，本研究基于一体化 PET/MR，比较 MRI 增强检查与 ^{18}F-FET-PET 显像在显示脑胶质瘤体积时的差异，为指导胶质瘤穿刺和手术提供依据。

资料与方法： 本研究纳入了 33 例经病理确诊，且 ^{18}F-FET-PET 显像及增强（contrast-enhanced，CE）MRI 检查均为阳性的脑胶质瘤患者，分别以肿瘤靶 / 本比值 1.6 为阈值和视觉评估，确定脑胶质瘤的 PET 图像定量体积（V_{PET}）和 MR 图像的体积（V_{CE}），并评估反映肿瘤空间分布一致性和差异性的 Dice 相似系数（Dice's coefficient，DSC）、重叠体积（overlap volume，OV）、非 VCE 内的 PET 代谢区域（discrepancy-PET）、非 VPET 内的 MRI 强化区域体积（discrepancy-CE）。

研究结果： 31 例（93.94%）脑胶质瘤患者的 ^{18}F-FET-PET 定量体积显著大于 CE MRI 体积 [（77.84±51.74）cm³ *vs.*（34.59±27.07）cm³，$P < 0.05$]，二者呈正相关（图 1-1-72）。^{18}F-FET-PET 和 CE MRI 显示脑胶质瘤的空间范围不一致，其中 7 例患者进行立体定向导航下穿刺活检，共取得 24 例活检样本。21 例样本取自 ^{18}F-FET-PET 显示摄取明显升高部位，病理证实均为肿瘤组织或肿瘤细胞浸润，其中仅 13 例样本的 CE MRI 表现为明显强化。另有 3 例样本取自 ^{18}F-FET-PET 显示摄取无明显升高，且 CE MRI 表现未见明显强化，但 T_2-FLAIR 可见异常高信号的部位，其中 1 例样本病理显示有肿瘤细胞浸润，其余 2 例均为正常脑组织（图 1-1-73）。

研究结论： 一体化 PET/MR 同步获得脑胶质瘤患者氨基酸代谢和 MRI 结构信息，可更精确显示肿瘤病灶范围，对脑肿瘤个体化精准治疗方案制订具有重要价值。

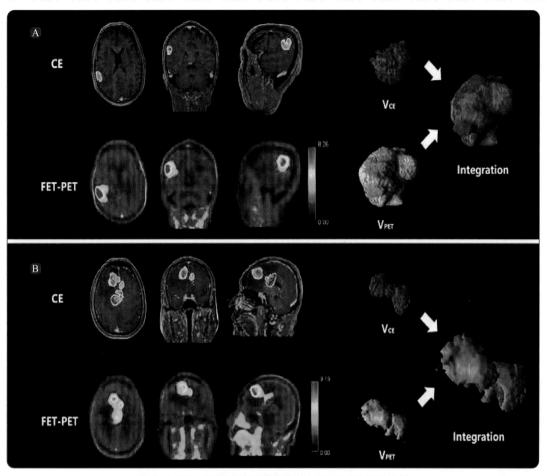

图 1-1-72　两例脑胶质瘤患者的 VPET 和 VCE 比较

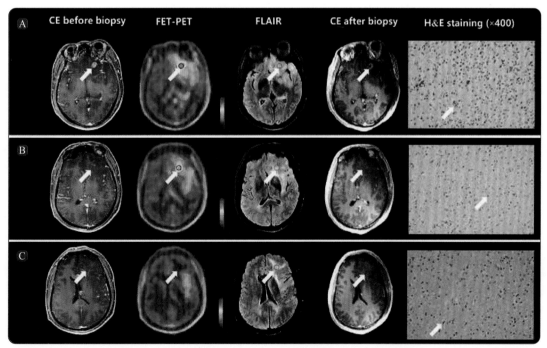

A. 脑胶质瘤 CE MRI 强化且 FET 高代谢的活检部位；B.CE MRI 未强化且 FET 高代谢的活检部位；C.CE MRI 未强化且 FET 低代谢的活检部位的 CE MRI、FET-PET、FLAIR、活检后的 CE MRI 和病理 HE 染色，证实 FET-PET 高代谢而 CE MRI 未强化的区域为肿瘤组织。

图 1-1-73

European Journal of Nuclear Medicine and Molecular Imaging (2020) 47:1458–1467
https://doi.org/10.1007/s00259-019-04656-2

ORIGINAL ARTICLE

Simultaneous FET-PET and contrast-enhanced MRI based on hybrid PET/MR improves delineation of tumor spatial biodistribution in gliomas: a biopsy validation study

Shuangshuang Song[1,2] · Ye Cheng[3] · Jie Ma[4] · Leiming Wang[5] · Chengyan Dong[6] · Yukui Wei[3] · Geng Xu[3] · Yang An[3] · Zhigang Qi[1,2] · Qingtang Lin[3] · Jie Lu[1,2,4]

Received: 25 October 2019 / Accepted: 9 December 2019 / Published online: 9 January 2020
© The Author(s) 2019

Abstract

Purpose Glioma treatment planning requires precise tumor delineation, which is typically performed with contrast-enhanced (CE) MRI. However, CE MRI fails to reflect the entire extent of glioma. O-(2-^{18}F-fluoroethyl)-L-tyrosine (^{18}F-FET) PET may detect tumor volumes missed by CE MRI. We investigated the clinical value of simultaneous FET-PET and CE MRI in delineating tumor extent before treatment planning. Guided stereotactic biopsy was used to validate the findings.

Methods Conventional MRI and ^{18}F-FET PET were performed simultaneously on a hybrid PET/MR in 33 patients with histopathologically confirmed glioma. Tumor volumes were quantified using a tumor-to-brain ratio ≥ 1.6 (V_{PET}) and a visual threshold (V_{CE}). We visually assessed abnormal areas on FLAIR images and calculated Dice's coefficient (DSC), overlap volume (OV), discrepancy-PET, and discrepancy-CE. Additionally, several stereotactic biopsy samples were taken from "matched" or "mismatched" FET-PET and CE MRI regions.

Results Among 31 patients (93.94%), FET-PET delineated significantly larger tumor volumes than CE MRI (77.84 ± 51.74 cm^3 vs. 34.59 ± 27.07 cm^3, $P < 0.05$). Of the 21 biopsy samples obtained from regions with increased FET uptake, all were histopathologically confirmed as glioma tissue or tumor infiltration, whereas only 13 showed enhancement on CE MRI. Among all patients, the spatial similarity between V_{PET} and V_{CE} was low (average DSC 0.56 ± 0.22), while the overlap was high (average OV 0.95 ± 0.08). The discrepancy-CE and discrepancy-PET were lower than 10% in 28 and 0 patients, respectively. Eleven patients showed V_{PET} partially beyond abnormal signal areas on FLAIR images.

Conclusion The metabolically active biodistribution of gliomas delineated with FET-PET significantly exceeds tumor volume on CE MRI, and histopathology confirms these findings. Our preliminary results indicate that combining the anatomic and

---

Shuangshuang Song and Ye Cheng contributed equally to this work.

This article is part of the Topical Collection on Oncology–Brain.

Electronic supplementary material The online version of this article (https://doi.org/10.1007/s00259-019-04656-2) contains supplementary material, which is available to authorized users.

✉ Qingtang Lin
   kingsang2002@hotmail.com

✉ Jie Lu
   imaginglu@hotmail.com

   Shuangshuang Song
   song2222shuang@163.com

   Ye Cheng
   chengye.1990@163.com

[1] Department of Radiology, Xuanwu Hospital, Capital medical University, Beijing, China

[2] Beijing Key Laboratory of Magnetic Resonance Imaging and Brain Informatics, Beijing, China

[3] Department of Neurosurgery, Xuanwu Hospital, Capital Medical University, Beijing, China

[4] Department of Nuclear Medicine, Xuanwu Hospital, Capital Medical University, Beijing, China

[5] Department of Pathology, Xuanwu Hospital, Capital Medical University, Beijing, China

[6] GE Healthcare, Beijing, China

⌀ Springer

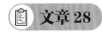

WANG J, SHAN Y, DAI J, et al.Altered coupling between resting-state glucose metabolism and functional activity in epilepsy.Ann Clin Transl Neurol, 2020, 7(10): 1831-1842.

【研究简介】

研究背景： 伴海马硬化内侧颞叶癫痫（medial temporal lobe epilepsy due to hippocampal sclerosis，mTLE-HS）是成年人难治性癫痫的常见类型，研究发现伴海马硬化内侧颞叶癫痫发作与皮层和皮层下大脑区域广泛的异常放电有关，与正常人相比，此类患者脑功能活动异常且代谢减低，但是癫痫反复发作是否干扰生物信息耦合及其与预后的关系尚不清楚。本研究通过一体化 PET/MR 同步扫描探究伴海马硬化内侧颞叶癫痫代谢和静息态功能活动之间的耦联机制，并进一步揭示耦联性与患者预后之间的关系。

资料与方法： 本研究纳入了 26 例经病理证实为难治性伴海马硬化内侧颞叶癫痫的患者，术后每年进行随访，使用 Engel 分级对患者预后进行评估，其中 2 例患者失访。本研究招募了健康对照组 26 例。12 例左侧海马硬化患者的图像进行了左右反转，使致痫灶显示在右侧（图 1-1-74）；使用 WFU PickAtlas 工具获取双侧海马，提取对应的 SUVR、fALFF、ReHo；使用配对 t 检验样本评估半球之间的差异，双样本 t 检验评估患者组与健康对照组之间的差异；全脑逐像素分析伴海马硬化内侧颞叶癫痫患者功能代谢耦联性改变及其与预后之间的关联。

研究结果： 伴海马硬化内侧颞叶癫痫患者和健康对照组均显示 SUVR 和 rsfMRI 指标之间存在显著正相关性；与健康对照组相比，伴海马硬化内侧颞叶癫痫患者的 SUVR 和 fMRI 衍生的灰质指标之间的空间相关性显著更高（fALFF/SUFR，$P < 0.001$；ReHo/SUVR，$P=0.022$）（图 1-1-75）；术后 Engel ⅠA 级患者的 fALFF-SUVR 耦联度高于其他级别患者（$P=0.025$），而 ReHo/SUVR 耦联率无显著差异（$P=0.097$）（图 1-1-76）。

研究结论： 伴海马硬化内侧颞叶癫痫患者海马网络内的代谢与功能活动耦合发生了改变，并且与预后相关，可能为发现伴海马硬化内侧颞叶癫痫的发病机制及指导癫痫手术提供新思路。

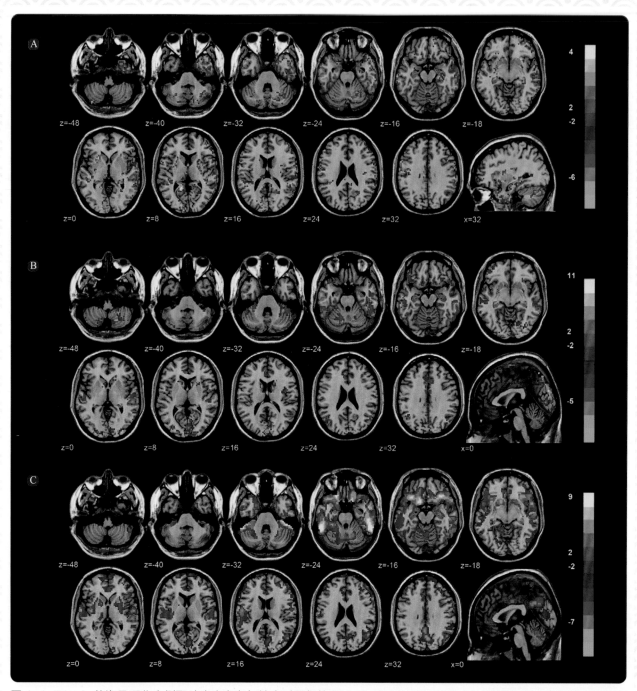

图 1-1-74　A. 伴海马硬化内侧颞叶癫痫患者与健康对照组的 SUVR；B.fALFF；C.ReHo 组间差异。暖色调表示伴海马硬化内侧颞叶癫痫患者影像参数显著增加，冷色调表示显著减低

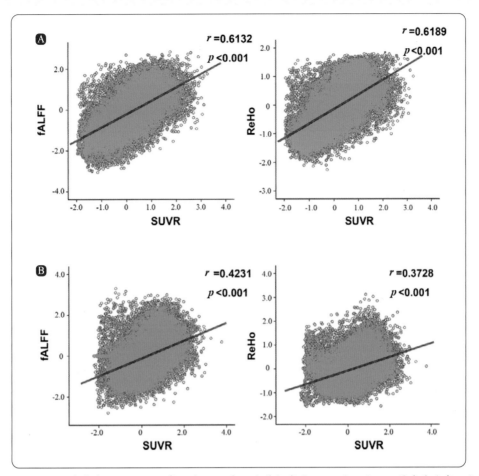

A. 伴海马硬化内侧颞叶癫痫患者，男性，32岁，病程15年，发作频率为3～4次/月；B. 健康受试者，女性，30岁。

图 1-1-75　基于同侧海马网络的体素间 SUVR 与 fALFF、ReHo 相关性耦联散点图

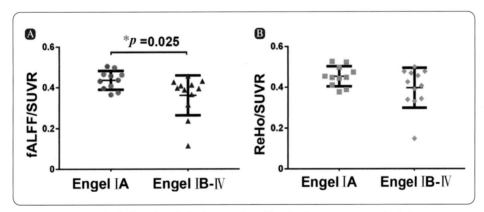

A. 术后无癫痫发作（Engel ⅠA级）患者和其他患者（Engel ⅠB～Ⅳ级）的 fALFF/SUVR 相关性；B.ReHo/SUVR 相关性。

图 1-1-76　伴海马硬化内侧颞叶癫痫患者灰质体素内的 SUVR 与 fMRI 参数的相关性分析

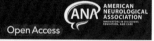

RESEARCH ARTICLE

Altered coupling between resting-state glucose metabolism and functional activity in epilepsy

Jingjuan Wang[1] , Yi Shan[2,3] , Jindong Dai[4,5] , Bixiao Cui[1] , Kun Shang[1] , Hongwei Yang[1] , Zhongwei Chen[6] , Baoci Shan[7,8,9] , Guoguang Zhao[10] & Jie Lu[1,2,3]

[1]Department of Nuclear Medicine, Xuanwu Hospital Capital Medical University, Beijing, China
[2]Department of Radiology, Xuanwu Hospital Capital Medical University, Beijing, China
[3]Key Laboratory of Magnetic Resonance Imaging and Brain Informatics, Beijing, China
[4]Department of Neurosurgery, Beijing Haidian Section of Peking University Third Hospital, Beijing, China
[5]Department of Functional Neurosurgery, Xuanwu Hospital Capital Medical University, Beijing, China
[6]GE Healthcare, Beijing, China
[7]Division of Nuclear Technology and Applications, Institute of High Energy Physics, Chinese Academy of Sciences, Beijing, China
[8]Beijing Engineering Research Center of Radiographic Techniques and Equipment, Beijing, China
[9]CAS Centre for Excellence in Brain Science and Intelligent Technology, Shanghai, China
[10]Department of Neurosurgery, Xuanwu Hospital, Capital Medical University, Beijing, China

Correspondence
Jie Lu, No.45 Changchun Street, Xicheng District, 100053, Beijing, China. Tel: +8610-8319-8379; Fax: +86 10 83198379; E-mail: imaginglu@hotmail.com
Guoguang Zhao, No.45 Changchun Street, Xicheng District, 100053, Beijing, China. Tel: +8610-8319-8252; Fax: +86 10 63012833; E-mail: ggzhao@vip.sina.com

Funding Information
This work was supported by the National Key Research and Development Program of China (grant numbers 2016YFC0103909); the National natural science foundation of china [grant numbers 81671662]; and Beijing Municipal Administration of Hospitals Ascent Plan [grant numbers DFL20180802].

Received: 12 May 2020; Revised: 22 June 2020; Accepted: 30 July 2020

Annals of Clinical and Translational Neurology 2020; 7(10): 1831–1842

doi: 10.1002/acn3.51168

Abstract

Objective: Altered functional activities and hypometabolism have been found in medial temporal lobe epilepsy patients with hippocampal sclerosis (mTLE-HS). Hybrid PET/MR scanners provide opportunities to explore the relationship between resting-state energy consumption and functional activities, but whether repeated seizures disturb the bioenergetic coupling and its relationship with seizure outcomes remain unknown. **Methods:** ^{18}F-FDG PET and resting-state functional MRI (rs-fMRI) scans were performed with hybrid PET/MR in 26 patients with mTLE-HS and in healthy controls. Energy consumption was quantified by ^{18}F-FDG standardized uptake value ratio(SUVR) relative to cerebellum. Spontaneous neural activities were estimated using regional homogeneity (ReHo), fractional amplitude of low frequency fluctuations (fALFF) from rs-fMRI. Between-group differences in SUVR and rs-fMRI derived metrics were evaluated by two-sample t test. Voxel-wise spatial correlations were explored between SUVR and ReHo, fALFF across gray matter and compared between groups. Furthermore, the relationships between altered fALFF/SUVR and ReHo/SUVR coupling and surgical outcomes were evaluated. **Results:** Both the patients and healthy controls showed significant positive correlations between SUVR and rs-fMRI metrics. Spatial correlations between SUVR and fMRI-derived metrics across gray matter were significantly higher in patients with mTLE-HS compared with healthy controls (fALFF/SUVR, $P < 0.001$; ReHo/SUVR, $P = 0.022$). Higher fALFF/SUVR couplings were found in patients who had Engel class IA after surgery than all other ($P = 0.025$), while altered ReHo/SUVR couplings ($P = 0.097$) were not. **Conclusion:** These findings demonstrated altered bioenergetic coupling across gray matter and its relationship with seizure outcomes, which may provide novel insights into pathogenesis of mTLE-HS and potential biomarkers for epilepsy surgery planning.

Introduction

Medial temporal lobe epilepsy (mTLE-HS) is a common type of refractory epilepsy in adults, characterized by repeated seizures originating from hippocampus and related mesial temporal lobe structures.[1] EEG studies have found extensively abnormal discharge in cortical and subcortical brain regions, which are associated with seizure

ZHANG L, SONG T, MENG Z, et al.Correlation between apparent diffusion coefficients and metabolic parameters in hypopharyngeal squamous cell carcinoma: A prospective study with integrated PET/MRI.Eur J Radiol, 2020, 129: 109070.

【研究简介】

研究背景： 下咽鳞状细胞癌（hypopharyngeal squamous cell carcinoma，HSCC）是头颈部鳞状细胞癌（head and neck squamous cell carcinomas，HNSCC）预后最差的肿瘤之一，5年生存率为30%～35%。MRI可以显示头颈部肿瘤并评估局部肿瘤的扩散和侵袭性，PET反映葡萄糖代谢水平，已成为头颈部肿瘤早期分期和治疗监测的首选技术。本研究利用一体化PET/MR对下咽鳞状细胞癌患者进行前瞻性研究，探讨ADC值（ADC_{mean}和ADC_{min}）与^{18}F-FDG PET代谢参数SUV_{max}、SUV_{mean}、肿瘤代谢体积（metabolic tumor volume，MTV）和糖酵解总量（total lesion glycolysis，TLG）的相关性。

资料与方法： 本研究纳入了27例经活检证实的下咽鳞状细胞癌患者，进行颈部^{18}F-FDG PET/MR检查，其中包括梨状窝癌15例、下咽后壁癌9例、环后区癌3例（图1-1-77）。ADC图手动测量下咽鳞状细胞癌的ADC_{mean}和ADC_{min}（图1-1-78），PET图像自动计算下咽鳞状细胞癌的代谢参数，包括SUV_{max}、SUV_{mean}、MTV和TLG；评估下咽鳞状细胞癌肿瘤的ADC值与代谢参数之间的相关性，以及不同组织学分级、临床分期和解剖亚区肿瘤组间的关系。

研究结果： 下咽鳞状细胞癌患者ADC_{mean}和MTV之间呈显著负相关（r=-0.556，P=0.003）（图1-1-79），ADC_{min}和^{18}F-FDG PET代谢参数无显著相关性；ADC_{mean}和下咽鳞状细胞癌的MTV之间呈显著负相关（图1-1-79）；低分化组、Ⅳ期组或非梨状窝癌组的ADC值与^{18}F-FDG PET代谢参数无显著相关。

研究结论： 下咽鳞状细胞癌患者ADC_{mean}与MTV之间呈显著负相关，且和组织学分级、临床分期和解剖部位有关。

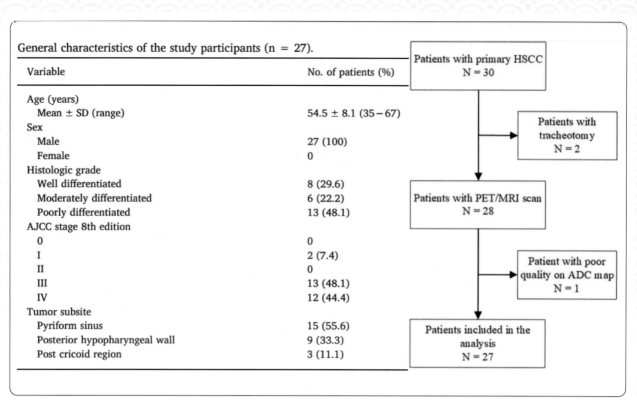

General characteristics of the study participants (n = 27).

Variable	No. of patients (%)
Age (years)	
Mean ± SD (range)	54.5 ± 8.1 (35−67)
Sex	
Male	27 (100)
Female	0
Histologic grade	
Well differentiated	8 (29.6)
Moderately differentiated	6 (22.2)
Poorly differentiated	13 (48.1)
AJCC stage 8th edition	
0	0
I	2 (7.4)
II	0
III	13 (48.1)
IV	12 (44.4)
Tumor subsite	
Pyriform sinus	15 (55.6)
Posterior hypopharyngeal wall	9 (33.3)
Post cricoid region	3 (11.1)

Patients with primary HSCC N = 30

Patients with tracheotomy N = 2

Patients with PET/MRI scan N = 28

Patient with poor quality on ADC map N = 1

Patients included in the analysis N = 27

图 1-1-77　入组下咽鳞状细胞癌患者临床资料及流程

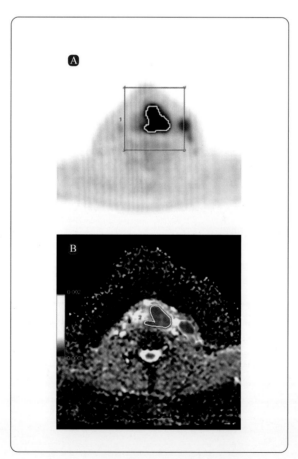

PET 图像的肿瘤 ROI（白色，图 A），与 PET 图像相同层面的 ADC 图像的肿瘤 ROI（白色，图 B）。

图 1-1-78　PET 和 ADC 图像的肿瘤 ROI

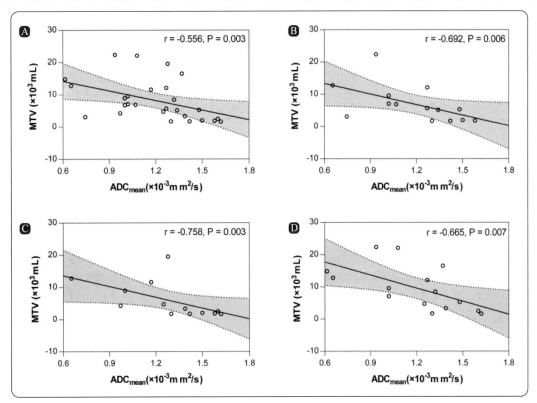

图 1-1-79　下咽鳞状细胞癌组（图 A）、中度至高度分化下咽鳞状细胞癌组（图 B）、Ⅲ 期下咽鳞状细胞癌组（图 C）和梨状窝下咽鳞状细胞癌组（图 D）的 ADC_{mean} 与肿瘤的 MTV 相关性分析

European Journal of Radiology 129 (2020) 109070

Contents lists available at ScienceDirect

European Journal of Radiology

journal homepage: www.elsevier.com/locate/ejrad

Correlation between apparent diffusion coefficients and metabolic parameters in hypopharyngeal squamous cell carcinoma: A prospective study with integrated PET/MRI

Lingyu Zhang[a,1], Tianbin Song[b,1], Zhaoting Meng[a], Caiyun Huang[a], Xiaohong Chen[c], Jie Lu[b,d,e,**], Junfang Xian[a,*]

[a] Department of Radiology, Beijing Tongren Hospital, Capital Medical University, Beijing, China
[b] Department of Nuclear Medicine, Xuanwu Hospital, Capital Medical University, Beijing, China
[c] Department of Otolaryngology, Head and Neck Surgery, Beijing Tongren Hospital, Capital Medical University, Beijing, China
[d] Department of Radiology, Xuanwu Hospital, Capital Medical University, Beijing, China
[e] Beijing Key Laboratory of Magnetic Resonance Imaging and Brain Informatics, Beijing, China

ARTICLE INFO

Keywords:
Hypopharynx
Squamous cell carcinoma
PET/MRI
Multimodal imaging

ABSTRACT

Purpose: Apparent diffusion coefficients (ADCs) derived from diffusion-weighted magnetic resonance imaging (DW-MRI) and metabolic parameters derived from ^{18}F-FDG positron emission tomography (PET) are promising prognostic indicators for head and neck squamous cell carcinoma (SCC). However, the relationship between them remains unclear. This study aimed to investigate the relationship between ADCs and metabolic parameters in hypopharyngeal SCC (HSCC) using integrated PET/MRI.

Materials and methods: Twenty-seven patients with biopsy-proven HSCC underwent integrated ^{18}F-FDG neck PET/MRI. ADCs of HSCC, including the mean and minimum ADC values (ADC_{mean} and ADC_{min}), were measured manually on ADC maps. Metabolic parameters of HSCC, including maximum and mean standardized uptake values (SUV_{max} and SUV_{mean}), metabolic tumor volume (MTV), and total lesion glycolysis (TLG), were calculated automatically on PET images. Spearman correlation coefficients were used to assess the relationships between ADCs and metabolic parameters in HSCC tumors as well as in tumor groups with different histological grading, clinical staging, and anatomical subsites. P values < 0.05 were considered statistically significant.

Results: No significant correlation was observed between ADCs and ^{18}F-FDG PET metabolic parameters in the entire cohort, except for a significant inverse correlation between ADC_{mean} and MTV (r = -0.556, P = 0.003). Furthermore, a significant inverse correlation was observed between ADC_{mean} and MTV of HSCC in the moderately to well differentiated group ($r_{ADCmean/MTV}$ = -0.692, P = 0.006), stage III group ($r_{ADCmean/MTV}$ = -0.758, P = 0.003), and pyriform sinus group ($r_{ADCmean/MTV}$ = -0.665, P = 0.007), whereas no significant correlation was observed in the poorly differentiated group, stage IV group, or non-pyriform sinus group.

Conclusions: Inverse correlation between ADC_{mean} and MTV in the HSCC population was observed and the correlativity depended on histological grading, clinical staging, and anatomical subsites of HSCC.

1. Introduction

Hypopharyngeal squamous cell carcinoma (HSCC) has one of the poorest prognosis among the head and neck squamous cell carcinomas (HNSCCs) with an overall 5-year survival rate of approximately 30 %–35 % [1]. Magnetic resonance imaging (MRI) is routinely used to image head and neck tumors owing to its superior soft tissue contrast. It allows for better assessment of local tumor spread and invasiveness [2,3]. Positron emission tomography (PET) is useful for reflecting in vivo metabolism and has become the technique of choice for initial

* Corresponding author at: Department of Radiology, Beijing Tongren Hospital, Capital Medical University, No.1 Dongjiaominxiang Street, Dongcheng District, Beijing 100730, China.
** Corresponding author at: Department of Nuclear Medicine and Radiology, Xuanwu Hospital, Capital Medical University, No.45 Changchunjie, Xicheng District, Beijing 100053, China.
E-mail addresses: imaginglu@hotmail.com (J. Lu), cjr.xianjunfang@vip.163.com (J. Xian).
[1] Lingyu Zhang and Tianbin Song contributed equally to this work.

https://doi.org/10.1016/j.ejrad.2020.109070
Received 19 January 2020; Received in revised form 3 May 2020; Accepted 9 May 2020

HUANG C, SONG T, MUKHERJI SK, et al.Comparative study between integrated positron emission tomography/magnetic resonance and positron emission tomography/computed tomography in the T and N Staging of hypopharyngeal cancer: an initial result. J Comput Assist Tomogr, 2020, 44(4): 540-545.

【研究简介】

研究背景：下咽部鳞状细胞癌是头颈部肿瘤预后最差类型之一，其中 75% 的下咽癌患者表现为 Ⅲ~Ⅳ B 期，5 年生存率约 25%～40%。NCCN 指南提示 CT、MRI 和 PET/CT 作为一线影像学手段评估头颈癌分期和再分期情况，本研究旨在比较 PET/MR、PET/CT、MRI 对下咽部鳞状细胞癌患者 T 分期和 N 分期的准确性。

资料与方法：本研究共纳入了 20 例活检确诊下咽癌的男性患者，平均年龄为 55.5±6.1 岁，所有患者行一体化 PET/MR、PET/CT 和 MRI 检查。肿瘤位置包括梨状窝（$n=16$）、环状软骨后区（$n=2$）、咽后壁（$n=2$）。在 PET/MR 完成 14±l2 分钟后进行 PET/CT 扫描，MRI 扫描序列包括 T_1WI、T_2WI 和 DWI（$b=0$ 和 $b=800$）。PET 扫描参数为：10 分钟 / 床位，利用 TOF 技术重建图像，OSEM 重建，2 次迭代，28 个子集，FWHM 为 5.0 mm。比较 PET/MR、PET/CT 和 MRI 三种检查手段诊断下咽癌的敏感度、特异度、PPV 和 NPV 的一致性（图 1-1-80，图 1-1-81）。

研究结果：PET/MR、PET/CT 和 MRI 对下咽癌患者 T 分期的准确率分别为 81.8%、63.6% 和 72.7%。PET/MR 检测转移淋巴结的敏感度和特异度分别为 88.2% 和 98.2%，PET/CT 为 76.5% 和 98.3%，MRI 为 64.7% 和 94.7%。

研究结论：PET/MR 评估下咽癌的转移淋巴结和 T 分期优于 PET/CT，可作为临床评估的重要检查。

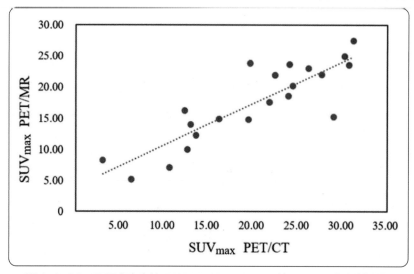

图 1-1-80 下咽癌患者的 PET/MR 和 PET/CT 的 SUV_{max} 相关性分析

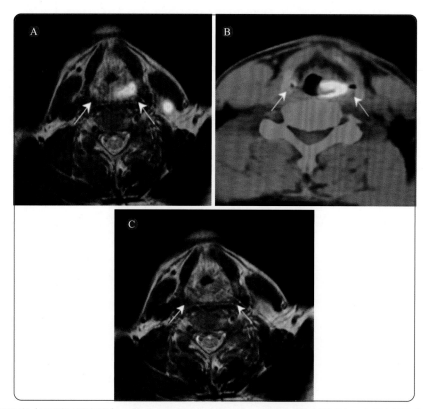

图 1-1-81 下咽癌（双侧梨状窝癌）一体化 PET/MR（图 A）、PET/CT（图 B）、MRI（图 C），箭头示肿瘤

ORIGINAL ARTICLE

Comparative Study Between Integrated Positron Emission Tomography/Magnetic Resonance and Positron Emission Tomography/Computed Tomography in the T and N Staging of Hypopharyngeal Cancer: An Initial Result

Caiyun Huang, MD,* Tianbin Song, MD,† Suresh Kumar Mukherji, MD, MBA, FACR,‡ Lingyu Zhang, MD,* Jie Lu, MD, PhD,†§∥ Xiaohong Chen, MD, PhD,¶ and Junfang Xian, MD, PhD*

Objective: To compare the diagnostic accuracy of positron emission tomography/magnetic resonance (PET/MR) versus PET/computed tomography (PET/CT) for T and N staging of hypopharyngeal cancer.

Methods: Integrated PET/MR and PET/CT examinations were performed in 20 patients with hypopharyngeal cancer after same-day single injection. Eleven of 20 patients underwent surgery with histologic findings directly compared with imaging findings. Statistical analysis included Spearman correlation and McNemar test.

Results: Accuracy of PET/MR, PET/CT, and MRI for T staging was 81.8%, 63.6%, and 72.7%, respectively. Sensitivity and specificity for detecting metastatic lymph nodes was 88.2% and 98.2% on PET/MR, 76.5% and 98.3% on PET/CT, and 64.7% and 94.7% on MRI.

Conclusions: The PET/MR and PET/CT provide comparable results for assessing hypopharyngeal carcinoma and detecting metastatic lymph nodes.

Key Words: hypopharyngeal cancer, integrated PET/MR, PET/CT, initial tumor staging, maximum standard uptake value

(*J Comput Assist Tomogr* 2020;44: 540–545)

S quamous cell carcinoma of the hypopharynx has one of the poorest prognosis among the head and neck cancers.[1] About 75% of patients present with stage III–IVB disease,[2] with an overall 5-year survival rate between 25% and 40%.[1] The National Comprehensive Cancer Network guidelines list computed tomography (CT), magnetic resonance imaging (MRI), and positron emission tomography (PET)/CT as the first-line radiological evaluations for staging and restaging of head and neck cancers.[3]

From the *Department of Radiology, Beijing Tongren Hospital, †Department of Nuclear Medicine, Xuanwu Hospital, Capital Medical University, Beijing, China; ‡Clinical Professor: Marian University, Director of Head & Neck Radiology Pro Scan Imaging, Indianapolis, IN; §Department of Radiology, Xuanwu Hospital, Capital Medical University; ∥Beijing Key Laboratory of Magnetic Resonance Imaging and Brain Informatics; and ¶Department of Otolaryngology, Head and Neck Surgery, Beijing TongRen Hospital, Capital Medical University, Beijing, China.

Received for publication December 10, 2019; accepted March 17, 2020.
Correspondence to: Junfang Xian, MD, PhD, Department of Radiology, Beijing Tongren Hospital, Capital Medical University, No. 1 Dongjiaominxiang St, Dongcheng District, Beijing 100730, China (e-mail: cjr.xianjunfang@vip.163.com); Xiaohong Chen, MD, PhD, Department of Otolaryngology, Head and Neck Surgery, Beijing TongRen Hospital, Capital Medical University, No. 1 Dongjiaominxiang St, Dongcheng District, Beijing 100730, China (e-mail: trchxh@163.com).
This study was supported by Beijing Municipal Administration of Hospitals Clinical Medicine Development of Special Funding Support (ZYLX201704), Beijing Municipal Administration of Hospitals' Ascent Plan (DFL20190203, DFL20180802), High Level Health Technical Personnel of Bureau of Health in Beijing (2014-2-005), National Key Research and Development Program of China (2016YFC0103000), the National Natural Science Foundation of China (81671662).

Magnetic resonance imaging is widely used to image head and neck tumors due to its superior soft-tissue contrast resolution compared with CT.[4,5] The PET/CT is routinely used for both initial staging and treatment monitoring for head and neck squamous cell carcinoma. The PET/MR gaining acceptance for initial evaluation for head and neck squamous cell carcinoma (HNSCC), but very few studies have been performed directly comparing PET/CT with PET/MR for individual subsites of the head and neck. Previous studies of head and neck cancer have been limited in suprahyoid lesions, such as oral squamous cell carcinoma, nasopharyngeal carcinoma, parotid gland tumor, and so on.[6,7] The purpose of our study was to investigate the correlation of maximum standard uptake value (SUV_{max}) of hypopharyngeal cancer derived from PET/MR with that of PET/CT, and prospectively compare the diagnostic accuracy of PET/MR with PET/CT and MRI for T and N staging in patients with squamous cell carcinoma of the hypopharynx.

MATERIALS AND METHODS

Patients

This study was approved by the institutional review board at our institution and written informed consent was obtained from all subjects before enrollment. Our study consisted of 20 patients with biopsy-proven hypopharyngeal carcinoma who underwent PET/MR, PET/CT and MRI between February 2017 and December 2018. The tumor locations included the pyriform sinus (n = 16), postcricoid region (n = 2), posterior pharyngeal wall (n = 2). All patients had a Karnofsky score greater than 60 with a blood glucose level less than 8 mmol/L. Patients were excluded if they had a prior history of radiation or chemotherapy for a prior cancer.

PET/CT Imaging Protocol

All patients were fasted for at least 6 hours before examination, and then underwent a dedicated head and neck PET/CT scan and a PET/CT whole-body scan. Positron emission tomography/computed tomography was performed on a 96-loop uMI510 whole-body scanner (United Imaging, China). A dedicated head and neck scan was performed from skull base to the aortic arch (slice thickness 3 mm) and initiated 81.3 ± 33 minutes after intravenous injection of ^{18}F-FDG with a target fixed dose of 0.1 mCi/kg. To minimize artifacts, the patient's arms were placed beside the body. Afterward, the patients were encouraged to place the arms over their head for the following whole-body examinations. The scan ranged from the vertex to midthigh (slice thickness 5 mm). The PET scanning parameters were as follows using 3D mode: 4 minutes/bed in the head and neck area and for 3 minutes/bed (5 beds) in the rest of the whole body with images reconstructed using TOF technology. The PET reconstruction parameters were as follows: ordered subset expectation maximization with 2 iterations, 24 subsets, Gaussian

第一章 一体化 PET/MR 科研成果

首都医科大学宣武医院一体化 PET/MR 成果集

WANG YH, AN Y, FAN XT, et al.Comparison between simultaneously acquired arterial spin labeling and ^{18}F-FDG PET in mesial temporal lobe epilepsy assisted by a PET/MR system and SEEG.Neuroimage Clin, 2018, 19: 824-830.

【研究简介】

研究背景： 内侧颞叶癫痫（medial temporal lobe epilepsy，MTLE）的治疗结果与识别致痫区的准确密切相关。^{18}F-FDG PET 是在癫痫发作间期进行手术前评估的主要手段，尤其是针对 MRI 阴性的难治性癫痫患者。磁共振 ASL 是一种定量测量脑灌注的 MRI 成像技术，可用于评估癫痫患者的脑功能改变。一体化 PET/MR 在同一生理状态下进行 ASL 和 PET 成像，能够更准确地探索内侧颞叶癫痫多模态影像之间的相关性及其与立体脑电图（stereoelectroencephalography，SEEG）、内侧颞叶癫痫临床治疗结果之间的相关性，阐述 PET 与 ASL 在定位偏侧性内侧颞叶癫痫起始发作区（seizure onset zone，SOZ）的有效性。

材料与方法： 回顾分析了 12 例确诊为单纯单侧内侧颞叶癫痫患者的 PET/MR 多模态影像数据。提取并定量计算双侧海马的 ASL 值和 PET 值，以立体脑电图发现和临床结果作为内侧颞叶癫痫定位的"金标准"，计算双侧不对称指数以评估 PET 和 ASL 之间的相关性。

研究结果： 立体脑电图结果显示 12 例患者发作间期一系列异常放电，发作时在近中颞区观察到快速脑电变化，10 例患者出现异常放电，2 例患者伴随双侧异常放电。立体脑电图记录了植入的 85 个电极的脑电图，没有显示任何向对侧颞区或颞叶外结构的传播放电（图 1-1-82）。PET/MR 结果显示 12 例患者的同侧海马代谢和灌注较低，视觉评价分析发现 PET 显示的低代谢区域大于 ASL 显示的灌注减低区域（图 1-1-83），ASL 显示内侧颞叶癫痫患者的 SOZ 偏侧化改变，与立体脑电图记录的结果一致（图 1-1-84）。

研究结论： 与 PET 相比，ASL 能够更好地实现内侧颞叶癫痫单侧病灶定位，可作为单侧内侧颞叶癫痫病灶定位的替代工具，实现致痫灶的精准定位并指导临床精准治疗。

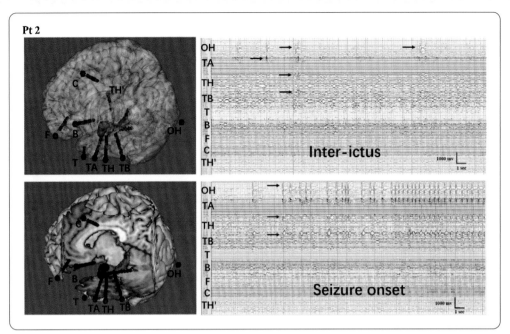

图 1-1-82 左内侧颞叶癫痫患者的重建图像和立体脑电图

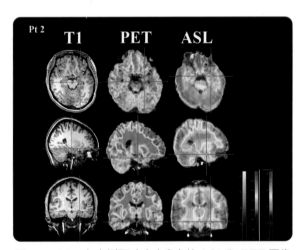

图 1-1-83 左内侧颞叶癫痫患者的 ASL 和 PET 图像

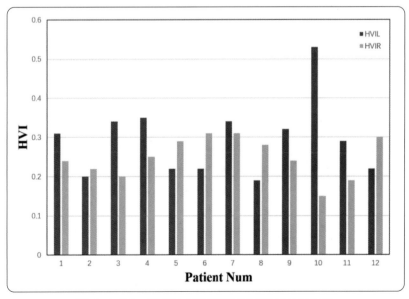

图 1-1-84 12 例内侧颞叶癫痫患者海马体积指数

NeuroImage: Clinical 19 (2018) 824–830

Contents lists available at ScienceDirect

NeuroImage: Clinical

journal homepage: www.elsevier.com/locate/ynicl

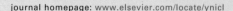

Comparison between simultaneously acquired arterial spin labeling and ^{18}F-FDG PET in mesial temporal lobe epilepsy assisted by a PET/MR system and SEEG

Yi-He Wang[a,1], Yang An[a,1], Xiao-Tong Fan[a], Jie Lu[b,c], Lian-Kun Ren[d], Peng-Hu Wei[a], Bi-Xiao Cui[c], Jia-Lin Du[d], Chao Lu[a], Di Wang[d], Hua-Qiang Zhang[a], Yong-Zhi Shan[a,*], Guo-Guang Zhao[a,e,*]

[a] Department of Neurosurgery, Xuanwu Hospital, Capital Medical University, Beijing 100053, China
[b] Department of Radiology, Xuanwu Hospital, Capital Medical University, Beijing 100053, China
[c] Department of Nuclear Medicine, Xuanwu Hospital, Capital Medical University, Beijing 100053, China
[d] Department of Neurology, Xuanwu Hospital, Capital Medical University, Beijing 100053, China
[e] Center of Epilepsy, Beijing Institute for Brain Disorder, Beijing 100069, China

ARTICLE INFO

Keywords:
Arterial spin labeling (ASL)
^{18}F-FDG PET
PET/MR
SEEG
Epilepsy

ABSTRACT

Objective: In the detection of seizure onset zones, arterial spin labeling (ASL) can overcome the limitations of positron emission tomography (PET) with ^{18}F-fluorodeoxyglucose (^{18}F-FDG), which is invasive, expensive, and radioactive. PET/magnetic resonance (MR) systems have been introduced that allow simultaneous performance of ASL and PET, but comparisons of these techniques with stereoelectroencephalography (SEEG) and comparisons among the treatment outcomes of these techniques are still lacking. Here, we investigate the effectiveness of ASL compared with that of SEEG and their outcomes in localizing mesial temporal lobe epilepsy (MTLE) and assess the correlation between simultaneously acquired PET and ASL.

Methods: Between October 2016 and August 2017, we retrospectively studied 12 patients diagnosed with pure unilateral MTLE. We extracted and quantitatively computed values for ASL and PET in the bilateral hippocampus. SEEG findings and outcome were considered the gold standard of lateralization. Finally, the bilateral asymmetry index (AI) was calculated to assess the correlation between PET and ASL.

Results: Our results showed that hypoperfusion in the hippocampus detected using ASL matched the SEEG-defined epileptogenic zone in this series of patients. The mean normalized voxel value of ASL in the contralateral hippocampus was 0.97 ± 0.19, while in the ipsilateral hippocampus, it was 0.84 ± 0.14. Meanwhile, significantly decreased perfusion and metabolism were observed in these patients (Wilcoxon, $p < 0.05$), with a significant positive correlation between the AI values derived from PET and ASL (Pearson's correlation, $r = 0.74$, $p < 0.05$).

Significance: In our SEEG- and outcome-defined patients with MTLE, ASL could provide significant information during presurgical evaluation, with the hypoperfusion detected with ASL reliably lateralizing MTLE. This non-invasive technique may be used as an alternative diagnostic tool for MTLE lateralization.

1. Introduction

During presurgical evaluation of mesial temporal lobe epilepsy (MTLE), a significant relationship between treatment outcome and accuracy in identifying the epileptogenic zone has been recognized (Hardy et al., 2003). Conventional non-invasive presurgical evaluation includes semiology, electroencephalography (EEG), structural imaging, and functional imaging (Chavakula and Cosgrove, 2017; Duncan, 2010; Fisher et al., 1997; Rosenow and Luders, 2001). In recent years, ^{18}F-fluorodeoxyglucose positron emission tomography (^{18}F-FDG PET) has been considered as the leading functional imaging option for presurgical evaluation during the interictal phase, particularly in patients with structural imaging-negative refractory epilepsy. This is because high consistency has been observed between regional hypometabolism and the epileptogenic zone (Rathore et al., 2014). However, there remain some limitations in the use of ^{18}F-FDG PET in clinical practice: 1) it is invasive and expensive, 2) it involves exposure to radiation, 3) it is unavailable in many epilepsy centers.

* Corresponding authors at: Department of Neurosurgery, Xuan Wu Hospital, Capital Medical University, No. 45, Changchun Street, Xuanwu District, Beijing 100053, China.
  E-mail addresses: shanyongzhi@xwhosp.org (Y.-Z. Shan), ggzhao@vip.sina.com (G.-G. Zhao).
[1] Yi-He Wang and Yang An contributed equally to the study.

https://doi.org/10.1016/j.nicl.2018.06.008
Received 19 December 2017; Received in revised form 2 June 2018; Accepted 4 June 2018
Available online 07 June 2018

SONG T, CUI B, YANG H, et al.Diffusion-weighted imaging as a part of PET/MR for small lesion detection in patients with primary abdominal and pelvic cancer, with or without TOF reconstruction technique.Abdom Radiol (NY), 2019, 44(7): 2639-2647.

【研究简介】

研究背景： 一体化 PET/MR 同时获得 PET 和 MR 图像的综合信息，有助于提高肿瘤评估的准确性。DWI 在一体化 TOF PET/MR 检查中的应用价值具有争议，本研究评估 DWI 在 TOF 及 noTOF 技术的一体化 PET/MR 检查中对腹盆腔恶性肿瘤患者小病灶（≤ 10 mm）的检出价值。

资料与方法： 本研究纳入了 20 例患者［女性 11 例，男性 9 例，平均年龄为（67.23 ± 12.90）岁］，均经病理证实为腹盆腔恶性肿瘤，应用一体化 PET/MR 进行分期检查及术后复查。DWI 和 T$_2$WI 序列发现的 64 个高度怀疑转移的体部小病灶（长径 ≤ 30 mm），分为两组（≤ 10 mm 和 10 ~ 30 mm），比较 TOF PET、noTOF PET、DWI 图像上小病灶（长径 ≤ 30 mm 和长径 ≤ 10 mm）的视觉评分和可检测性。

研究结果： DWI 图像上所有小病灶（≤ 10mm 和 10 ~ 30 mm）的视觉评分均高于 TOF PET 和 noTOF PET 图像（$P < 0.01$），DWI 和 noTOF PET 图像上微小病灶（≤ 10 mm）的漏诊率均为 9.1%（图 1-1-85）。Logistic 回归分析结果显示 TOF PET 能检出 ≤ 10 mm 的微小病灶，而 noTOF PET 需结合 DWI 补充诊断；DWI、TOF PET、noTOF PET 对 10 ~ 30 mm 小病灶的检出效能相当（图 1-1-86）。

研究结论： DWI 能够明显提高 noTOF 技术的一体化 PET/MR 检出的微小病灶能力，一体化 TOF PET/MR 可精简临床扫描流程，以节省扫描时间。

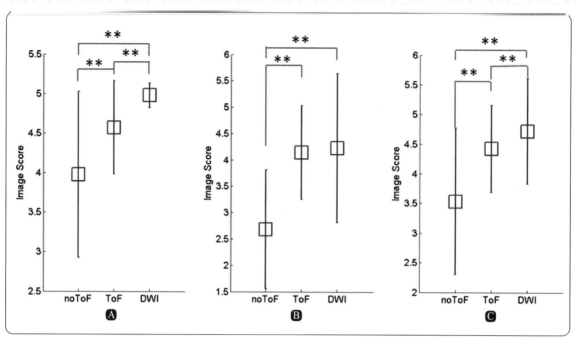

图 1-1-85 DWI、TOF PET 和 noTOF PET 图像上微小病灶视觉评分比较

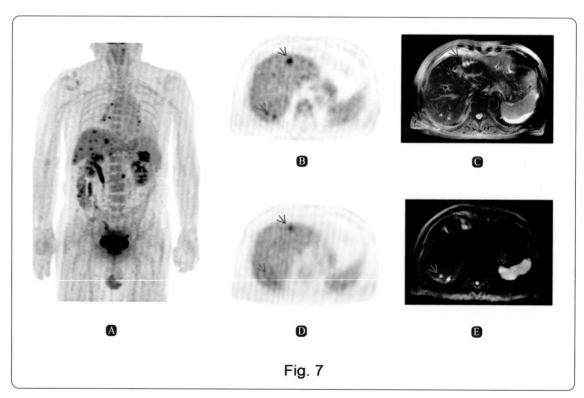

Fig. 7

A.PET MIP；B.TOF PET；C.T$_2$WI；D.noTOF PET；E.DWI。一体化 PET/MR 显示肝脏多发病灶，TOF PET 和 DWI 显示位于 S$_3$ 的小病灶图像质量优于 noTOF PET 图像（红箭头），TOF PET、T$_2$WI、DWI 可见两个 ≤ 10 mm 的微小病灶（蓝箭头），noTOF PET 图像上未见显示。

图 1-1-86 胰腺癌多发肝转移的一体化 PET/MR 检查

Abdominal Radiology
https://doi.org/10.1007/s00261-019-01980-x

PRACTICE

Diffusion-weighted imaging as a part of PET/MR for small lesion detection in patients with primary abdominal and pelvic cancer, with or without TOF reconstruction technique

Tianbin Song[1] · Bixiao Cui[1] · Hongwei Yang[1] · Jie Ma[1] · Dongmei Shuai[1] · Zhongwei Chen[2] · Zhigang Liang[1] · Yun Zhou[3] · Jie Lu[1,4,5]

Abstract

Objectives To investigate the value of diffusion-weighted imaging (DWI) in detection of small lesions (≤ 10 mm) in patients with primary abdominal and pelvic cancer in hybrid PET/MR with or without time-of-flight (TOF) technique.

Materials and methods Twenty patients (11 females and 9 males, mean age 67.23 ± 12.90 years) with histologically confirmed primary abdominal and pelvic cancer underwent hybrid PET/MR examination. A total of 64 small lesions were included in this study, which were divided into two groups (≤ 10 mm and 10–30 mm). Visual scores of small lesion detection ability were rated by five-point ordinal scale. The visual scores and detectability of small lesions on TOF PET image, noTOF PET image, and DWI sequences of hybrid PET/MR examination with or without TOF technique were analyzed. Logistic regression model was established for analysis in the value of DWI in hybrid PET/MR examination with or without TOF technique in detection of the small lesions between two groups.

Results The visual evaluation revealed the small lesion (≤ 10 mm) visual scores of DWI (mean $\pm$ SD: 4.23 ± 1.41), TOF PET image (mean $\pm$ SD: 4.14 ± 0.89), and noTOF PET image (mean $\pm$ SD: 2.68 ± 1.13);.and the visual scores of small lesions (10–30 mm) on DWI (mean $\pm$ SD: 4.98 ± 0.15), TOF PET image (mean $\pm$ SD: 4.57 ± 0.59), and noTOF PET image (mean $\pm$ SD: 3.98 ± 1.05). The visual scores of all small lesions on DWI were higher than that on TOF PET data and noTOF PET data in both two groups (**$P < 0.01$). The missed diagnosis rates of small FDG avid lesions (≤ 10 mm) of DWI and noTOF PET image were 9.1% and 9.1%, respectively. However, the TOF PET-based clinical diagnosis detected all small lesions (≤ 30 mm). DWI was of great importance in detection of small lesions (≤ 10 mm) in the absence of TOF technique in PET/MR examination (**$P < 0.01$). DWI's effect on detection of small lesions(10-30 mm) has shown no difference between PET/MR examinations with TOF and without TOF techniques ($P > 0.05$).

Conclusion DWI has significant value in the detection of small lesions (≤ 10 mm) in hybrid PET/MR examination without TOF technique for patients with primary abdominal and pelvic cancer. However, it had less detection benefits in the small lesions (≤ 10 mm) in hybrid PET/MR examination with TOF PET image.

Keywords Diffusion-weighted imaging (DWI) · Hybrid positron emission tomography/magnetic resonance (PET/MR) · Time of flight (TOF) · FDG

Introduction

Hybrid positron emission tomography/magnetic resonance (PET/MR) improves the accuracy in assessment of tumor, based on the combined information of simultaneously obtained PET and MR images. Diffusion-weighted imaging (DWI) and PET are both functional modalities presenting biological characteristics of malignant tumor. PET/MR provides a new generation of multimodal imaging, combining PET data of tumor metabolism with structural and functional information of MRI [1, 2].

Not only the superior anatomic contrast of MR may help provide more accurate location of PET positive lesions, but also the functional information provided by MR, such as DWI and perfusion imaging, may further

---

✉ Jie Lu
    imaginglu@hotmail.com

Extended author information available on the last page of the article

Published online: 12 March 2019

 Springer

SHANG K, WANG J, FAN X, et al.Clinical value of hybrid TOF-PET/MR imaging-based multiparametric imaging in localizing seizure focus in patients with MRI-negative temporal lobe epilepsy.AJNR Am J Neuroradiol, 2018, 39(10): 1791-1798.

【研究简介】

研究背景：难治性颞叶癫痫早期手术治疗优于长期药物治疗，术前致痫区的精准定位可提高患者预后。^{18}F-FDG PET 在 MRI 阴性或电生理结果与影像结果不一致时有助于癫痫患者定侧或定位病灶，ASL 是一种非对比灌注技术，癫痫患者在发作期血流灌注增加，发作后血流灌注减少。本研究旨在评估基于一体化 TOF PET/MR 成像的多参数成像在常规 MRI 阴性的颞叶癫痫中的定位价值。

资料与方法：本研究纳入 20 例术前 MRI 阴性的颞叶癫痫患者和 10 例健康对照，所有受试者接受 TOF PET/MR 扫描，同时获取 PET 和 ASL 数据。首先由 2 名医师视觉判断 20 例 MRI 阴性颞叶癫痫患者的代谢和血流减低区，计算相应脑区的 SUVR 和 CBF，通过 ROC 曲线和 Logistic 回归模型预测 PET 和 ASL 的定位价值；最后进行体素分析，比较患者组和正常组的 SUVR、CBF、代谢不对称性区和血流不对称性区之间的差异。

研究结果：20 例 MRI 阴性的颞叶癫痫患者中 12 例患者的 ^{18}F-FDG PET、ASL 和病理结果在定位致痫灶方面完全一致；8 例患者的 ^{18}F-FDG PET 和 ASL 可以提供互补性信息。ROC 曲线显示 PET、ASL 及二者结合对病灶定位的敏感度、特异度分别为 100% 和 81.8%、83.3% 和 54.5%、100% 和 90.9%（图 1-1-87）。体素分析结果显示，与正常组相比，患者组代谢减低区、代谢不对称性区和血流不对称性区均位于颞叶（$P < 0.001$），与病理结果一致（图 1-1-88）。

研究结论：基于一体化 TOF PET/MR 成像的多参数成像 ASL 和 PET 及其不对称性，对于常规 MRI 阴性的颞叶癫痫定位具有重要价值。

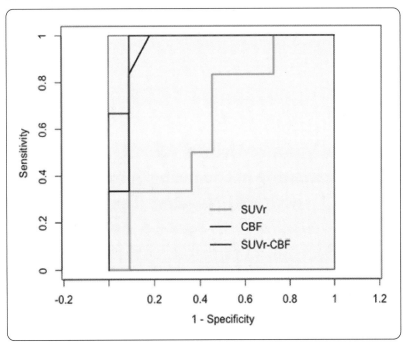

图 1-1-87　SUVR、CBF 和 SUVR-CBF 对于癫痫致痫灶定位的 ROC 曲线

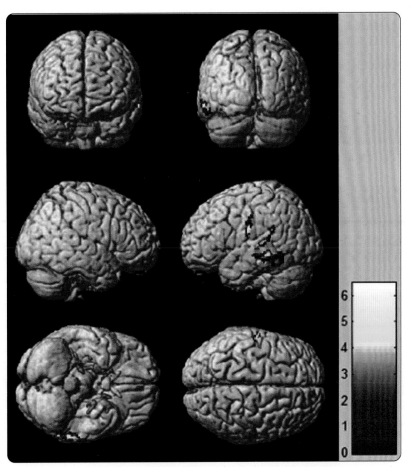

图 1-1-88　MRI 阴性颞叶癫痫患者低代谢区主要位于颞中回

首
都
医
科
大
学
宣
武
医
院
一
体
化
PET/MR
成
果
集

Clinical Value of Hybrid TOF-PET/MR Imaging–Based Multiparametric Imaging in Localizing Seizure Focus in Patients with MRI-Negative Temporal Lobe Epilepsy

K. Shang, J. Wang, X. Fan, B. Cui, J. Ma, H. Yang, Y. Zhou, G. Zhao, and J. Lu

ABSTRACT

BACKGROUND AND PURPOSE: Temporal lobe epilepsy is the most common type of epilepsy. Early surgical treatment is superior to prolonged medical therapy in refractory temporal lobe epilepsy. Successful surgical operations depend on the correct localization of the epileptogenic zone. This study aimed to evaluate the clinical value of hybrid TOF-PET/MR imaging–based multiparametric imaging in localizing the epileptogenic zone in patients with MR imaging-negative for temporal lobe epilepsy.

MATERIALS AND METHODS: Twenty patients with MR imaging-negative temporal lobe epilepsy who underwent preoperative evaluation and 10 healthy controls were scanned using PET/MR imaging with simultaneous acquisition of PET and arterial spin-labeling. On the basis of the standardized uptake value and cerebral blood flow, receiver operating characteristic analysis and a logistic regression model were used to evaluate the predictive value for the localization. Statistical analyses were performed using statistical parametric mapping. The values of the standardized uptake value and cerebral blood flow, as well as the asymmetries of metabolism and perfusion, were compared between the 2 groups. Histopathologic findings were used as the criterion standard.

RESULTS: Complete concordance was noted in lateralization and localization among the PET, arterial spin-labeling, and histopathologic findings in 12/20 patients based on visual assessment. Concordance with histopathologic findings was also obtained for the remaining 8 patients based on the complementary PET and arterial spin-labeling information. Receiver operating characteristic analysis showed that the sensitivity and specificity of PET, arterial spin-labeling, and combined PET and arterial spin-labeling were 100% and 81.8%, 83.3% and 54.5%, and 100% and 90.9%, respectively. When we compared the metabolic abnormalities in patients with those in healthy controls, hypometabolism was detected in the middle temporal gyrus ($P < .001$). Metabolism and perfusion asymmetries were also located in the temporal lobe ($P < .001$).

CONCLUSIONS: PET/MR imaging–based multiparametric imaging involving arterial spin-labeling may increase the clinical value of localizing the epileptogenic zone by providing concordant and complementary information in patients with MR imaging-negative temporal lobe epilepsy.

ABBREVIATIONS: AI = asymmetry index; ASL = arterial spin-labeling; EZ = epileptogenic zone; FCD = focal cortical dysplasia; HS = hippocampal sclerosis; SPM = statistical parametric mapping; SUV = standardized uptake value; SUVr = standardized uptake value ratio; TLE = temporal lobe epilepsy

Epilepsy is a common chronic neurologic disorder characterized by recurrent spontaneous seizures. It has an incidence of 50 per 100,000 persons per year.[1] Temporal lobe epilepsy (TLE) is the most common type of epilepsy. A published randomized trial reported that early surgical treatment is superior

to prolonged medical therapy in refractory TLE.[2] Successful operations depend on the correct localization of the epileptogenic zone (EZ). MR imaging is a powerful tool in identifying the lesions causing epilepsy, such as hippocampal sclerosis (HS). However, approximately 16% of patients with TLE have a normal MR imaging appearance.[3] Histopathologic studies have shown that many focal cortical dysplasias (FCDs) are small or subtle and are difficult to identify visually using MR imaging.[4] FCDs are identified as the most common histo-

Received April 4, 2018; accepted after revision July 18.

From the Departments of Nuclear Medicine (K.S., J.W., B.C., J.M., H.Y., J.L.), Neurosurgery (X.F., G.Z.), and Radiology (J.L.), Xuanwu Hospital, Capital Medical University, Beijing, China; and Department of Radiology (Y.Z.), Johns Hopkins University, Baltimore, Maryland.

This work was supported by the National Natural Science Foundation of China (Grant No. 81522021) and the National Key Research and Development Program of China (Grant No. 2016YFC0103000).

Paper previously presented, in part, at: Annual Meeting of the Society of Nuclear Medicine and Molecular Imaging, June 10–14, 2017; Denver, Colorado.

Please address correspondence Jie Lu, MD, Department of Nuclear Medicine, Xuanwu Hospital, Capital Medical University, 45 Changchunjie, Xicheng District, Beijing 100053, China; e-mail: imaginglu@hotmail.com

Indicates open access to non-subscribers at www.ajnr.org

http://dx.doi.org/10.3174/ajnr.A5814

AJNR Am J Neuroradiol 39:1791–98   Oct 2018   www.ajnr.org   **1791**

HE Y, XIE F, YE J, et al.1-(4-[^{18}F] Fluorobenzyl)-4-[(tetrahydrofuran-2-yl)methyl] piperazine: a novel suitable radioligand with low lipophilicity for imaging σ 1 receptors in the brain.J Med Chem, 2017, 60(10): 4161-4172.

【研究简介】

研究背景： σ₁ 受体由 223 个氨基酸组成，分子量为 25kDa，该受体能够与质膜、内质网、线粒体甚至胞质中的其他功能蛋白相互作用。σ₁ 受体参与许多人类疾病的病理生理学，包括阿尔茨海默病、帕金森病、肌萎缩侧索硬化症等。

材料与方法： 从 4-（*n*，*n*，*n* 三甲基氨基）苯甲醛碘化物开始使用两步程序制备放射性示踪剂，通过取代三甲基碘化铵基团从前体制备 4-[^{18}F] 氟苯甲醛，使用 NaBH$_3$CN 作为还原剂和 CH$_3$COOH 作为催化剂，将 ^{18}F 标记的产出化合物与 4-[^{18}F] 氟苯甲醛还原胺化获得示踪剂产物。采用半制备型高效液相色谱（high pressure chromatography，HPLC）测定不同时间点的放化纯度，评价化合物的 ^{18}F 在生理盐水和小鼠血清中的体外稳定性。应用体外放射自显影研究评价 ^{18}F 在 ICR 鼠的不同脑区的分布情况，为进一步评估 ^{18}F 在大脑中的动力学和特异性结合，在 Sprague-Dawley 大鼠中进行 PET/MR 动态成像研究。最后使用 σ₁- 选择性激动剂 SA4503 进行了阻断研究确定 ^{18}F 标记的新型 σ₁ 受体 PET 示踪剂在体内的结合特异性。

研究结果： 本研究设计的新型 σ₁ 受体示踪剂总合成时间约 80 分钟，放射化学产率 20% ~ 30%，放射化学纯度 > 99%，比活度为 54 ~ 86 GBq/μmol。鼠的体外放射自显影发现放射性示踪剂浓聚于颞皮层听觉区域，在中脑、红核等高水平 σ₁ 受体的脑区也观察到高水平的 ^{18}F 摄取（图 1-1-89）。图 1-1-90 展示 Sprague-Dawley 大鼠静脉注射新型 PET 示踪剂后 15 ~ 30 分钟、30 ~ 45 分钟、45 ~ 60 分钟和 60 ~ 75 分钟的动态 PET 成像。图 1-1-91 的 TAC 曲线表明新型 σ₁ 受体示踪剂能快速进入大脑，在 2 分钟内达到峰值浓度，然后随着时间的推移稳定地被洗出，与生物分布研究的结果一致。选择性激动剂 SA4503 阻断研究发现在注射放射性示踪剂后 15 分钟、30 分钟和 60 分钟，大脑中放射性示踪剂的累积水平显著降低，分别为 79%、88% 和 86%，表明新型示踪剂与体内 σ₁ 受体实现了高度特异性结合。

研究结论： 新型 σ₁ 受体 PET 示踪剂，对 σ₁ 受体具有纳摩尔亲和力及良好的亚型选择性，对 VAChT 和其他受体具有高选择性，是一种可为阿尔茨海默病、帕金森病等神经系统疾病提供早期诊断的特异性 PET 示踪剂。

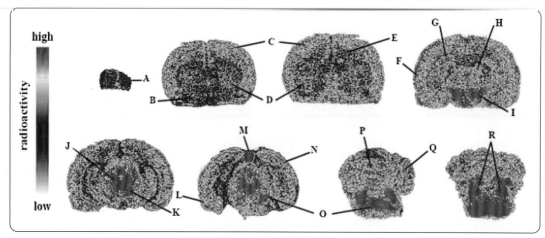

图 1-1-89　静脉注射 [^{18}F] 新型 σ$_1$ 受体示踪剂（0.4 mL，24.9 MBq）后 30 分钟鼠冠状脑切片的放射自显影

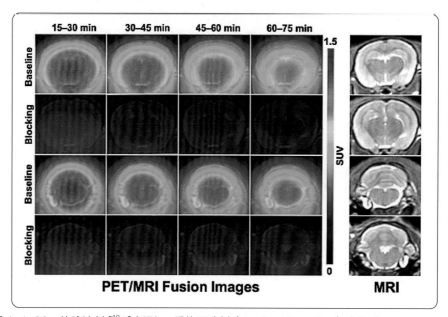

图 1-1-90　静脉注射 [^{18}F] 新型 σ$_1$ 受体示踪剂（22.1～23.7 MBq）大鼠脑 PET/MR 图像

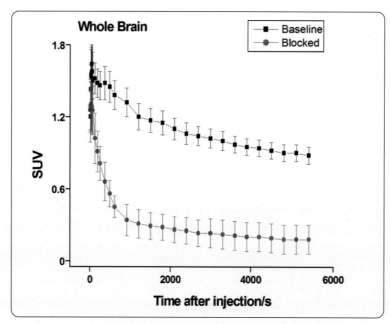

图 1-1-91　大鼠全脑动态 PET 图像的时间－活性曲线（TACs）

Journal of

Medicinal Chemistry

Article

pubs.acs.org/jmc

1-(4-[18F]Fluorobenzyl)-4-[(tetrahydrofuran-2-yl)methyl]piperazine: A Novel Suitable Radioligand with Low Lipophilicity for Imaging σ_1 Receptors in the Brain

Yingfang He,[†] Fang Xie,[†] Jiajun Ye,[†] Winnie Deuther-Conrad,[‡] Bixiao Cui,[§] Liang Wang,[†] Jie Lu,[†] Jörg Steinbach,[‡] Peter Brust,[‡] Yiyun Huang,[∥] Jie Lu,*,[§] and Hongmei Jia*,[†]

[†]Key Laboratory of Radiopharmaceuticals (Beijing Normal University), Ministry of Education, College of Chemistry, Beijing Normal University, Beijing, China

[‡]Helmholtz-Zentrum Dresden-Rossendorf, Institute of Radiopharmaceutical Cancer Research, Department of Neuroradiopharmaceuticals, 04318 Leipzig, Germany

[§]Department of Nuclear Medicine, Xuanwu Hospital Capital Medical University, Beijing, China

[∥]Yale PET Center, Department of Radiology and Biomedical Imaging, Yale University School of Medicine, New Haven, Connecticut 06520-8048, United States

⑤ *Supporting Information*

ABSTRACT: We have designed and synthesized novel piperazine compounds with low lipophilicity as σ_1 receptor ligands. 1-(4-Fluorobenzyl)-4-[(tetrahydrofuran-2-yl)methyl]piperazine (**10**) possessed a low nanomolar σ_1 receptor affinity and a high selectivity toward the vesicular acetylcholine transporter (>2000-fold), σ_2 receptors (52-fold), and adenosine A_{2A}, adrenergic α_2, cannabinoid CB_1, dopamine D_1, D_{2L}, γ-aminobutyric acid A (GABA$_A$), NMDA, melatonin MT_1, MT_2, and serotonin 5-HT_1 receptors. The corresponding radiotracer [18F]**10** demonstrated high brain uptake and extremely high brain-to-blood ratios in biodistribution studies in mice. Pretreatment with the selective σ_1 receptor agonist SA4503 significantly reduced the level of accumulation of the radiotracer in the brain. No radiometabolite of [18F]**10** was observed to enter the brain. Positron emission tomography and magnetic resonance imaging confirmed suitable kinetics and a high specific binding of [18F]**10** to σ_1 receptors in rat brain. *Ex vivo* autoradiography showed a reduced level of binding of [18F]**10** in the cortex and hippocampus of the senescence-accelerated prone (SAMP8) compared to that of the senescence-accelerated resistant (SAMR1) mice, indicating the potential dysfunction of σ_1 receptors in Alzheimer's disease.

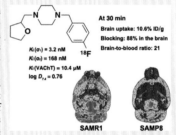

At 30 min
Brain uptake: 10.6% ID/g
Blocking: 88% in the brain
Brain-to-blood ratio: 21

$Ki(\sigma_1) = 3.2$ nM
$Ki(\sigma_2) = 168$ nM
$Ki(VAChT) = 10.4$ μM
$\log D_{7.4} = 0.76$

SAMR1   SAMP8

■ INTRODUCTION

The σ_1 receptor consists of 223 amino acids with a molecular weight of 25 kDa.[1] Contrary to the prevailing model of two transmembrane segments,[2] the recently reported crystal structures of the human σ_1 receptor revealed a trimeric architecture with a single transmembrane domain in each protomer.[3] Most importantly, this receptor is a unique "ligand-operated receptor chaperone"[4] and interacts with other functional proteins in the plasma membrane, endoplasmic reticulum, mitochondria, and even cytosol.[5] A growing body of evidence has indicated the involvement of the σ_1 receptors in the pathophysiology of a number of human diseases, including Alzheimer's disease (AD), Parkinson's disease (PD), amyotrophic lateral sclerosis (ALS), Huntington's disease, stroke/ischemia, pain/neuropathic pain, cocaine addiction, myocardial hypertension, and cancers.[5−12] Molecular probes with appropriate affinity, high selectivity, and specificity for σ_1 receptors will be useful in the understanding and monitoring of σ_1 receptor-related diseases using noninvasive imaging techniques such as positron emission tomography (PET) and single photon emission computed tomography (SPECT).

In the past several decades, many PET and SPECT radiotracers for σ_1 receptors have been reported.[13] However, to date, there have been no suitable σ_1 receptor radiotracers for clinical use. Among the existing radiotracers investigated thus far in humans, [18F]FPS ([18F]**2**)[14] and [123I]TPCNE ([123I]**3**)[15] (Figure 1) displayed irreversible kinetics in the brain. [11C]SA4503 [[11C]**1** (Figure 1)], as the first useful PET radiotracer for imaging σ_1 receptors in humans,[16−18] possessed nanomolar affinity for σ_1 receptors and high selectivity toward 36 other receptors, ion channels, and second-messenger systems.[19] However, the use of [11C]**1** needs an on-site cyclotron because of the short half-life of ^{11}C ($t_{1/2}$ = 20 min). More recently, [18F]FTC-146 ([18F]**4**)[20−22] has been reported to be a promising PET radiotracer for visualizing σ_1 receptors. However, further investigation is still required for its clinical

Received: November 24, 2016
Published: April 14, 2017

ACS Publications   4161   DOI: 10.1021/acs.jmedchem.6b01723
J. Med. Chem. 2017, 60, 4161−4172

SHANG K, CUI B, MA J, et al.Clinical evaluation of whole-body oncologic PET with time-of-flight and point-spread function for the hybrid PET/MR system.Eur J Radiol, 2017, 93: 70-75.

【研究简介】

研究背景： 一体化 PET/MR 可以同时采集结构信息和功能信息，本研究评估飞行时间（time of flight，TOF）和点扩散函数（point spread function，PSF）对临床患者 PET/MR 图像中小病灶的检出价值。

资料与方法： 本研究纳入了 14 例接受一体化 ^{18}F-FDG PET/MR 检查的体部恶性肿瘤患者，直径 < 30 mm 的病灶共 54 个。分别对 PET 图像进行 OSEM、OSEM+PSF、OSEM+TOF 和 OSEM+TOF+PSF 重建，对 PET 图像质量和小病灶进行视觉评估，用 3 分评分法进行评分，并定量分析小病灶的平均和最大标准化摄取值（SUV_{mean} 和 SUV_{max}）。根据病灶直径和位置分别将病灶分为两组，并用每种重建算法进行评估。

研究结果： OSEM+TOF+PSF 测量小病灶的 SUV 值最高，OSEM+TOF 和 PSF 的视觉评估和定量分析值均较 OSEM 更高。TOF 联合 PSF 将 SUV 平均值提高了 26.6%，SUV 最大值提高了 30.0%。对于 OSEM+TOF+PSF 模型，直径 < 10 mm 的病灶的 SUV_{mean} 和 SUV_{max} 变化分别为 31.9% 和 35.8%，直径为 10～30 mm 的病灶的 SUV_{mean} 和 SUV_{max} 变化分别为 24.5% 和 27.6%。在 TOF 和（或）PSF 图像上，腹部病变的 SUV 高于胸部病变（图 1-1-92）。图 1-1-93 展示一例患者腹部小病灶的一体化 PET/MR 表现。

研究结论： 本研究表明 TOF 和 PSF 的应用显著提高了 PET/MR 图像中小病灶的 SUV，提高了小病灶的检测。

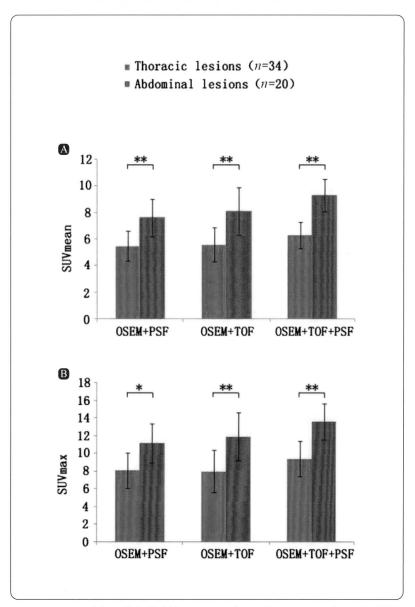

图 1-1-92　胸部和腹部病变的 SUV$_{mean}$（图 A）和 SUV$_{max}$（图 B）比较

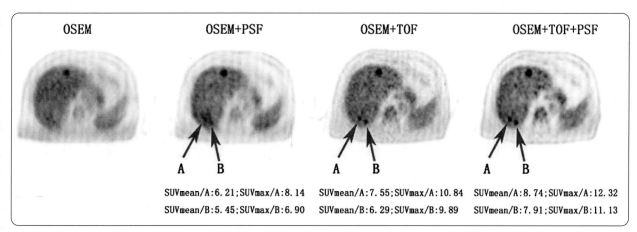

图 1-1-93　胰腺癌肝转移患者，每种重建算法 PET 腹部图像比较

左侧竖排：首都医科大学宣武医院一体化 PET/MR 成果集

European Journal of Radiology 93 (2017) 70–75

Contents lists available at ScienceDirect

European Journal of Radiology

journal homepage: www.elsevier.com/locate/ejrad

Research papers

Clinical evaluation of whole-body oncologic PET with time-of-flight and point-spread function for the hybrid PET/MR system

CrossMark

Kun Shang[a], Bixiao Cui[a], Jie Ma[a], Dongmei Shuai[a], Zhigang Liang[a], Floris Jansen[c], Yun Zhou[d], Jie Lu[a,*], Guoguang Zhao[a,b]

[a] Department of Nuclear Medicine, Xuanwu Hospital of Capital Medical University, Beijing, China
[b] Department of Neurosurgery, Xuanwu Hospital of Capital Medical University, Beijing, China
[c] GE Healthcare, Waukesha, WI, USA
[d] Department of Radiology, Johns Hopkins University, Baltimore, MD, USA

ARTICLE INFO

Keywords:
Time-of-flight
Point-spread function
Hybrid PET/MR
Small lesion detection

ABSTRACT

Purpose: Hybrid positron emission tomography/magnetic resonance (PET/MR) imaging is a new multimodality imaging technology that can provide structural and functional information simultaneously. The aim of this study was to investigate the effects of the time-of-flight (TOF) and point-spread function (PSF) on small lesions observed in PET/MR images from clinical patient image sets.

Materials and methods: This study evaluated 54 small lesions in 14 patients who had undergone ^{18}F-fluorodeoxyglucose (FDG) PET/MR. Lesions up to 30 mm in diameter were included. The PET data were reconstructed with a baseline ordered-subsets expectation-maximization (OSEM) algorithm, OSEM + PSF, OSEM + TOF and OSEM + TOF + PSF. PET image quality and small lesions were visually evaluated and scored by a 3-point scale. A quantitative analysis was then performed using the mean and maximum standardized uptake value (SUV) of the small lesions (SUV_{mean} and SUV_{max}). The lesions were divided into two groups according to the long-axis diameter and the location respectively and evaluated with each reconstruction algorithm. We also evaluated the background signal by analyzing the SUV_{liver}.

Results: OSEM + TOF + PSF provided the highest value and OSEM + TOF or PSF showed a higher value than OSEM for the visual assessment and quantitative analysis. The combination of TOF and PSF increased the SUV_{mean} by 26.6% and the SUV_{max} by 30.0%. The SUV_{liver} was not influenced by PSF or TOF. For the OSEM + TOF + PSF model, the change in SUV_{mean} and SUV_{max} for lesions < 10 mm in diameter was 31.9% and 35.8%, and 24.5% and 27.6% for lesions 10–30 mm in diameter, respectively. The abdominal lesions obtained the higher SUV than those of chest on the images with TOF and/or PSF.

Conclusion: Application of TOF and PSF significantly increased the SUV of small lesions in hybrid PET/MR images, potentially improving small lesion detectability.

1. Introduction

Hybrid positron emission tomography/magnetic resonance (PET/MR) imaging is a new multimodality imaging technology that can provide structural and functional information simultaneously [1–3]. This new technology has the potential to expand the success of hybrid imaging modality, such as PET/computed tomography (CT), particularly for oncologic indications [4]. MR is considered as the first-line imaging procedure in the diagnosis and staging of various cancers due to the superior soft tissue contrast compared with CT [5,6]. However, the spatial resolution of PET is relatively low. Incorporation of time-of-flight (TOF) and point-spread function (PSF) information during image

reconstruction has been shown to improve the spatial resolution and signal-to-noise ratio (SNR) of PET images [7–10].

The first attempt at TOF PET dated back to the 1980s, and the first TOF PET scanners were based on cesium fluoride (CsF) and barium fluoride (BaF_2). It was not until the development of lutetiumoxyorthosilicate (LSO) and lutetium–yttrium oxyorthosilicate (LYSO) that the TOF PET scanner was successful and introduced commercially. The TOF information provides a difference in arrival times between a pair of coincidence photons and localizes the annihilation points along the line-of-response (LOR). Using this information during reconstruction can reduce image noise and improve contrast [11]. Now, PET/CT systems with advanced TOF capability are available widely. The first

* Corresponding author at: Department of Nuclear Medicine, Xuanwu Hospital of Capital Medical University, 45 Changchunjie, Xicheng District, Beijing 100053, China.
E-mail address: imaginglu@hotmail.com (J. Lu).

http://dx.doi.org/10.1016/j.ejrad.2017.05.029
Received 23 February 2017; Received in revised form 18 May 2017; Accepted 22 May 2017

第二节　统计源期刊收录文章

截至 2022 年 12 月，首都医科大学宣武医院团队共发表 33 篇统计源期刊收录文章，其中神经系统 14 篇（脑血管病 6 篇、脑功能 3 篇、癫痫 2 篇、脑胶质瘤 2 篇和痴呆 1 篇）、体部肿瘤 2 篇、技术 9 篇、护理 4 篇、规范与专家共识 4 篇。

1. 发表文章列表

[1] 郭坤，尚琨，崔碧霄，等. ^{18}F-FDG PET/MR对MRI阴性药物难治性癫痫患者致痫灶的定位价值. 中华核医学与分子影像杂志，2021，41（7）：410-414.

[2] 张越，卢洁. 颈动脉粥样硬化斑块稳定性评估正电子发射断层扫描/磁共振研究进展. 首都医科大学学报，2021，42（1）：31-36.

[3] 崔亚莹，白玫. MR磁场对一体化PET/MR系统灵敏度的影响. 中国医学装备，2021，18（07）：6-9.

[4] 杨宏伟，崔碧霄，宋天彬，等. Q. Static运动校正技术对一体化PET/MR胸腹部成像质量的影响研究. 医学影像学杂志，2021，31（8）：1301-1305.

[5] 胡鹏程，赵军，杨志，等. . 肝胆系统PET/MR成像检查规范专家共识. 中国临床医学，2020，27（5）：881-885.

[6] 陈曙光，胡鹏程，樊卫，等. PET/MR全身显像工作流及协议规划专家共识. 中国临床医学，2020，27（4）：713-721.

[7] 单艺，李静，许潇尹. 缺血性脑卒中的脑功能与分子成像研究——卢洁教授. 首都医科大学学报，2020，41（5）：788-794.

[8] 宋双双，齐志刚，王雷明，等. 间变性多形性黄色星形细胞瘤1例. 医学影像学杂志，2020，30（9）：1586-1591.

[9] 田德峰，杨宏伟，庄静文，等. 选择一体化PET/MR小病灶图像重建方案. 中国医学影像技术，2020，36（04）：596-600.

[10] 马蕾，帅冬梅，宋双双，等. 规范化护理在脑肿瘤患者一体化^{18}F-FET PET/MR检查中的应用. 医学影像学杂志，2020，30（07）：1322-1324.

[11] 郭坤，李云波，卢洁. 韧带样纤维瘤病18F-FDG PET/MR误诊为输尿管癌1例. 医学影像学杂志，2020，30（12）：2312-2316.

[12] 李再升，宋双双，曾天翼，等. PET-MRI脑部定量准确性对比研究：MRI与PET脑分区对SUVR计算的影响. 核技术，2020，43（5）：16-25.

[13] 崔碧霄，张苗，马杰，等. 一体化^{18}F-FDG PET/MR评估缺血性脑血管病. 中国医学影像技术，2019，35（12）：1817-1822.

[14] 郭坤，卢洁. MRI、^{18}F-FDG PET以及PET/MRI在难治性癫痫术前精准定位中的价值. 癫痫杂志，2019，5（5）：372-375.

[15] 宋天彬，崔碧霄，杨宏伟，等. 一体化PET/MR检查中"热气管征"伪影探讨. 中国医学影像技

术，2019，35（11）：1727-1732.

[16] 田德峰，杨宏伟，庄静文，等.一体化PET/MR不同衰减校正方式定量准确性分析及图像质量评估.中国医学装备，2019，16（6）：16-19.

[17] 吴萍，吴天棋，白玫.重建矩阵对一体化PET/MR图像质量的影响.中国医学装备，2019，16（3）：43-47.

[18] 帅冬梅，卢洁，李秋萍.一体化PET/MR受检者护理需求及影响因素调查.医学影像学杂志，2019，29（7）：1209-1212.

[19] 闫少珍，卢洁，李坤成.一体化正电子发射断层显像磁共振在阿尔茨海默病的研究进展.中华老年心脑血管病杂志，2018，20（12）：1336-1338.

[20] 张越，杨旗，卢洁.正电子发射断层显像与磁共振成像联合评价颈动脉易损斑块的研究进展.中华老年心脑血管病杂志，2018，20（4）：440-442.

[21] 董硕，李东，吴天棋，等.一体化PET-MR设备中飞行时间技术和点扩展函数技术对PET图像质量的影响.中国医学装备，2018，15（2）：1-5.

[22] 马蕾，卢洁，帅冬梅，等.护理因素对一体化TOF PET/MR图像质量影响的原因分析.医学影像学杂志，2018，28（12）：2107-2108.

[23] 卢洁，张苗，方继良，等.一体化PET/MR颅脑成像检查规范（2017版）.中国医学影像技术，2017，33（5）：791-794.

[24] 韩斌如，帅冬梅，方继良，等.一体化PET/MR检查临床护理操作规范（2017版）.中国医学影像技术，2017，33（5）：795-798.

[25] 王静娟，崔碧霄，杨宏伟，等.一体化PET/MR分析脑默认网络工作机制.中国医学影像技术，2017，33（11）：1620-1623.

[26] 王静娟，卢洁.一体化PET/MR在脑功能方面的研究进展.医学影像学杂志，2017，27（9）：1798-1799+1802.

[27] 单艺，卢洁，李坤成.一体化PET/MR评估脑血流量的研究进展.中国医学影像技术，2017，33（8）：1269-1272.

[28] 赵永瑞，徐建堃.PET/MRI在高级别脑胶质瘤放射治疗中的应用.实用肿瘤学杂志，2017，31（6）：564-568.

[29] 宋天彬，卢洁，崔碧霄，等.TOF-PET/MR和TOF-PET/CT在体部恶性肿瘤SUV_{max}值的比较.中国医学影像技术，2017，33（9）：1401-1406.

[30] 庄静文，谢峰，吴天棋，等.不同重建条件对一体化PET-MR图像空间分辨率影响的研究.中国医学装备，2017，14（11）：12-15.

[31] 臧玉峰，冯逢，霍力，等.PET/fMRI对异常脑活动的精准定位：研究进展与展望.中华核医学与分子影像杂志，2017，37（12）：802-808.

[32] 卢洁，刘振宇，李亚明.一体化TOF PET/MR影像技术实现精准定量脑血流量.中华核医学与分子影像杂志，2016，36（6）：547-548.

[33] 帅冬梅，卢洁，梁志刚，等.一体化PET/MRI检查的护理配合.中日友好医院学报，2016，30（4）：258-260.

2. 附列表中文章原文首页

文章 1

· 410 · 中华核医学与分子影像杂志 2021 年 7 月第 41 卷第 7 期　Chin J Nucl Med Mol Imaging, Jul. 2021, Vol. 41, No. 7

· PET/MR ·

^{18}F-FDG PET/MR 对 MRI 阴性药物难治性癫痫患者致痫灶的定位价值

郭坤[1]　尚琨[1]　崔碧霄[1]　侯亚琴[1]　杨宏伟[1]　樊晓彤[2]　帅冬梅[1]　卢洁[3]
[1]首都医科大学宣武医院核医学科,北京　100053;[2]首都医科大学宣武医院神经外科,北京　100053;[3]首都医科大学宣武医院放射科,北京　100053
通信作者:卢洁,Email:imaginglu@ hotmail.com

【摘要】　目的　探讨^{18}F-脱氧葡萄糖(FDG)PET/MR 对常规 MRI 阴性的药物难治性癫痫患者术前致痫灶的定位价值。方法　回顾性分析 2016 年 8 月至 2018 年 12 月间在首都医科大学宣武医院接受手术治疗的 57 例[男 36 例、女 21 例,年龄(24.0±10.3)岁]常规 MRI 阴性的药物难治性癫痫患者资料。所有患者术前均行发作间期^{18}F-FDG PET/MR 扫描,采用视觉及半定量方法综合定位致痫灶。术后 1 年随访,根据 Engel 分级评价手术疗效,以手术切除病变及术后随访结果为定位诊断的"金标准",计算^{18}F-FDG PET/MR 定位致痫灶的灵敏度、特异性和准确性。结果　89.5%(51/57)的患者^{18}F-FDG PET/MR 表现为 1 处或多处葡萄糖代谢减低,10.5%(6/57)的患者未见异常葡萄糖代谢改变。18 例(31.6%,18/57)常规 MRI 阴性的药物难治性癫痫患者^{18}F-FDG PET/MR 图像上检出微小结构异常。46 例患者获得术后 1 年随访,癫痫症状改善者(Engel Ⅰ～Ⅲ级)占 84.8%(39/46)。^{18}F-FDG PET/MR 定位致痫灶的灵敏度、特异性、准确性分别为 90.0%(27/30)、3/16、65.2%(30/46)。结论　对于常规 MRI 阴性药物难治性癫痫患者,^{18}F-FDG PET/MR 有助于致痫灶术前定位,为手术治疗提供可靠信息。
【关键词】　癫痫;正电子发射断层显像术;体层摄影术;X 线计算机;磁共振成像;脱氧葡萄糖
基金项目:北京市医院管理局"登峰"计划专项(DFL20180802)
DOI:10.3760/cma.j.cn321828-20200302-00083

Preoperative localization of ^{18}F-FDG PET/MR in refractory epilepsy patients with negative MRI
Guo Kun[1], Shang Kun[1], Cui Bixiao[1], Hou Yaqin[1], Yang Hongwei[1], Fan Xiaotong[2], Shuai Dongmei[1], Lu Jie[3]
[1]Department of Nuclear Medicine, Xuanwu Hospital, Capital Medical University, Beijing 100053, China;
[2]Department of Neurosurgery, Xuanwu Hospital, Capital Medical University, Beijing 100053, China;
[3]Department of Radiology, Xuanwu Hospital, Capital Medical University, Beijing 100053, China
Corresponding author: Lu Jie, Email: imaginglu@hotmail.com
【Abstract】　Objective　To explore the accuracy of ^{18}F-fluorodeoxyglucose (FDG) PET/MR in preoperative localization of refractory epilepsy patients with conventional MRI negative. Methods　From August 2016 to December 2018, 57 refractory epilepsy patients (36 males, 21 females, age (24.0±10.3) years) with conventional MRI negative who underwent surgery in Xuanwu Hospital were retrospectively enrolled. All patients received interictal ^{18}F-FDG PET/MR before surgery and the epileptogenic foci were determined by using visual and semi-quantitative methods. Patients were followed up for 1 year and the surgical outcome was evaluated according to Engel classification. The sensitivity, specificity and accuracy of ^{18}F-FDG PET/ MR in locating epileptogenic foci were calculated according to surgical resection and followed-up results as the "gold standard". Results　Of 57 patients, 51(89.5%, 51/57) showed single or multiple hypo-metabolism focus on ^{18}F-FDG PET/MR, and 6(10.5%, 6/57) showed no abnormal metabolism changes. The microstructure abnormality was found in 18 patients (31.6%, 18/57) on ^{18}F-FDG PET/MR images. Follow-up results were obtained from 46 patients, and 84.8%(39/46) with seizure improvement (Engel Ⅰ-Ⅲ). The sensitivity, specificity and accuracy of ^{18}F-FDG PET/MR in preoperative localization of epileptic foci was 90.0%(27/30), 3/16 and 65.2%(30/46), respectively. Conclusion　^{18}F-FDG PET/MR is helpful for the detection of epileptic foci in patients with MRI-negative refractory epilepsy, and can provide reliable information for further surgical treatment.
【Key words】　Epilepsy; Positron-emission tomography; Tomography, X-ray computed; Magnetic resonance imaging; Deoxyglucose
Fund program: Project of Beijing Municipal Administration of Hospitals' Ascent Plan (DFL 20180802)
DOI:10.3760/cma.j.cn321828-20200302-00083

第一章　一体化 PET/MR 科研成果

2021年 2月
第42卷 第1期

首都医科大学学报
Journal of Capital Medical University

Feb. 2021
Vol. 42 No. 1

[doi: 10.3969/j.issn.1006-7795.2021.01.006]

· 核医学基础与临床 ·

颈动脉粥样硬化斑块稳定性评估正电子发射断层扫描/磁共振研究进展

张 越¹ 卢 洁¹,²*

(1. 首都医科大学宣武医院放射与核医学科, 北京100053; 2. 磁共振成像脑信息学北京市重点实验室, 北京100053)

【摘要】 颈动脉粥样硬化斑块破裂是导致脑梗死的主要原因, 探索斑块进展的病理生理机制, 尽早发现易损斑块是国际研究热点。研究显示炎性反应与斑块发生、发展、破裂密切相关, 但炎性反应过程及其与预后关系的病理生理机制尚不清楚。高分辨磁共振成像(high-resolution magnetic resonance imaging, HR-MRI)和正电子发射断层扫描(positron emission tomography, PET)是评价颈动脉粥样硬化斑块的有力手段, HR-MRI能提供斑块形态学信息, PET能提供斑块内炎性反应的巨噬细胞代谢信息。本文重点对HR-MRI、PET及一体化PET/MR成像在颈动脉粥样硬化斑块稳定性评估的研究进展进行综述, 阐明颈动脉斑块易损性的病理生理机制, 以期进行早期影像学预警, 有效预防脑梗死。

【关键词】 动脉粥样硬化; 颈动脉斑块; 高分辨磁共振成像; 正电子发射断层扫描; 一体化PET/MR

【中图分类号】 R445

Research progresses in evaluating the stability of carotid atherosclerotic plaque with positron emission tomography/computed tomography

Zhang Yue¹, Lu Jie¹,²*

(1. *Department of Radiology and Nuclear Medicine, Xuanwu Hospital, Capital Medical University, Beijing* 100053, *China*; 2. *Beijing Key Laboratory of Magnetic Resonance Imaging and Brain Informatics, Beijing* 100053, *China*)

【Abstract】 Rupture of carotid atherosclerotic plaque is the primary cause of cerebral infarction. It is a cutting edge in atherosclerosis to investigate the pathophysiological mechanism of vulnerable plaque progression for early detection. Recent studies have revealed that inflammation may cause the occurrence, development, and rupture of atherosclerotic plaque, however, its physiological mechanism and relationship with the outcome of atherosclerotic plaque are poorly understood. High-resolution magnetic resonance imaging(HR-MRI) and positron emission tomography(PET) are the non-invasive imaging technology and increasingly applied to evaluate atherosclerotic plaque. As HR-MRI is used for imaging morphology of carotid plaque with high spatial resolution, PET can be used for quantitative imaging macrophages metabolism of response to inflammation with high sensitivity and specificity. In this work, we reviewed the research progresses in the evaluation of carotid atherosclerotic plaque stability with HR-MRI, PET and simultaneous PET/MR imaging to reveal the physiological mechanism of inflammation and plaque stability and provide early imaging warning of vulnerable plaques, and develop more effective treatment strategies. It may play an important role in effectively preventing the occurrence of cerebral infarction.

【Key words】 atherosclerosis; carotid plaque; high-resolution magnetic resonance imaging(HR-MRI); positron emission tomography(PET); simultaneous PET/MR

　　脑卒中是严重威胁人类健康的重大疾病之一, 具有高发病率、高病死率和高复发率的特点[1-2], 颈动脉粥样硬化是导致我国人群缺血性脑卒中的主要原因, 约70%的缺血性脑卒中由颈动脉斑块破裂所致[3-5]。因此, 早期识别易损斑块, 评价斑块的稳定性, 对于预防和控制缺血性脑卒中事件的发生尤为重要[3]。

　　目前影像学检查为颈动脉斑块提供了重要的诊断依据, 对于临床早期预警和指导治疗具有重要价值。传统血管影像学检查方法包括: 颈部血管彩色多普勒超声、数字减影血管造影(digital subtraction angi-

基金项目: 国家自然科学基金面上项目(81974261)。This study was supported by National Natural Science Foundation of China (81974261).
* Corresponding author, E-mail: imaginglu@ hotmail. com
网络出版时间: 2021 - 01 - 19 13:23 网络出版地址: https://kns.cnki.net/kcms/detail/11.3662.R.20210119.1000.012.html

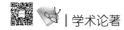 学术论著

中国医学装备2021年7月第18卷第7期 China Medical Equipment 2021 July Vol.18 No.7

MR磁场对一体化PET/MR系统灵敏度的影响*

崔亚莹① 白玫①*

[文章编号] 1672-8270(2021)07-0006-04 [中图分类号] R318.6 [文献标识码] A

[摘要] 目的：研究核磁共振(MR)射频线圈及不同强度的主磁场对一体化正电子发射断层扫描(PET)/MR系统灵敏度的影响。方法：利用基于蒙特卡罗工具的文本工程通用架构(GATE)软件建立GE Signa PET/MR仿真模型，在有无射频线圈的情况下选取不同强度磁场，依据美国电器制造商协会(NEMA)NU2-2012标准对系统灵敏度进行测量，分析不同强度磁场及射频线圈对一体化PET/MR系统灵敏度的影响；并与体模实验结果对比，验证仿真实验的准确性。结果：仿真实验与体模实验结果偏差＜3%；磁场从0T增加到7T，系统灵敏度最多降低4%；同等静磁场条件下，射频线圈的存在使系统灵敏度降低20.57%～23.5%。当时间分辨率为2.25 ns、能窗下限为300 keV时，将能量分辨率从20%优化为11%，系统灵敏度提升0.5%；当时间分辨率为2.25 ns、能窗下限为450 keV时，将能量分辨率从20%优化为11%，系统灵敏度提升16.2%。在能量分辨率为11%时，将能窗下限从450 keV降低到300 keV时，系统灵敏度提高21.2%；能量分辨率为20%时，将能窗下限从450 keV降低到300 keV时，系统灵敏度提高40.2%。当时间分辨率从2.25 ns优化至0.4 ns时，系统灵敏度整体高于时间分辨率为2.25 ns时的灵敏度，但提高程度在1%左右。结论：磁场增大PET的系统灵敏度有所降低，但程度较小；射频线圈会大幅度降低PET的系统灵敏度。降低能量阈值，优化时间分辨率以及能量分辨率有助于提高系统灵敏度。
[关键词] 正电子发射断层扫描(PET)；核磁共振(MR)；文本工程通用架构(GATE)；主磁场；射频线圈；灵敏度

DOI: 10.3969/J.ISSN.1672-8270.2021.07.002

The influences of MR magnetic field on the sensitivity of integrated PET/MR system/CUI Ya-ying, BAI Mei// China Medical Equipment,2021,18(7):6-9.

[Abstract] Objective: To study the influences of magnetic resonance radio frequency (MR RF) coil and mainly magnetic fields with different strengths on the sensitivity of integrated positron emission tomography/magnetic resonance (PET/MR) system. Methods: Generic architecture of text engineering (GATE) software based on Monte Carlo tool was adopted to establish GE Signa PET/MR simulation model so as to select the sizes of different magnetic field. The sensitivity of this system was measured according to NU2-2012 standard of national electrical manufacturers association (NEMA). And then, the influences of magnetic field with different strengthen and RF coil on the sensitivity of integrated PET/MR system were further analyzed. The accuracy of simulation experiment was verified by comparing with the results of phantom experiment. Results: The results deviation between simulation experiment and phantom experiment was less than 3%, and the sensitivity of system decreased 4% at most when the magnetic field was increased from 0T to 7T. Under the same condition of static magnetic field, the RF coil reduced the sensitivity of system from 20.57%-23.5%. The energy resolution was optimized from 20% to 11% and the sensitivity of system was increased 0.5% when the time resolution was 2.25 ns and the lower limit of energy window was 300keV. And the energy resolution was optimized from 20% to 11% and the sensitivity of system was increased 16.2% when the time resolution was 2.25 ns and the lower limit of energy window was 450keV. The lower limit of energy window was reduced from 450 keV to 300 keV and the sensitivity of system was increased 21.2% when energy resolution was 11%. And the lower limit of energy window was reduced from 450 keV to 300 keV and the sensitivity of system was increased 40.2% when energy resolution was 20%. When the time resolution was optimized from 2.25ns to 0.4ns, the sensitivity of system was overall higher than that of the time resolution of 2.25ns, but the degree of improvement was approximately 1%. Conclusion: The sensitivity of the PET system decreases with the increasing of the magnetic field strength, but the extent is smaller. The RF coil can reduce sensitivity of PET system by a large margin. The reduction of energy threshold value, the optimization of the time resolution and energy resolution can contribute to improve the sensitivity of the system.
[Key words] Positron emission tomography/magnetic resonance (PET/MR); Generic architecture of text engineering (GATE); Mainly magnetic field; Radio frequency coil; Sensitivity

[First-author's address] Department of Medical Engineering, Xuanwu Hospital Capital Medical University, Beijing 100053, China.

正电子发射断层成像(positron emission tomography，PET)与磁共振成像(magnetic resonance imaging，MRI)的双模态融合(PET/MR)，在过去的20年中一直是医学影像的研究热点[1]。MRI高分辨率的解剖信息以及运动信息改善了PET的图像质量[2]。然而，MR磁场及MR元件的存在都可能会对PET的性能产生影响[1,3]。本研究通过利用基于蒙特卡罗仿真工具GATE[4]软件对PET及MR射频线圈进行仿真，

*基金项目：国家重点研发计划(2016YFC1307201)"适宜临床使用的抑郁障碍客观诊断指标体系的构建"；国家重点研发计划数字诊疗装备研发专项课题(2016YFC0103909)"PET/MR在神经系统疾病中的高级临床应用"；
①首都医科大学宣武医院医学工程处 北京 100053
*通信作者：jswei65@163.com
作者简介：崔亚莹，女，(1996-)，硕士研究生，从事医学影像设备图像质量控制研究工作。

医学影像学杂志 2021 年第 31 卷第 8 期　　J Med Imaging Vol. 31 No. 8 2021

Q. Static 运动校正技术对一体化 PET/MR 胸腹部成像质量的影响研究

杨宏伟[1]　崔碧霄[1 2]　宋天彬[1]　宋双双[2 3]　马　杰[1]　马　蕾[1]　卢　洁[1 2 3]

1. 首都医科大学宣武医院核医学科　北京　100053　2. 首都医科大学宣武医院放射科　北京　100053　3. 磁共振成像脑信息学北京市重点实验室　北京　100053

【摘　要】　目的　探讨一体化 PET/MR 的 Q. Static 运动校正技术对胸腹部病灶 PET 成像质量的影响。方法　选取并分析 22 例行一体化 PET/MR 检查肿瘤患者的 Q. Static、Gated 及 Static 模式 PET 图像 比较三种模式下病灶感兴趣区体积 volume of interest VOI 、最大标准摄取值 maximum standardized uptake value SUVmax 、平均标准摄取值 mean standardized uptake value SUVmean 和信噪比 signal-to-noise ratio SNR 的差异。结果　22 例患者共检出 60 个 ^{18}F-FDG 阳性病灶 VOI 均 > 1 cm^3 Q. Static 模式测量病灶 VOI 最小值 较 Static 模式减少 12.91% P < 0.01 Q. Static 模式测量病灶 SNR 较 Gated 模式提高 91.55% P < 0.01 与 Static 模式比较差异无统计学意义 P > 0.05 Q. Static 模式测量病灶 SUVmax 较 Static 模式和 Gated 模式 SUVmax 分别提高 13.43% P < 0.01 和 6.52% P < 0.05 SUVmean 较 Static 模式和 Gated 模式分别提高 13.83% P < 0.01 和 8.47% P < 0.01 。结论　一体化 PET/MR 的 Q. Static 运动校正技术能减少胸腹部呼吸运动伪影 提高胸腹部的 PET 图像质量。

【关键词】　正电子发射型计算机断层显像　磁共振成像　门控　标准化摄取值　图像质量

中图分类号 R445.2 R734　　文献标识码 A　　文章编号 1006-9011 2021 08-1301-05

Effect of Q. Static motion correction mode based on integrated PET / MR on thoracoabdominal imaging

YANG Hongwei[1] CUI Bixiao[1 2] SONG Tianbin[1] SONG Shuangshuang[2 3] MA Jie[1] MA Lei[1] LU Jie[1 2 3]

1. Department of Nuclear Medicine Xuanwu Hospital Capital Medical University Beijing 100053 P. R. China
2. Department of Radiology Xuanwu Hospital Capital Medical University Beijing 100053 P. R. China
3. Beijing Key Laboratory of Magnetic Resonance Imaging and Brain Informatics Beijing 100053 P. R. China

【Abstract】　Objective　To investigate the effect of Q. Static motion correction technology on thoracoabdominal lesions of PET image on integrated PET/MR. Methods　This study was a retrospective analysis of 22 patients on Q. Static Gated and Static PET images of integrated PET/MR examination. Volume of interest VOI maximum standardized uptake value SUVmax mean standardized uptake value SUVmean and signal-to-noise ratio SNR of these lesions were compared. Results　A total of 60 ^{18}F-FDG positive lesions were detected in 22 patients both VOI was greater than 1 cm^3. The minimum VOI of the lesions measured on Q. Static mode was less than that of Static mode P < 0.01 which was 12.91%. The SNR of the lesions measured on Q. Static mode was higher than that of Gated mode P < 0.01 which was 91.55%. There were no statistical differences between Q. Static mode and Static mode P > 0.05. The SUVmax of the lesions measured on Q. Static mode was higher than that of Static and Gated mode P < 0.01 P < 0.05 which was 13.43% and 6.52% respectively. The SUVmean of the lesions measured on Q. Static mode was higher than that of Static and Gated mode P < 0.01 P < 0.01 which was 13.83% and 8.47% respectively. Conclusion　The Q. Static motion correction technology on integrated PET/MR can reduce artifacts caused by respiratory motion and improve the PET image quality.

【Key words】　Positron emission computed tomography Magnetic resonance imaging Gated Standardized uptake value Image quality

　　近几年出现的一体化 PET/MR 将高灵敏度 PET 和高软组织分辨力的 MRI 有机融合 可以同步获得患者功能与结构信息 对疾病诊断具有重要价值[1-3]。一体化 PET/MR 检查可能出现伪影 如 "热气管征" 伪影、呼吸运动伪影等 研究[4] 已经发现飞行时间技术 time of flight TOF 可以消除 "热气管征" 伪影 而呼吸运动伪影导致 PET 图像胸腹部器官和病灶边界显示不清楚、高估病灶体积、与 MR 图

基金项目 北京市医院管理局 "登峰" 计划专项经费资助 编号 DFL20180802

作者简介 杨宏伟 1993- 男 技师 主要从事 PET/MR 技术工作

通信作者 卢洁　E-mail imaginglu@ hotmail.com

1301

DOI:10.12025/j.issn.1008-6358.2020.20201571

·标准与规范·

肝胆系统 PET/MR 成像检查规范专家共识

胡鹏程[1]，赵　军[2]，杨　志[3]，王雪梅[4]，赵长久[5]，高永举[6]，卢　洁[7]，王　峰[8]，莫　逸[9]，樊　卫[10]，杜雪梅[11]，陈曙光[1]，张　政[12]，石洪成[1]*

1. 复旦大学附属中山医院核医学科,上海　200032
2. 同济大学附属东方医院核医学科,上海　200120
3. 北京大学肿瘤医院核医学科,北京　100142
4. 内蒙古医科大学附属医院核医学科,呼和浩特　010050
5. 哈尔滨医科大学附属第一医院核医学科,哈尔滨　150001
6. 河南省人民医院核医学科,郑州　450003
7. 首都医科大学宣武医院核医学科,北京　100053
8. 南京医科大学附属南京医院核医学科,南京　210029
9. 湖南省肿瘤医院核医学科,长沙　410013
10. 中山大学附属肿瘤医院核医学科,广州　510060
11. 大连医科大学附属第一医院核医学科,大连　116011
12. 上海联影医疗科技有限公司,上海　201807

［关键词］　腹部;肝胆系统;正电子发射体层摄影术;磁共振成像;PET/MR;共识
［中图分类号］　R 816.5　　　［文献标志码］　B

Expert consensus on standardization of PET/MR imaging examination of hepatobiliary system

HU Peng-cheng[1], ZHAO Jun[2], YANG Zhi[3], WANG Xue-mei[4], ZHAO Chang-jiu[5], GAO Yong-ju[6], LU Jie[7], WANG Feng[8], MO Yi[9], FAN Wei[10], DU Xue-mei[11], CHEN Shu-guang[1], ZHANG Zheng[12], SHI Hong-cheng[1]*

1. Department of Nuclear Medicine, Zhongshan Hospital, Fudan University, Shanghai 200032, China
2. Department of Nuclear Medicine, Dongfang Hospital Affiliated to Tongji University, Shanghai 200120, China
3. Department of Nuclear Medicine, Peking University Cancer Hospital, Beijing 100142, China
4. Department of Nuclear Medicine, Affiliated Hospital of Inner Mongolia Medical University, Hohhot 010050, Inner Mongolia, China
5. Department of Nuclear Medicine, the First Affiliated Hospital of Harbin Medical University, Harbin 150001, Heilongjiang, China
6. Department of Nuclear Medicine, Henan Provincial People's Hospital, Zhengzhou 450003, Henan, China
7. Department of Nuclear Medicine, Xuan Wu Hospital, Capital Medical University, Beijing 100053, China
8. Department of Nuclear Medicine, Nanjing Hospital Affiliated to Nanjing Medical University, Nanjing 210029, Jiangsu, China
9. Department of Nuclear Medicine, Hunan Cancer Hospital, Changsha 410013, Hunan, China
10. Department of Nuclear Medicine, Sun Yat-sen University Cancer Center, Guangzhou 510060, Guangdong, China
11. Department of Nuclear Medicine, the First Affiliated Hospital of Dalian Medical University, Dalian 116011, Liaoning, China
12. Shanghai United Imaging Medical Technology Co., Ltd, Shanghai 201807, China

［Key Words］　abdomen; hepatobiliary system; positron emission tomography; magnetic resonance imaging;

［收稿日期］　2020-07-13　　　［接受日期］　2020-09-30
［基金项目］　国家重点研发计划"数字诊疗装备研发"重点专项(2016YFC0103900),上海市科学技术委员会"科技创新行动计划"产学研医合作领域项目(19DZ1930700),上海市临床重点专科核医学科项目(shslczdzk03401). Supported by National Key Research and Development Plan "Digital Diagnosis and Treatment Equipment Research And Development" Key Specialty (2016YFC0103900), Shanghai Science and Technology Commission "Science and Technology Innovation Action Plan" in the Field of Cooperation of Industry, Education, Research, Medicine (19DZ1930700), and Programme of Shanghai Municipal Key Clinical Specialty(shslczdzk03401).
［作者简介］　胡鹏程,博士,主治医师. E-mail: hpc0210@126.com
* 通信作者(Corresponding author). Tel: 021-64041990, E-mail: shi.hongcheng@zs-hospital.sh.cn

第一章　一体化 PET/MR 科研成果

DOI：10.12025/j. issn. 1008-6358. 2020. 20201589

· 标准与规范 ·

PET/MR 全身显像工作流及协议规划专家共识

陈曙光[1]，胡鹏程[1]，樊　卫[2]，莫　逸[3]，王　峰[4]，卢　洁[5]，高永举[6]，杨　志[7]，赵　军[8]，杜雪梅[9]，张　政[10]，
石洪成[1]*

1. 复旦大学附属中山医院核医学科，上海　200032
2. 中山大学附属肿瘤医院核医学科，广州　510060
3. 湖南省肿瘤医院核医学科，长沙　410013
4. 南京市第一医院核医学科，南京　210029
5. 首都医科大学宣武医院核医学科，北京　100053
6. 河南省人民医院核医学科，郑州　450003
7. 北京大学肿瘤医院核医学科，北京　100142
8. 同济大学附属东方医院核医学科，上海　200120
9. 大连医科大学附属第一医院核医学科，大连　116011
10. 上海联影医疗科技有限公司，上海　201807

　　[摘要]　正电子发射计算机断层成像/核磁共振（PET/MR）作为一款创新型医疗设备，其价值尚未得到临床广泛认可。设备使用方法、图像的扫描重建、图像后处理技术等依赖生产厂家提供的软硬件平台，因而近年 PET/MR 进入临床常规检查面临不少挑战。2018 年起，国内十多家医疗机构陆续安装了联影一体化 PET/MR 设备，各主要装机医院和联影研发人员进行了深度交流与合作。针对设备特点，就 PET/MR 临床检查规范、全身扫描床位规划、全身扫描协议组规划、时空一体扫描和图像质量控制等达成共识，为后续 PET/MR 临床工作开展提供建议和参考。

　　[关键词]　操作规范；显像协议；正电子发射体层摄影术；磁共振成像；PET/MR；共识
　　[中图分类号]　R 445.2　　　[文献标志码]　B

Expert consensus on PET/MR whole body imaging workflow and protocol planning

CHEN Shu-guang[1]，HU Peng-cheng[1]，FAN Wei[2]，MO Yi[3]，WANG Feng[4]，LU Jie[5]，GAO Yong-ju[6]，YANG Zhi[7]，
ZHAO Jun[8]，DU Xue-mei[9]，ZHANG Zheng[10]，SHI Hong-cheng[1]*

1. Department of Nuclear Medicine, Zhongshan Hospital, Fudan University, Shanghai 200032, China
2. Department of Nuclear Medicine, Sun Yat-Sen University Cancer Center, Guangzhou 510060, Guangdong, China
3. Department of Nuclear Medicine, Hunan Cancer Hospital, Changshan 410013, Hunan China
4. Department of Nuclear Medicine, Nanjing First Hospital, Nanjing 210029, Jiangsu, China
5. Department of Nuclear Medicine, Xuan Wu Hospital, Capital Medical University, Beijing 100053, China
6. Department of Nuclear Medicine, Henan Provincial People's Hospital, Zhengzhou, 450003, Henan China
7. Department of Nuclear Medicine, Beijing Cancer Hospital, Beijing 100142, China
8. Department of Nuclear Medicine, Shanghai East Hospital, Tongji University School of Medicine, Shanghai 200120, China
9. Department of Nuclear Medicine, the First Affiliated Hospital of Dalian Medical University, Dalian 116011, LiaoningChina
10. Shanghai United Imaging Medical Technology Co. , Ltd, Shanghai 201807, China

　　[Abstract]　PET/MR faces many challenges in entering clinical routine examination. As an innovative medical device,

[收稿日期]　2020-07-15　　　　[接受日期]　2020-08-25
[基金项目]　国家重点研发计划"数字诊疗装备研发"重点专项（2016YFC0103900），上海市科学技术委员会"科技创新行动计划"产学研医合作领域项目（19DZ1930700），上海市临床重点专科核医学科（shslczdzk03401）. Supported by National Key Research and Development Plan "digital diagnosis and treatment equipment research and development" Key Specialty（2016YFC0103900），Shanghai Science and Technology Commission "Science and Technology Innovation Action Plan" in the field of cooperation in the field of industry, education and research （19DZ1930700），Shanghai Municipal Key Clinical Specialty（shslczdzk03401）.
[作者简介]　陈曙光，硕士，主管技师. E-mail：tc99m@sina.com
* 通信作者（Corresponding author）. Tel：021-64041990，E-mail：shi. hongcheng@zs-hospital. sh. cn

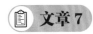
2020 年 10 月
第 41 卷 第 5 期

首都医科大学学报
Journal of Capital Medical University

Oct. 2020
Vol. 41 No. 5

[doi: 10.3969/j. issn. 1006-7795. 2020. 05. 013]

· 国家优秀青年科学基金获得者 ·

缺血性脑卒中的脑功能与分子成像研究
——卢洁教授

单 艺 李 静 许潇尹

(首都医科大学宣武医院放射科,北京 100053)

【摘要】 卢洁教授是国家"万人计划"科技创新领军人才、国家优秀青年基金获得者,长期围绕"缺血性脑卒中"这一国际前沿重大医学研究领域,运用新型一体化正电子发射型计算机断层摄影(positron emission computer tomography, PET)/磁共振成像(magnetic resonance imaging,MRI)融合脑功能与分子成像技术,引领国内本领域的发展。

【关键词】 脑功能成像;分子成像;缺血性脑卒中

【中图分类号】 R445

Functional and molecular imaging of ischemic stroke
——Professor Lu Jie

Shan Yi, Li Jing, Xu Xiaoyin

(Department of Radiology, Xuanwu Hospital, Capital Medical University, Beijing 100053, China)

【Abstract】 Professor Lu Jie is the member of the National High-level Talents Program. She was supported by the National Science Fund for Outstanding Young Scholars. She has been focusing on the major problem of ischemic stroke and advancing the development of imaging in ischemic stroke by applying the new integrated positron emission computer tomography(PET)/magnetic resonance imaging(MRI) on brain function and molecular imaging.

【Key words】 functional imaging; molecular imaging; ischemic stroke

1 个人简介

卢洁教授(图1),1975 年 11 月 24 日出生于中国北京,首都医科大学宣武医院副院长、放射科主任、核医学科副主任、党支部支委。自 2004 年在首都医科大学获得医学博士学位后,于首都医科大学宣武医院放射科工作至今,期间围绕"缺血性脑卒中"这一国际前沿重大医学研究领域,开展从基础到临床的全链条脑功能与分子影像研究,分别于 2011、2013、2016 年晋升主任医师、教授、博士生导师,于 2016 年度获批国家优秀青年科学基金项目,2019 年获国家"万人计划"科技创新领军人才称号、中华医学会放射学分会杰出青年奖等。

卢洁教授作为首都医科大学宣武医院影像科的学术带头人,依托国家老年疾病临床医学研究中心、教育部神经变性病重点实验室、磁共振成像脑信息学北京市重点实验室,与所带领团队针对缺血性脑卒中发病不同阶段临床诊疗存在的重大问题,突破脑功能

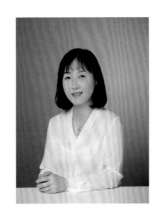

图 1 卢洁教授

成像技术个体化应用的技术瓶颈,在国内率先运用新型一体化正电子发射型计算机断层摄影(positron emission computer tomography, PET)/磁共振成像(magnetic resonance imaging,MRI)融合脑功能与分子成像技术,研究成果对患者的早期诊断、个体化诊疗

第一章 一体化 PET/MR 科研成果

医学影像学杂志 2020 年第 30 卷第 9 期　J Med Imaging Vol. 30 No.9 2020

4　余小情　丛阳　唐蕾 等. 术前超声漏诊甲状腺癌颈部淋巴结转移的原因分析 J . 中国超声医学杂志 2017 2 101-103.

5　黄芸谦　陶玲玲　樊金芳 等. 甲状腺结节的常规超声和弹性成像联合诊断方法研究 J . 中国医学计算机成像杂志 2017 23 1 86-90.

6　樊金芳　陶玲玲　王怡 等. 可疑甲状腺结节超声造影和细针穿刺的临床价值探讨 J . 中国医学计算机成像杂志 2017 23 2 179-184.

7　张桦. 超声弹性成像与造影联合应用诊断甲状腺结节的临床价值 J . 医学影像学杂志 2017 27 6 1060-1062.

8　张斌　余秀华　施红 等. 常规超声、超声造影及弹性成像在甲状腺结节良恶性鉴别中的价值 J . 医学影像学杂志 2018 28 6 913-916.

9　Moon HJ　Kim EK　Yoon JH　et al. Clinical implication of elas-tography as a prognostic factor of papillary thyroid microcarcinoma J . Ann surg Oncol 2012 19 7 2279-2287.

10　李美　宁春平　房世保. 弹性成像技术对甲状腺癌颈部淋巴

结转移诊断价值 J . 齐鲁医学杂志 2016 2 165-167.

11　Deng J　Zhou P　Tian SM　et al. Comparison of diagnostic effi-cacy of contrast-enhanced ultrasound acoustic radiation force im-pulse imaging and their combined use in differentiating focal sol-id thyroid nodules J . PLoS One 2014 9 3 90674-90680.

12　陶玲玲　黄芸谦　樊金芳 等. 不同医师对甲状腺结节超声造影定量分析的诊断价值 J . 临床超声医学杂志 2016 18 12 826-829.

13　陶玲玲　吴敏　陆采蔚 等. Bcl-2 与甲状腺乳头状癌超声造影模式的相关性研究 J . 中国医学计算机成像杂志 2016 22 6 564-568.

14　樊秋兰　陈薇　于春洋 等. 普通超声及超声造影预测甲状腺微小乳头状癌中央区淋巴结转移的价值 J . 中国超声医学杂志 2016 32 12 1060-1062.

15　Hu Y　Ping L　Jiang S　et al. Quantitative analysis of suspicious thyroid nodules by contrast—enhanced ultrasonography J . Int J Clin Exp Med 2015 8 7 11786-11793.

收稿日期 2019-08-22

间变性多形性黄色星形细胞瘤 1 例

Anaplastic pleomorphic xanthoastrocytoma one case report

宋双双[1][2]　齐志刚[1][2]　王雷明[3]　卢　洁[1][2][4]

1. 首都医科大学宣武医院放射科　北京　100053 2. 磁共振成像脑信息学北京市重点实验室　北京　100053 3. 首都医科大学宣武医院病理科　北京　100053 4. 首都医科大学宣武医院核医学科　北京　100053

基金项目 北京市医院管理局"登峰"人才培养计划专项经费资助 编号 DFL20180802

通信作者 卢洁 主任医师 教授 E-mail imaginglu@ hotmail.com

【关键词】 间变性多形性黄色星形细胞瘤 磁共振成像 影像诊断

中图分类号 R739.41 R445　　　文献标识码 B　　　文章编号 1006-9011 2020 09-1586-02

患者　女 21 岁。左侧肢体活动不利半年 于 2019 年 1 月 3 日入院。半年前洗澡时突发一过性左上肢麻木、无力 表现为抬举困难 左手指屈曲状态、伸开困难 4 个月前感左下肢活动后疼痛 3 个月前学校体能训练跳远后不能并腿 下楼时左下肢不稳感 就诊于我院治疗。

术前于一体化[18]F-FET PET/MR GE SIGNA 行颅脑多模态影像检查。MRI 平扫示右侧额叶-基底节区团块状长 T_1 图 1 稍长 T_2 信号影 图 2 病灶左侧见点状 T_1 高信号 FLAIR 为稍高信号 图 3 DWI 为高信号 图 4 其内信号较均匀 周围见指状长 T_1 长 T_2 信号影 MRI 增强扫描病变明显强化不均匀强化 图 5 较大病变下方见小结节样强化信号 边界清楚。[18]F-FET-PET/MR 增强融合图显示病变区域[18]F-FET 摄取明显增高 图 6 7 SUVmax 为 3.35 SUVmean 为 2.10 肿瘤靶本比 tumor-to-brain ratio TBR 最大值为 4.19 TBRmean 为 2.63。术前诊断 右额叶深部占位性病变 考虑

淋巴瘤或胶质瘤。行手术切除术后病理 间变性多形性黄色星形细胞瘤 镜下 HE×400 见肿瘤细胞弥漫性浸润性生长 部分细胞胞浆丰富、红染 部分胞浆泡沫状 可见双核 具有异型性 部分细胞呈梭形 可见小灶坏死及血管内皮增生 局部伴钙化 血管周围淋巴袖套形成 图 8 免疫组化及特殊染色示 GFAP + Olig-2 + Ki-67 约 30% + IDH-1R132H - p53 个别 + ATRX 部分 + H3K27M - MGMT + EGFR 灶 + EGFRv Ⅲ - Vimentin + CD68 + CD34 血管 + 网织纤维 局部 + 。

讨论 多形性黄色星形细胞瘤好发于儿童和青年人 在所有神经胶质肿瘤中比例不足 1% 是发生于中枢神经系统星形细胞源性的罕见特殊类型胶质瘤 约 15% ~ 20% 的多形性黄色星形细胞瘤表现出间变特征[1] 2016 版 WHO 中枢神经系统胶质源性肿瘤针对其分类做出明显改变 将"间变型

下转 1591 页

· 596 ·
中国医学影像技术 2020 年第 36 卷第 4 期　Chin J Med Imaging Technol,2020,Vol 36,No 4

❖影像技术学

Selection of integrated PET/MR image reconstruction scheme for small lesions

TIAN Defeng[1,2], *YANG Hongwei*[3], *ZHUANG Jingwen*[4], *YAN Hanmin*[4], *LU Jie*[1,2,3]*
*(1. Department of Radiology, 3. Department of Nuclear Medicine, 4. Department of
Biomedical Engineering, Xuanwu Hospital, Capital Medical University,
Beijing 100053, China; 2. Beijing Key Laboratory of Magnetic
Resonance Imaging and Brain Informatics, Beijing 100053, China)*

[Abstract]　Objective　To explore the impacts of different reconstruction combinations on image quality of different sized lesions, so as to propose the optimal reconstruction scheme for smaller lesions on integrated PET/MR. Methods　SIGNA TOF PET/MR system was used for scanning of PET image quality (IQ) emission phantom designed taken standards of the International Electrotechnical Commission (IEC) recommendations. Then the list mode raw data of PET were reconstructed using time of flight(TOF)－ordered subsets expectation maximization(OSEM) under different conditions, including the maximum expected value of the ordered subset (the iterative subset: 28, the number of iterations: 1—9 times), the reconstruction matrix (128×128, 192×192, 256×256), Gaussian low-pass filter full width at half maximum (FWHM) (1—6 mm), time-of-flight (TOF) technology alone (TOF＋NOTOF), separate point spread function (PSF) (PSF＋NOPSF), both TOF and PSF (TOF＋PSF), as well as neither TOF nor PSF (NOTOF＋NOPSF). Imaging quality was assessed under different reconstruction conditions using parameters including contrast recovery (CR), background variability (BV) and signal-to-noise ratio (SNR). Results　Balls with 10 and 13 mm diameters simulating small lesions in the OSEM (3 iterations, 28 subsets), 192×192 matrix, 2 mm Gaussian low-pass filter full width at half maximum and TOF＋PSF reconstruction combination achieved the highest SNR, which was 13.31% and 21.73%, 13.31% and 21.73%, 25.74% and 35.8% as well as 26.25% and 46.01%, respectively. Conclusion　Using reconstruction combination as 3 iterations, 28 subsets, 192×192 matrix and TOF＋PSF, the best image quality of small lesions can be obtained under the above mentioned conditions.
[Keywords]　positron-emission tomography; magnetic resonance imaging; reconstruction condition; image quality
DOI:10.13929/j.issn.1003-3289.2020.04.029

选择一体化 PET/MR 小病灶图像重建方案

田德峰[1,2]，杨宏伟[3]，庄静文[4]，严汉民[4]，卢　洁[1,2,3]*
(1.首都医科大学宣武医院放射科,3.核医学科,4.医学工程科,北京　100053,
2.磁共振成像脑信息学北京市重点实验室,北京　100053)

[摘　要]　目的　观察不同重建条件组合对不同大小病灶图像质量的影响,提出一体化 PET/MR 对于小病灶的最佳图像重建方案。方法　采用 GE SIGNA TOF PET/MR 系统对符合国际电工协会(IEC)推荐标准的 PET 图像质量(IQ)发射体模进行扫描,并对列表模式 PET 原始数据按照以下条件分别组合进行重建:有序子集最大期望值(迭代子集:28;选

[基金项目]　北京市医院管理局"登峰"计划专项经费资助(DFL20180802)、国家重点研发项目(2016YFC0103909)。
[第一作者]　田德峰(1989—),男,山东济南人,硕士,技师。研究方向:医学影像设备图像质量控制。E-mail:18660984603@163.com
[通信作者]　卢洁,首都医科大学宣武医院放射科,核医学科,100053;磁共振成像脑信息学北京市重点实验室,100053。
　　E-mail:imaginglu@hotmail.com
[收稿日期]　2019-04-19　　[修回日期]　2019-10-19

化,慢性期血肿包膜可呈环形强化。

　　总之,多期增强 CT 对鉴别肾上腺节细胞神经瘤与皮质腺瘤具有重要意义,肿瘤形态呈卵圆形或水滴状、平扫呈等密度影及动脉期 CT 值增加小于15.3HU 是肾上腺节细胞神经瘤的 CT 影像特征。部分皮质腺瘤平扫为等密度,动脉期及静脉期轻度强化,与节细胞神经瘤鉴别较困难。

参考文献:

[1] Rondeau G, Nolet S, Latour M, et al. Clinical and biochemical features of seven adult adrenal ganglioneuromas [J]. Clin Endo-erinol Metab, 2010, 97(7): 3118-3125.

[2] Morelli V, Reimondo G, Giordano R, et al. Long-term follow-up in adrenal incidentalomas: an Italian multicenter study [J]. J Clin Endocrinol Metab, 2014, 99(3): 827-834.

[3] 范谋海,王永军,熊艾平,等.肾上腺节细胞神经瘤的 CT 、MRI 表现及病理对照[J].放射学实践,2014,29(1):85-87.

[4] 赵平山,沈训泽,赵峰.肾上腺节细胞神经瘤 CT 表现与病理对照[J].医学影像学杂志,2015,25(5):853-856.

[5] 周建军,曾维新,周康荣,等.肾上腺节细胞神经瘤的 CT 诊断价值[J].中华放射学杂志,2002,40(10):1021-1023.

[6] 杨国美,孙骏,胡晓华,等.肾上腺节细胞神经瘤的 CT 诊断[J].医学影像学杂志,2015,25(2):293-295.

[7] 王洁,陈宏伟,方向明.肾上腺节细胞神经瘤的 CT 表现[J].临床放射学杂志,2014,33(4):544-547.

[8] 聂思,李海军,聂晓,等.肾上腺节细胞神经瘤与腺瘤的 CT 鉴别诊断[J].实用放射学杂志,2016,32(4):642-644.

[9] 郭应坤,杨志刚,张梅,等.肾上腺皮质小腺瘤的 CT 表现与临床及病理的关系[J].中国医学影像学杂志,2004,12(4):259-261.

[10] 姜蕾,陈敏,周意明,等.肾上腺肿瘤的平扫 CT 值与磁共振化学移位成像反相位信号丢失程度相关性的研究[J].中国医学影像技术,2007,23(3):417-420.

(收稿日期:2019-05-22)

规范化护理在脑肿瘤患者一体化[18]F-FET PET/MR 检查中的应用

Application of standardized nursing in hybrid ^{18}F-FET PET/MR examination of brain tumor patients

马　蕾[1],帅冬梅[1],宋双双[2,3],卢　洁[1,2,3]

首都医科大学宣武医院 1.核医学科;2.放射科　北京　100053;3.磁共振成像脑信息学北京市重点实验室　北京　100053

【摘　要】　目的　探讨规范化护理操作在脑肿瘤患者行一体化 FET-PET/MR 检查中的临床应用价值。方法　对就诊于首都医科大学宣武医院行一体化 FET-PET/MR 检查的 98 例患者在检查前、检查中和检查后进行规范护操作,总结其在PET/MR 检查中的经验。结果　90 例患者静态或动态[18]F-FET PET 检查顺利完成,8 例患者头动控制不佳。67 例行 MRI 增强检查的患者中,62 例顺利完成检查,5 例患者增强检查失败难以达到诊断目的。结论　规范化护理操作在提高脑肿瘤患者 FET-PET/MR 检查成功率、保证图像质量中具有重要作用。

【关键词】　PET/MR;脑肿瘤;护理

中图分类号:R815;R472.9　　文献标识码:A　　文章编号:1006-9011(2020)07-1322-03

　　随着医学影像检查技术的飞速发展,越来越多的医院引入了国际高端设备—一体化 PET/MR,其主要优势是可同步行 MRI 和 PET 多模态影像信息采集,获得可反映病变结构、血流、功能和代谢等全面信息,简化扫描流程,为临床工作和科研探索的开展提供更方便、精确的技术条件[1-3]。[18]F-FET 示踪剂在正常脑组织中呈低摄取,在脑肿瘤组织中不同程度摄取增高,与本底之间形成了较高的对比度,相较于常规示踪剂[18]F-FDG 在脑肿瘤的术前诊断、分级及分期、鉴别诊断、疗效及预后评估等方面具有显著优势[4-5]。我院作为最早应用一体化 PET/MR 的单位之一,自 2015 年至今在脑肿瘤患者检查前和检查中的护理工作中积累了丰富的经验,对提高脑肿瘤检查成功率、图像质量及患者舒适度有重要价值,现将规范化护理体会报告如下。

1　资料与方法

1.1　一般资料

　　回顾性分析 2018 年 12 月~2019 年 10 月于我院行一体化[18]F-FET PET/MR 检查的脑肿瘤患者 98 例,其中男性 64 例,女性 34 例,年龄 4~76 岁,平均年龄(48.5±13.5)岁。包括脑胶质瘤 80 例,脑转移瘤 8 例,淋巴瘤 7 例,脑膜瘤 2 例,松果体区未成

　　基金项目:国家科技部重点研发计划项目(编号:2016YFC0103000)
　　作者简介:马蕾(1975-),女,北京人,大专学历,初级护师,主要从事核医学护理研究工作
　　通信作者:卢洁　主任医师　E-mail: imaginglu@hotmail.com

医学影像学杂志2020年第30卷第12期　J Med Imaging Vol.30 No.12 2020

spective cohort study J . Medicine Baltimore 2017 96 10 1-7.

28 Saidha NK Aggarwal R Sen A. Identification of sentinel lymph nodes using contrast-enhanced ultrasound in breast cancer J . Indian J Surg Oncol 2018 9 3 355-361.

29 Wang Z Zhou Q Liu J et al. Tumor size of breast invasive ductal cancer measured with contrast-enhanced ultrasound predicts regional lymph node metastasis and N stage J . Int J Clin Exp Pathol 2014 7 10 6985-6991.

30 Wang XY Hu Q Fang MY et al. The correlation between HER-2 expression and the CEUS and ARFI characteristics of breast cancer J . PLoS One 2017 12 6 1786-1789.

31 Liu H Jiang Y Dai Q et al. Peripheral enhancement of breast cancers on contrast-enhanced ultrasound correlation with microvessel density and vascular endothelial growth factor expression J . Ultrasound Med Biol 2014 40 2 293-299.

收稿日期 2020-03-20

韧带样纤维瘤病[18]F-FDG PET/MR误诊为输尿管癌1例
Desmoid-type fibromatoses misdiagnosed as ureteral carcinoma with ^{18}F-FDG PET / MR one case report

郭　坤[1]　李云波[4]　卢　洁[1 2 3]

1.首都医科大学宣武医院核医学科　北京　100053 2.首都医科大学宣武医院放射科　北京　100053 3.磁共振成像脑信息学北京市重点实验室　北京　100053 4.空军军医大学第二附属医院核医学科　陕西　西安　710045

基金项目 北京市医院管理局"登峰"计划专项经费资助 编号 DFL20180802
通信作者 卢洁 主任医师 教授 博士生导师 E-mail imaginglu@hotmail.com

【关键词】 韧带样纤维瘤病 [18]氧脂氧葡萄糖 正电子发射计算机断层显像 磁共振成像
中图分类号 R737 R445　　文献标识码 B　　文章编号 1006-9011 2020 12-2312-02

患者　女 24 岁。因"发现左肾积水、左侧盆腔包块半年余"行 PET/MR 检查。半年前外院给予体外碎石术后疼痛略有好转 1 月前外院 MRI 检查示 盆腔左侧混杂信号肿块并左侧输尿管盆段扩张 考虑肿瘤性病变 不除外"子宫内膜异位症"给予药物规范治疗后效果不佳。为明确诊断收入我院泌尿外科。体格检查 T 36.3 ℃ 双侧脊肋角无压痛 双肾区叩击痛阴性 沿双侧输尿管走行区无压痛。左侧骶韧带区扪及 3 cm×3 cm 质硬包块 压痛阳性。实验室检查未见明显异常。超声提示 子宫略小 图像未见异常。双侧附件区未见明显异常。左肾积水伴左侧输尿管全程扩张 下段图像考虑实性占位性病变。[18]F-FDG PET/MR 西门子 Biography 德国 显像示 左肾盂、肾盏扩张 左侧输尿管下段团块状异常信号影 大小约 3.7 cm×3.7 cm 边界欠清晰 呈长 T_1、STIR 稍长信号 DWI 呈不均匀高信号 内见流空血管影 葡萄糖代谢轻度增高 SUVmax 2.0 与子宫阔韧带关系密切 病变近端输尿管扩张、迂曲 多考虑恶性病变 输尿管移行上皮癌可能性大 图 1 。遂行左侧盆腔肿瘤切除术 术中膀胱左外侧见一约 4 cm×4 cm 包块 与周围组织呈纤维索带粘连 血供丰富。术中冰冻报 间叶性肿瘤 无法区分良恶性 故排除原发性输尿管上皮癌。继续行左侧输尿管膀胱再植术。术后病理回报 间叶组织肿瘤 结合组织学特点及免疫学表型特征倾向韧带样纤维瘤病 desmoid-type fibromatoses DTF 部分细胞增生活跃并在周围组织中呈侵袭性生长 图 2 。

2312

讨论 DTF 是一种来源于纤维组织的罕见肿瘤 占纤维组织肿瘤的 1.19%[1] 病因不清 可能和创伤、内分泌及结缔组织生长调节缺陷等因素相关。肿瘤好发于腹前壁、腹直肌及其肌腱上 亦可发生于腹壁以外横纹肌处 最常见于妊娠及产后妇女 20～40 岁多见。一般无自觉症状 如压迫邻近神经可产生疼痛或麻木感。虽可局部呈侵袭性生长 累及周围组织或器官 极易复发 但不发生转移。

DTF 影像学报道相对较少 以往的研究主要集中在其临床和病理特征上。超声是 DTF 的重要影像学检查方法 声像图示深部肌层梭形、较均匀弱回声病灶 与肌束平行扫查时肿块边界不清 垂直时相对较清楚 血供不丰富 呈少许点线状。需要与结节性筋膜炎、肌内型血管瘤以及子宫内膜异位症等进行鉴别诊断。DTF 的 CT、MRI 影像学表现有一定的特征性 CT 平扫密度等或稍低于肌肉 多较均匀 MRI T_1WI 均呈等或稍低于肌肉信号 信号较均匀 T_2WI 呈不均匀稍高或较高信号 强化扫描以中等以上渐进性强化为主 强化可均匀或不均匀。Oka 等[2]认为扩散加权成像有助于鉴别纤维瘤病与其他恶性软组织肿瘤。解剖学的影像学技术有助于术前诊断 并显示病变的范围及周围结构受累情况。在 FDG PET 显像上 即使体积较大的 DTF 肿块也通常表现为中度过度代谢 而较小的肿瘤倾向于表现为低代谢 FDG PET 可用于评价肿瘤复发[3-5]。目前国内外尚无[18]F-FDG PET/MR 相关报道。

下转 2316 页

第 43 卷 第 5 期
2020 年 5 月

核 技 术
NUCLEAR TECHNIQUES

Vol.43，No.5
May 2020

PET-MRI脑部定量准确性对比研究：
MRI与PET脑分区对SUVR计算的影响

李再升[1,2,3]　宋双双[5,6]　曾天翼[1,3]　卢洁[5,6,7]　胡凌志[4]　陈群[2,4]

1（中国科学院上海高等研究院　上海 201210）

2（上海科技大学 信息科学与技术学院　上海 201210）

3（中国科学院大学　北京 100049）

4（上海联影医疗科技有限公司　上海 201807）

5（首都医科大学宣武医院放射科　北京 100053）

6（磁共振成像脑信息学北京市重点实验室　北京 100053）

7（首都医科大学宣武医院核医学科　北京 100053）

摘要　在正电子发射断层成像（Positron Emission Tomography，PET）的临床诊断和科研中，为了减小标准化摄取值（Standard Uptake Value，SUV）在不同受试者间的差异性，通常会以特定的参考区域为基准计算标准化摄取值比（Standard Uptake Value Ratio，SUVR）。由于PET图像无法反应脑部结构信息，从PET图像中无法准确分割出参考区域，从而影响了SUVR的准确性。本文利用一体化正电子发射断层成像/磁共振成像（Positron Emission Tomography-Magnetic Resonance Imaging，PET-MRI）同步采集年龄相近的健康志愿者的PET和MRI数据，基于准确反映脑部结构信息的MRI图像分割出参考区域，映射到对应的PET图像后再进行SUVR的计算，将其与利用PET图像分割参考区域算出的SUVR进行比较。结果显示：利用MRI分割参考区域算出的SUVR变异系数更小，离散程度更低，在相似的健康志愿者间具有更好的一致性，更好地消除了受试者间的个体差异。

关键词　标准化摄取值比，定量，正电子发射断层成像-磁共振成像，氟代脱氧葡萄糖

中图分类号　R445，TL99

DOI: 10.11889/j.0253-3219.2020.hjs.43.050301

A comparative study of PET-MRI brain quantitative accuracy: the effect of MRI based segmentation and PET based segmentation on SUVR calculation

LI Zaisheng[1,2,3]　SONG Shuangshuang[5,6]　ZENG Tianyi[1,3]　LU Jie[5,6,7]　HU Lingzhi[4]　CHEN Qun[2,4]

1(Shanghai Advanced Research Institute, Chinese Academy of Sciences, Shanghai 201210, China)

2(School of Information Science and Technology, ShanghaiTech University, Shanghai 201210, China)

3(University of Chinese Academy of Sciences, Beijing 100049, China)

4(Shanghai United Imaging Healthcare Co., Ltd., Shanghai 201807, China)

5(Department of Radiology, Xuanwu Hospital, Capital Medical University, Beijing 100053, China)

6(Beijing Key Laboratory of Magnetic Resonance Imaging and Brain Informatics, Beijing 100053, China)

7(Department of Nuclear Medicine, Xuanwu Hospital, Capital Medical University, Beijing 100053, China)

国家重点研发计划"数字诊疗装备研发"试点专项(No.2016YFC0103900)资助

第一作者：李再升，男，1994年出生，2016年毕业于南京航空航天大学，现为硕士研究生，研究领域为医学影像处理

通信作者：陈群，E-mail: qun.chen@united-imaging.com

收稿日期：2020-02-06，修回日期：2020-03-04

Supported by National Key Research and Development Program Digital Diagnostic Equipment R&D Pilot (No.2016YFC0103900)

First author: LI Zaisheng, male, born in 1994, graduated from Nanjing University of Aeronautics and Astronautics in 2016, master student, focusing on medical imaging processing

Corresponding author: CHEN Qun, E-mail: qun.chen@united-imaging.com

Received date: 2020-02-06, revised date: 2020-03-04

中国医学影像技术 2019 年第 35 卷第 12 期　Chin J Med Imaging Technol,2019,Vol 35,No 12　　　　　　　　　　　　·1817·

❖中枢神经影像学

Hybrid 18F-FDG PET/MR evaluation of ischemic cerebrovascular disease

CUI Bixiao[1], ZHANG Miao[2], MA Jie[1], YANG Hongwei[1], MA Yan[3],
JIAO Liqun[3], ZHAO Guoguang[3], LU Jie[1,2,4]*

(1. Department of Nuclear Medicine, 2. Department of Radiology, 3. Department of Neurosurgery,
Xuanwu Hospital, Capital Medical University, Beijing 100053, China; 4. Beijing Key
Laboratory of Magnetic Resonance Imaging and Brain Informatics,
Beijing 100053, China)

[Abstract]　Objective　To investigate the value of hybrid 18F-FDG PET/MR in patients with ischemic cerebrovascular disease. Methods　A total of 10 healthy volunteers and 17 patients with chronic unilateral internal carotid artery (ICA) or middle cerebral artery (MCA) occlusion underwent hybrid 18F-FDG PET/MR examination. The images were analyzed by two experienced physicians. The mean ADC value (ADC_{mean}), mean standardized uptake value (SUV_{mean}) and the maximum standardized uptake value (SUV_{max}) were analyzed between left and right brain regions of healthy volunteers. ADC_{mean}, SUV_{mean} and SUV_{max} of corresponding areas of the cerebral infarction and contralateral corresponding areas, the surrounding areas of the cerebral infarction and contralateral side of patients were also compared. Results　MRI of 10 healthy volunteers showed no abnormal performance. 18F-FDG images were clear and the metabolic distribution of each brain region was symmetrical. ADC_{mean}, SUV_{mean}, SUV_{max} were not statistically different between the left and right brain regions (all $P>0.05$). The cerebral infarctions were observed in MRI of 17 patients, and ADC_{mean}, SUV_{mean} and SUV_{max} significantly reduced on the affected side (all $P<0.01$), while ADC_{mean}, SUV_{mean} and SUV_{max} also significantly reduced in the surrounding areas of the cerebral infarction (all $P<0.01$). Conclusion　Hybrid 18F-FDG PET/MR examination can evaluate patients with chronic ischemic cerebrovascular disease and provide information of brain structure and brain metabolism.

[Keywords]　brain ischemia; cerebrovascular circulation; radionuclide imaging; fluorodeoxyglucose F 18; magnetic resonance imaging

DOI:10.13929/j.1003-3289.201905104

一体化18F-FDG PET/MR 评估缺血性脑血管病

崔碧霄[1],张　苗[2],马　杰[1],杨宏伟[1],马　妍[3],
焦力群[3],赵国光[3],卢　洁[1,2,4]*

(1.首都医科大学宣武医院核医学科,2.放射科,3.神经外科,北京　100053;
4.磁共振成像脑信息学北京市重点实验室,北京　100053)

[摘　要]　目的　探讨一体化18F-FDG PET/MR 显像对于慢性缺血性脑血管病的应用价值。方法　对 10 名成年健康志愿者及 17 例慢性单侧颈内动脉(ICA)或大脑中动脉(MCA)闭塞患者行一体化18F-FDG PET/MR 检查。由 2 名医师分析

[基金项目]　国家自然科学基金面上项目(81671662)、北京市医院管理局"登峰"计划专项经费(DFL20180802)。
[第一作者]　崔碧霄(1989—),男,内蒙古包头人,在读博士。研究方向:脑功能与分子影像学。E-mail:bixiao1311@163.com
[通信作者]　卢洁,首都医科大学宣武医院核医学科,放射科,100053;磁共振成像脑信息学北京市重点实验室,100053。
E-mail:imaginglu@hotmail.com
[收稿日期] 2019-05-13　　[修回日期] 2019-07-21

第一章　一体化 PET/MR 科研成果

首都医科大学宣武医院一体化 PET/MR 成果集

·综　述·

MRI、^{18}F-FDG PET 以及 PET/MRI 在难治性癫痫术前精准定位中的价值

郭坤[1]，卢洁[1, 2, 3]

1. 首都医科大学宣武医院 核医学科（北京 100053）
2. 首都医科大学宣武医院 放射科（北京 100053）
3. 磁共振成像脑信息学北京市重点实验室（北京 100053）

【摘要】　癫痫是多种病因引起的慢性脑部疾病，以脑部神经元过度放电所导致的突然、反复和短暂的中枢神经系统失常为特征，并伴有相应的认知、神经生物学以及心理学方面的障碍。对于药物难治性局灶性癫痫患者而言，手术治疗是控制发作最有效的方法。一体化正电子发射计算机断层显像（Positron emission tomography, PET）/核磁共振成像（MRI）在进行 MRI 的同时实现 PET 显像的所有功能，达到真正意义的同步扫描，结构影像和功能影像的有机结合成为可能。神经影像学的发展尤其是一体化 PET/MR 的问世增加了精准定位切除病灶的可能性。本文主要对目前最先进的分子影像学检查技术一体化 PET/MRI 在难治性癫痫术前精准定位中的价值作一综述，以期为相关疾病的临床诊疗提供建议。

【关键词】　难治性癫痫；正电子发射计算机断层显像；核磁共振；一体化

癫痫（Epilepsy）是多种病因引起的慢性脑部疾病，以脑部神经元过度放电所导致的突然、反复和短暂的中枢神经系统失常为特征，并伴有相应的认知、神经生物学以及心理学方面的障碍。在我国约有 900 万癫痫患者，患病率约为 0.9 ~ 4.8‰[1]。大部分患者通过药物治疗能控制发作，但仍有 25 ~ 30% 的患者对药物治疗效果不佳，称为难治性癫痫[2]。而对于药物难治性局灶性癫痫患者而言，手术治疗是控制发作最有效的方法，且术后患者的认知能力、行为学能力和生命质量可显著改善，尤其在儿童患者中更是如此。但外科手术治疗的疗效取决于患者的癫痫类型，潜在的病理学机制，以及多种临床体检、神经电生理学检查手段和神经影像学对脑部致痫灶的精准定位。本文主要综述目前最先进的分子影像学检查技术——一体化正电子发射计算机断层显像（Positron emission tomography, PET）/核磁共振成像（MRI）在难治性癫痫术前精准定位中的价值。

1　核磁共振成像在难治性癫痫术前定位中的价值

MRI 可多序列、多方位成像，提供远优于断层

DOI: 10.7507/2096-0247.20190060
基金项目：北京市医院管理局"登峰"计划专项经费资助（DFL20180802）
通信作者：卢洁，Email: imaginglu@hotmail.com

扫描（Computer tomography, CT）的软组织分辨率及更多的诊断信息，能够发现海马硬化、皮质发育不良及继发的皮质损害等多种 CT 扫描不能发现的细微结构改变，在癫痫病因诊断、术前定位与术后评估中发挥着重要作用，是难治性癫痫患者术前定位评估中重要的影像学检查项目。有学者提出如果 MRI 发现明确的孤立脑内病灶，就要高度怀疑该病灶与癫痫的发作存在关联，而且在这种情况下，仅仅依据解剖结构影像定位致痫灶的可靠性可达 70% 以上[3]。随着 MRI 扫描技术探索的逐渐深入，高分辨 MRI 成像方法可以明确大脑结构改变引起的癫痫，主要包括海马硬化、部分皮质发育不全、神经节神经胶质瘤、肉芽肿、海绵状血管瘤以及各类炎症等。

近年来，随着 MRI 技术的飞速发展，为弥补单纯解剖结构影像在癫痫术前定位中的不足，MRI 的高级功能序列逐渐用于癫痫术前的精准定位。弥散张量成像（Diffusion densor imaging, DTI）的原理是水分子在脑神经的扩散运动主要沿着神经纤维走向行进，通过采集多个弥散方向的信息，形成水分子在组织三维空间中的弥散特性成像。由于白质扩散的不等向性比灰质或是脑室更为明显，因此 DTI 可以直接反映白质纤维束的完整性，能较传统的 MRI 更敏感的发现白质异常。DTI 图像经过后处理可以产生纤维示踪图（fiber tractography）。该方法是目前唯一能在活体、无创的提供大脑白质纤

❖影像技术学

Investigation of "hot air spot" artifact in integrated PET/MR examination

SONG Tianbin[1], CUI Bixiao[1], YANG Hongwei[1], MA Jie[1], SHUAI Dongmei[1],
LIANG Zhigang[1], LU Jie[1,2,3*], ZHAO Guoguang[4,5]

(1. *Department of Nuclear Medicine*, 2. *Department of Radiology*, 4. *Department of Neurosurgery*,
Xuanwu Hospital, *Capital Medical University*, *Beijing* 100053, *China*; 3. *Beijing Key
Laboratory of Magnetic Resonance Imaging and Brain Informatics*, *Beijing*
100053, *China*; 5. *Center of Epilepsy*, *Beijing Institute for
Brain Disorder*, *Beijing* 100069, *China*)

[Abstract] **Objective** T To investigate the distribution and occurrence probability of artifact of "hot air spot" in integrated PET/MR examination, and the role of time of flight (TOF) in alleviating the artifact of "hot air spot ". **Methods** The occurrence sites and probability of artifact of "hot air spot" in 105 examinees who underwent integrated whole-body PET/MR examination were retrospectively analyzed, and the occurrence of heat organ sign in integrated PET/MR without TOF technology and TOF-PET/MR images were evaluated. **Results** The artifacts of "hot air spot" were distributed in sinus, trachea, gastric sinus, colon and rectum, and most commonly in trachea in the integrated PET/MR examination, and the incidence rates were 60.00%(63/105), 68.57%(72/105), 8.57%(9/105), 20.00%(21/105) and 16.19%(17/105), respectively. The SUV_{max} of different parts on PET/MR images without TOF technology were 4.09±2.17, 1.77±0.81, 1.75±0.85, 3.73±0.51 and 11.77±8.39, respectively. The SUV_{mean} of different parts on integrated TOF-PET/MR images were 3.19±1.87, 1.38±0.70, 1.44±0.85, 2.68±0.46 and 6.78±4.19, respectively. The SUV_{max} and SUV_{mean} of artifact of "hot air spot" on PET/MR images without TOF technology were higher than those on integrated TOF-PET/MR images (all $P<0.01$). **Conclusion** The artifact of "hot air spot " mainly exists in the sinuses, trachea and digestive tract in integrated whole-body PET/MR examination. The artifact of "hot air spot" in the trachea is the most commonly happened among them. TOF technology can obviously help to reduce the "hot air spot" artifact on the integrated PET/MR examination without TOF technology, thus significantly improving the quality of the integrated PET/MR image.

[Keywords] time of flight; integrated; magnetic resonance imaging; positron-emission tomography; artifacts; hot air spot

DOI:10.13929/j.1003-3289.201903212

一体化 PET/MR 检查中"热气管征"伪影探讨

宋天彬[1],崔碧霄[1],杨宏伟[1],马 杰[1],帅冬梅[1],梁志刚[1],卢 洁[1,2,3*],赵国光[4,5]

(1.首都医科大学宣武医院核医学科,2.放射科,4.神经外科,北京 100053;
3.磁共振成像脑信息学北京市重点实验室,北京 100053;5.北京脑重大疾病研究院癫痫所,北京 100069)

[基金项目] 国家重点研发项目(2016YFC0103909)、国家自然科学基金面上项目(81671662)、北京市医管局人才培养计划"登峰"项目(DFL20180802)、国家重点研发项目(2016YFC0103000)。

[第一作者] 宋天彬(1984—),男,山西阳泉人,在读博士,主治医师。研究方向:神经系统疾病及体部肿瘤一体化 PET/MR 研究。
E-mail: songtb_1984@163.com

[通信作者] 卢洁,首都医科大学宣武医院核医学科,首都医科大学宣武医院放射科,磁共振成像脑信息学北京市重点实验室,100053。
E-mail: imaginglu@hotmail.com

[收稿日期] 2019-03-28   [修回日期] 2019-06-27

学术论著　　中国医学装备2019年6月第16卷第6期 China Medical Equipment 2019 June Vol.16 No.6

一体化PET/MR不同衰减校正方式定量准确性分析及图像质量评估*

田德峰① 杨宏伟② 庄静文③ 崔碧霄② 马杰② 严汉民③ 卢洁①②*

[文章编号] 1672-8270(2019)06-0016-04　　[中图分类号] R814.42　[文献标识码] A

[摘要] 目的：探究基于MR的衰减校正(AC)和基于CT的衰减校正对于美国国家电气制造商协会(NEMA)IQ标准体模在一体化正电子发射计算机断层显像与磁共振(PET/MR)定量评估中的准确性，以及两种衰减校正方法下PET/MR重建图像质量的差异。方法：利用SIGNA PET/MR系统分析MR-AC和CT-AC条件下NEMA IQ图像μ-map的衰减系数，评估两种衰减校正方式在NEMA IQ体模质量控制实验中定量的准确性。参照NEMA NU 2-2007标准，根据其推荐的图像质量参数计算公式，以图像信噪比(SNR)作为评估图像质量的指标，对两种衰减校正方式下PET/MR矩阵(192×192、256×256)、迭代(2、3、4次)以及使用飞行时间(TOF)技术与否不同重建条件的图像质量进行评估。结果：体模质量控制实验中，基于MR的AC存在衰减系数分配错误，将肺和脂肪的衰减系数错误的分配给了肺部插件以及体模背景；在不同重建条件下基于CT-AC的图像SNR均高于基于MR-AC图像的SNR。结论：以MR-AC作为衰减校正方式的质量控制实验不足以作为PET/MR的定量标准，以CT-AC作为衰减校正方式的图像有更高的SNR，更优的图像质量。
[关键词] 正电子发射计算机断层显像；磁共振；质量控制；MR衰减校正；CT衰减校正；图像质量

DOI: 10.3969/J.ISSN.1672-8270.2019.06.005

Accuracy analysis and imaging quality assessment for the quantification of different AC modes of integration PET/MR/TIAN De-feng, YANG Hong-wei, ZHUANG Jing-wen, et al//China Medical Equipment,2019,16(6):16-19.
[Abstract] Objective: To investigate the accuracy of MR-based attenuation correction (AC) and CT-based AC for NEMA IQ standard phantom in quantitative assessment of integration positron emission tomography/magnetic resonance (PET/MR), and the differences of reconstructive PET/MR imaging quality under two AC methods. Methods: Using the SIGNA PET/MR system to analyze the attenuation coefficient of the NEMA IQ image μ-map under MR-AC and CT-AC conditions, and to assess the accuracy of quantification of two AC modes in quality control experiment of NEMA IQ phantom. Referring to the National Electrical Manufacturers Association (NEMA) NU 2-2007 standard, and according to the recommended calculation formula of image quality parameter, and using signal noise ratio (SNR) of imaging as indicator of assessing imaging quality to implement assessment for imaging quality with different reconstruction conditions included PET/MR matrix (192×192, 256×256), iteration (2, 3, 4 times) and whether used time of fly (TOF) under two AC modes. Results: In the quality control experiment of phantom, MR-based AC had an error that was the attenuation coefficients of lung and fat were incorrectly assigned to the lung insert and phantom background in the allocation of attenuation coefficients. The SNR of CT-AC based image was higher than that of MR-AC based image under different reconstruction conditions. Conclusion: The quality control experiment that uses MR-AC as the AC mode is not enough as the quantitative standard of PET/MR. And the image that uses CT-AC as the AC mode has higher SNR and better image quality.
[Key words] Positron emission tomography (PET); Magnetic resonance (MR); Quality control; MR-attenuation correction (MR-AC); CT-attenuation correction (CT-AC); Image quality

[First-author's address] Department of Radiotherapy, Beijing Key Laboratory of MRI and Brain Informatics, Xuanwu Hospital Capital Medical University, Beijing 100053, China.

在医学成像中，成像系统的性能需要定期测试和评估，以确保正常的功能和最佳的图像质量。对于正电子发射计算机断层显像(positron emission tomography，PET)扫描仪，美国国家电气制造商协会(National Electrical Manufactures Association，NEMA)制定了评估PET系统性能的标准[1]。当引入新系统时，这种图像质量控制测量还用于PET/MR成像中PET性能的测量，且在评估PET/MR成像性能的临床研究中比较依赖于NEMA IQ体模测量[2-4]。

Drzezga A等[5]提到PET/MR图像的剂量优化研究也依赖于NEMA IQ体模测量，所有这些研究均建立在体模精确的衰减校正(attenuation correction，AC)基础上。

为了获得定量准确的PET图像，用质量控制体模来确定扫描仪的性能参数，需要对所采集的PET数据进行校正，以减弱由扫描对象以及系统的硬件造成的光子衰减[4,6]。在PET/CT成像中，关于被扫描物体衰减特性的信息是从CT扫描本身获得；在PET/MR成

*基金项目：国家重点研发计划(2016YFC0103000、2016YFC0103909)"一体化TOFPET/MRI脑血流定量方法研究及在脑疾病的应用""PET/MR在神经系统疾病中的高级临床应用"；北京市医院管理局"登峰"计划专项经费资助(DFL20180802)
①首都医科大学宣武医院放射科 磁共振成像脑信息学北京市重点实验室 北京 100053
②首都医科大学宣武医院核医学科 北京 100053
③首都医科大学宣武医院医学工程科 北京 100053
*通信作者：imaginglu@hotmail.com
作者简介：田德峰，男，(1989—)，硕士，技师，研究方向：医学影像设备图像质量控制。

中国医学装备2019年3月第16卷第3期 China Medical Equipment 2019 March Vol.16 No.3

学术论著 |

重建矩阵对一体化PET/MR图像质量的影响*

吴萍① 吴天棋① 白玫①*

[文章编号] 1672-8270(2019)03-0043-05　　[中图分类号] R812　[文献标识码] A

[摘要] 目的：探讨不同矩阵大小对一体化PET/MR图像质量的影响。方法：依据美国电器制造商协会(NEMA)NU2-2007标准，对国际电工委员会(IEC)61675-1标准规定的PET图像质量体模进行扫描；分别在像素矩阵为128×128、192×192和256×256的3种不同条件下重建PET图像，分析对比度(Q)、背景变化率(N)、信噪比(SNR)、衰减和散射矫正精度(ΔC)等参数。结果：以像素矩阵128×128条件下重建结果为参考，使用飞行时间(TOF)技术和非TOF技术，对比度平均值分别增长11.45%、10.1%和7.14%、7.92%；背景变化率均值分别降低了0.04%、0.22%和0.27%、0.2%；信噪比均值分别提高了3.71、3.69和2.71、3.06；衰减和散射矫正精度均值分别增加了0.28%、0.28%和1.04%、0.33%。结论：增大图像重建矩阵可提高PET图像质量，两种较大矩阵之间的图像质量差异并不明显。

[关键词] 一体化PET/MR；矩阵；图像质量

DOI: 10.3969/J.ISSN.1672-8270.2019.03.012

The effects of reconstruction matrix on image quality of integrated PET/MR/WU Ping, WU Tian-qi, BAI Mei// China Medical Equipment,2019,16(3):43-47.

[Abstract] Objective: To explore the effects of different matrix sizes on image quality of integrated PET/MR. Methods: According to the NU 2-2007 protocol of NEMA, the PET image quality phantom that was stipulated by (IEC)61675-1 standard was scanned. Under different sizes of matrix (128×128, 192×192, 256×256), PET image were reconstructed. And then, the contrast recovery (Q), background variability (N), signal-to-noise ratio (SNR) and correction precision of attenuation and scattering (ΔC) were further analyzed. Result: The reconstructed result of the matrix size of 128×128 was used as reference. The means of Q were increased 11.45% and 10.1% under the condition of TOF technique and means were increased 7.14% and 7.92% under the condition of non-TOF. And the means of N were decreased 0.04% and0.22% with TOF, and those were decreased 0.27% and 0.2% with non-TOF. And the means of SNR were increased 3.71 and 3.69with TOF, and those were increased 2.71 and 3.06with non-TOF. Besides, the means of ΔC were increased 0.28% and 0.28%with TOF and those were 1.04% and 0.33% with non-TOF. Conclusion: Through enlarges the reconstructed image matrix can enhance image quality of PET. And the difference of image quality between the two larger matrixes was no significant.

[Key words] Integrated PET/MR; Matrix; Image quality

[First-author's address] Department of Medical Engineering, Xuanwu Hospital, Capital Medical University, Beijing 100053, China.

　　电子发射型计算机断层显像(positron emission computed tomography，PET)是通过对放射性核素在体内的聚集成像，反映生命代谢活动情况的设备，是核医学领域常用的影像检查技术；磁共振成像(magnetic resonance imaging，MRI)是利用磁共振现象从人体中获得电磁信号，通过图像重建获得人体结构成像的设备，是放射影像领域常用的检查技术之一[1]。一体化PET/MR设备[2-3]是同时进行PET和MR扫描，并将PET分子图像与MR结构图像结合在一起的全新医学影像设备，其内置飞行时间(time of flight，TOF)图像采集重建技术是基于镥素晶体和高性能的光电转化器的新技术[4-5]。

　　在图像后处理时，一般采用不同重建条件以获取高质量扫描图像，其中矩阵大小是一个重要的变量参数[6-7]。重建矩阵(reconstruction matrix)记作Mx(x为矩阵大小)，是反映重建图像大小的参数，一般认为和图像的空间分辨率等性能有关[8]。以灰度图像为例，其像素数据就是一个矩阵，矩阵的行对应图像的高(单位为像素)，矩阵的列对应图像的宽(单位为像素)，矩阵的元素对应图像的像素，矩阵元素的值就是像素的灰度值。本研究以图像矩阵大小为变量，探讨一体化PET/MR设备中PET图像质量的变化。

1 材料与方法

1.1 一体化PET/MR设备

　　本研究所用扫描设备为美国通用电气公司的一体化PET/MR设备，型号为SIGNA，图像处理为设备配套AW4.6工作站。该设备以3.0T静音磁共振设备作为平台，采用LBS镥闪烁晶体与全数字化固态阵列式光电转化器(SiPM)融合技术，PET探测器具有TOF技术；以零回波成像技术(zero echo time，ZTE)实现PET衰减矫正；时间分辨率<400ps，灵敏度>21cps/kBq，轴向视野25cm，能够实现PET与MR一体化同步扫描

*基金项目：国家重点研发计划(2016YFC0103909) "PET/MR在神经系统疾病中的高级临床应用"
①首都医科大学宣武医院医学工程处 北京 100053
*通信作者：jswei65@163.com

作者简介：吴萍，女，(1988-)，硕士，助理工程师，从事医疗设备管理工作。

第一章 一体化PET/MR科研成果

医学影像学杂志 2019 年第 29 卷第 7 期　J Med Imaging Vol. 29 No. 7 2019

一体化 PET/MR 受检者护理需求及影响因素调查

帅冬梅[1]，卢洁[1,2]，李秋萍[1]，宣萱[1]，马蕾[1]，候亚琴[1]

首都医科大学宣武医院　1. 核医学科；2. 放射科　北京　100053

【摘要】 目的　探讨一体化 PET/MR 受检者的护理需求及相关影响因素，满足不同层次受检者护理需求。方法　采用抽样法选取我院核医学科行一体化 PET/MR 受检者 44 例，男 20 例，女 24 例，年龄（51.16 ± 19.50）岁。对受检者护理需求进行问卷调查，受检者护理需求各维度得分及护理需求各条目需求率进行统计分析，并对受检者不同人口学护理需求进行比较。结果　44 例受检者问卷总分为 16 ~ 48（43.5 ± 6.59）分，护理需求得分第一为"PET/MR 检查后注意事项"（41/44，93.2%），第二为"有问必答，善于倾听"（40/44，90.9%），并列第三为"候诊室安静整洁"、"仪表端庄，微笑服务，耐心周到"（38/44，86.4%）。44 例受检者不同年龄、检查次数受检者护理需求总分比较差异无显著统计学意义（P > 0.05），不同性别及文化程度受检者护理需求总分比较差异有显著统计学意义（P < 0.05）。结论　护理人员应在充分评估一体化 PET/MR 受检者需求的前提下开展相应的护理实践活动，进一步提升优质护理服务质量。

【关键词】　护理需求；影响因素；一体化 PET/MR

中图分类号：R817.4；R47　　文献标识码：A　　文章编号：1006-9011（2019）07-1209-04

Survey of the needs and effects of nursing in the patients underwent hybrid PET/MR

SHUAI Dongmei[1], LU Jie[1,2], LI Qiuping[1], XUAN Xuan[1], MA Lei[1], HOU Yaqin[1]

1. Department of Nuclear Medicine, Xuanwu Hospital Capital Medical University, Beijing 100053, P. R. China

2. Department of Radiology, Xuanwu Hospital Capital Medical University, Beijing 100053, P. R. China

【Abstract】 Objective　To investigate the nursing needs and effecting factors in the patients underwent hybrid PET/MR, to provide evidence of clinical nursing so as to meet the demand of different client care. Methods　The convenience sampling method was adopted to select 44 cases (20 males and 24 females, average age was 51.16 ± 19.50 years) underwent hybrid PET/MR in our nuclear medicine department from August 2016 to December 2016. The patients were performed the survey of nursing needs of hybrid PET/MR. Each dimension score and rate of each entry requirements were analyzed. In addition, the different demographic nursing needs of the patients were compared. Results　The total scores of 44 questionnaires were 16 ~ 48(43.5 ± 6.59) points. The first was notice after PET/MR examination (41/44, 93.2%), the second was answering all the questions and was good at listening (40/44, 90.9%), the third was keep waiting room quiet, clean and tidy and personable, smiling service, patient and thoughtful (38/44, 86.4%). The nursing needs of 44 patients total scores had no statistical difference between different age and examination times (P > 0.05). However, there was statistical difference between different gender and degree of education (P < 0.05). Conclusion　The nursing work of hybrid PET/MR examination should be done after fully evaluating the patients needs, to further improving the quality of high quality nursing service.

【Key words】　Nursing needs; Effecting factors; Hybrid PET/MR

一体化 PET/MR 是将正电子发射计算机断层显像仪（positron emission tomography，PET）和 MRI 融合成一体化的大型新型影像诊断设备，是功能与分子影像学发展的前沿技术之一[1]。一体化 PET/MR 同时具有 PET 和 MR 的功能，两者的融合能达到最大意义上的优势互补。目前一体化 PET/MR 技术日趋成熟并已逐步应用于临床诊断[2]，但由于检查的特殊性、检查人群的多样性，为确保检查安全和最大限度地满足患者的需求，体现"以患者为中心"的护理理念，本文旨在探讨一体化 PET/MR 受检者的护理需求及相关影响因素，为临床护理实践提供依据，进一步满足不同层次受检者护理需求，提升护理质量。

基金项目：国家科技部十三五重点研发项目资助（编号：2016YFC0103000）

作者简介：帅冬梅（1973-），女，四川人，毕业于首都医科大学，主管护师，专科学历，主要从事核医学护理工作

通信作者：卢洁　教授，主任医师　E-mail：imaginglu@ hotmail.com

1　资料与方法

· 1336 ·　　　　中华老年心脑血管病杂志2018年12月 第20卷 第12期　 Chin J Geriatr Heart Brain Vessel Dis,Dec 2018,Vol 20,No.12

·综述·

一体化正电子发射断层显像磁共振在阿尔茨海默病的研究进展

闫少珍,卢洁,李坤成

关键词:正电子发射断层显像术;磁共振波谱学;阿尔茨海默病;认知障碍;淀粉样β蛋白;早期诊断

阿尔茨海默病(Alzheimer's disease,AD)是一种以进行性认知功能障碍和行为损害为主要特征的神经退行性疾病,是老年痴呆中最常见的一种类型。轻度认知功能障碍(mild cognitive impairment,MCI)是处于正常老化与痴呆之间的一种认知状态,具有转化为AD或其他痴呆类型的高风险。目前诊断AD的影像技术主要是功能MRI和正电子发射断层显像(positron emission tomography,PET)。近年来研究表明,一体化PET/MR能够同时提供形态学、功能及分子水平成像信息,为AD患者的早期诊断和鉴别诊断提供了新的价值。本研究重点就一体化PET/MR在AD患者的研究进展进行综述。

1　PET在AD的应用

PET是采用同位素示踪剂标记放射性核素进行分子显像技术,能够从¹⁸F-脱氧葡萄糖(¹⁸F-fluorode-oxyglucose,¹⁸F-FDG)代谢显像、β淀粉样蛋白(β-amyloid,Aβ)显像和tau显像等多方面对AD进行研究。¹⁸F-FDG-PET通过¹⁸F标记FDG的代谢评价神经元功能状态,是最常用的PET示踪剂。¹⁸F-FDG-PET可以显示早期AD患者颞顶叶、扣带回和海马等部位¹⁸F-FDG的摄取减少,并且后扣带回葡萄糖代谢减低较颞叶和额叶皮质明显[1]。MCI患者主要表现为后扣带回和海马低代谢。而额颞叶痴呆则主要表现为额颞叶皮质代谢降低,典型额颞叶痴呆患者易于与AD鉴别。路易体痴呆在顶颞联合区、后扣带回、枕叶代谢出现降低,特别是初级视觉皮质代谢下降较AD更明显。¹⁸F-FDG-PET不仅能够鉴别AD与其他类型痴呆,而且还能预测MCI患者是否转化为AD,并具有较高的敏感性和特异性,对于监测疾病进展具有重要的作用[2-3]。研究还发现,¹¹C标记的匹茨堡化合物(¹¹C-Pittsburgh compound-B,¹¹C-PIB)、¹⁸F-AV等Aβ显像剂以及¹⁸F-AV1451、¹⁸F-THK5351等tau显像剂已逐渐应用于临床或科学研究[4-6]。其中,¹¹C-PIB是目前研究最多的Aβ分子探针,属于硫磺素衍生物类,可与Aβ特异性结合。Villemagne等[7]研究发现,AD患者痴呆症状出现前17年就发现Aβ沉积。另外,tau配体与AD患者神经原纤维缠结高度结合,tau-PET可以显示脑内tau沉积,对揭示患者神经退行性病变、认知功能损害的机制具有重要作用[8]。研究显示,tau沉积和认知功能障碍紧密相关,其中颞叶tau沉积有助于预测认知功能变化[5]。但由于¹¹C-PIB半衰期只有20

DOI:10.3969/j.issn.1009-0126.2018.12.028
基金项目:国家重点研发计划(2016YFC0103000,2016YFC0107107)
作者单位:100053 北京,首都医科大学宣武医院放射科

min以及tau-PET对临床诊断的作用有待更多的研究证实,因此临床应用受限。

2　静息态功能MRI在AD的应用

静息态功能MRI是一种简便、无创的脑功能成像方法,能够获取人脑的功能信息,已广泛应用于AD等疾病的研究。AD患者研究最多的是默认网络,默认网络与AD病理学典型的好发部位相似,主要包括后扣带回、楔前叶、内侧颞叶、颞顶叶和内侧前额叶皮质等。AD患者楔前叶、后扣带回默认网络内功能连接减少,MCI患者功能连接值介于正常受试者与AD患者之间[9]。AD患者默认网络连接存在一个动态变化,即疾病早期后部默认网络连接开始减少,而前部和腹侧默认网络连接则增强,随着疾病进展所有网络连接均降低[10]。纵向研究发现,海马亚区功能连接有助于鉴别MCI和AD患者(敏感性83.3%,特异性83.3%)[11]。除了以上集中在默认网络区域的研究外,以往大部分研究认为,小脑在AD患者中不易被累及,而Bai等[12]研究发现,小脑功能连接的改变可能与遗忘型MCI发病机制有关,但尚需更多的研究证实小脑在AD中的作用。此外,局部一致性(regional homogeneity,ReHo)以及低频振幅波动(amplitude of low-frequency fluctuation,ALFF)也是比较常用的研究方法。其中,ReHo可用于检测全脑局部活动相关性。He等[13]研究发现,AD患者后扣带回和楔前叶的ReHo值减低,MCI患者中左侧顶下小叶ReHo值显著增加,这可能是一种代偿性改变。而且,计算ReHo值能够以85%的正确率把AD患者从MCI和正常对照组区分开来。ALFF是通过脑部功能活动的血氧水平依赖信号相对基线的变化幅度来观察脑部神经元自发性活动的方法。AD患者在双侧后扣带皮质、楔前叶、顶下小叶及多个楔区较正常对照组ALFF值下降,在双侧海马、海马旁回、颞中回和颞下回皮质ALFF值升高[14]。另有学者并未发现轻度AD患者ALFF值增高。这些研究结果的差异可能与AD处于不同疾病时期有关。特别指出的是,在早期MCI阶段就可以检测到明显改变的ALFF活动,并且独立于年龄、性别和脑萎缩,提示ALFF异常是早期诊断AD的潜在生物标志物。但是,静息态功能MRI易受多种因素的影响,尚需更深一步的研究去了解静息态功能MRI的神经基础。

3　一体化PET MR在AD的应用

3.1　一体化PET MR

一体化PET/MR是将PET探测器与MR体线圈整合在一起,将PET和MR技术融合,是目前最先进的新型影像设备。一体化PET/MR真正实现了同步

· 440 ·　　　中华老年心脑血管病杂志2018年4月第20卷第4期　Chin J Geriatr Heart Brain Vessel Dis,Apr 2018,Vol 20,No.4

·综述·

正电子发射断层显像与磁共振成像联合评价
颈动脉易损斑块的研究进展

张越,杨旗,卢洁

关键词:正电子发射断层显像术;磁共振成像;颈动脉损伤;动脉粥样硬化

　　脑卒中是严重危害人类生命和健康的主要原因,其发病率和死亡率在发展中国家均已位居首列[1]。颈动脉粥样硬化中易损斑块(vulnerable plaque)与缺血性脑卒中密切相关[2]。因此,早期识别易损斑块,评价斑块的稳定性,对于预防和控制缺血性脑卒中事件的发生尤为重要。目前,在该领域,超声、CT、MRI以及单光子发射计算机断层摄影(SPECT)、正电子发射断层显像(PET)均能提供相应的部分信息,但各有优劣,从而融合影像应运而生。近年来,PET、CT作为多模态成像技术,已经较为成熟地应用于临床。然而,随着影像技术的进一步发展,PET、MR设备走向市场,其相对于PET、CT的优势主要在于提高软组织分辨率和减少辐射损伤。现对PET与MRI联合在颈动脉易损斑块的识别及其临床应用研究进展综述如下。

1　易损斑块

　　介入心脏病和心血管病理学家将导致急性缺血性脑卒中的斑块视为"罪犯"斑块,而不论其病理学特征。为了进行前瞻性评估,临床医师需要更精确的术语来描述危险事件发生前的斑块。2003年Naghavi等将"所有有破裂倾向、容易血栓形成和(或)进展迅速的危险斑块"统一命名为易损斑块。其诊断的主要标准:活动性炎症,单核细胞及巨噬细胞浸润,有时可有T细胞浸润;薄纤维帽伴大脂质坏死核心;内皮磨损伴表面血小板聚集;斑块裂隙形成;管腔狭窄>90%。次要标准:斑块表面钙化结节;镜下黄亮斑块;斑块内出血;内皮功能障碍;正性重构。可见,易损斑块并不完全是软斑块,非钙化斑块,美国心脏协会Ⅳ型斑块和非狭窄斑块[3]。富含脂质的坏死核心、薄纤维帽和斑块内出血是易损斑块的代表性特征[3]。表面溃疡及血栓形成均易导致斑块破裂,从而导致缺血性脑卒中事件的发生[4]。

2　MR血管壁成像技术对易损斑块的无创性识别

2.1　MR血管壁成像技术的应用

高分辨MRI作为颈动脉斑块常用的扫描方法,采用小视野、大矩阵,对于易损斑块的识别有很高的敏感性和特异性。MR血管壁"黑血"和"亮血"成像技术以及MR动态增强扫描成像等技术,能够增加管腔内血液与斑块对比度,清晰显示颈动脉管壁与斑块的结

DOI:10.3969/j.issn.1009-0126.2018.04.028
基金项目:国家自然科学基金(81671662);国家重点研发计划项目(2016YFC1301702,2016YFC0103000)
作者单位:100053北京,首都医科大学宣武医院放射科
通信作者:卢洁,Email:imaginglu@hotmail.com

构,准确判定管腔狭窄程度和斑块稳定性[5]。"黑血"技术常规序列包括T1WI、T2WI和质子密度加权成像,能够清晰显示管壁细微结构;"亮血"技术的三维时间飞跃(3D-TOF)序列可直观显示富含脂质的坏死核心、纤维帽和钙化,二者技术互补结合,可明显提高易损斑块的检出效力。对比增强MRI可判断脂核的存在以及纤维帽的厚度,评估纤维帽与脂核的比例,但因其时间分辨率较差,不能定量斑块内部新生血管及炎性反应程度,故较难进行易损斑块的准确定位。MR动态增强扫描成像通过对比剂时间-增强信号曲线,计算斑块血浆的容积分数和容积传输参数来测定特定斑块区域组织的微血流变化,评估其灌注情况及渗透特性,从而对易损斑块进行定量分析。

　　近年来,三维颈动脉斑块MRI的特殊序列飞速发展,包括三维磁化准备快速梯度回波成像序列、三维多回波重组梯度回波序列、三维多组织对比序列、三维反转恢复准备的快速扰相梯度回波序列、三维扰相梯度召回回波脉冲序列等,具有更高的空间分辨率和信噪比,能敏感的显示斑块内出血,从而更好地评估斑块的稳定性[6]。

2.2　颈动脉易损斑块的MR信号特征

(1)脂质核心T1WI呈等或稍高信号,3D-TOF呈等信号,质子密度加权成像呈等或低信号,T2WI依内部成分不同而呈现出不同信号特点,若以甘油三酯为主,T2WI呈低信号,若以胆固醇为主,T2WI呈高信号[7]。(2)纤维帽因富含胶原纤维和平滑肌细胞,T1WI呈等信号,T2WI呈稍高信号,3D-TOF呈低信号。脂核内部因缺乏新生血管,对比增强T1WI序列基本不强化,而纤维帽内部因新生血管丰富而明显强化,通过对比增强检测新生血管,判断脂核与纤维帽的比例,可作为评估不稳定斑块的可靠指标。(3)活动性炎症是易损斑块的核心特征。有研究发现,动态增强MRI能定量新生毛细血管,分析炎性细胞活性,斑块的灌注强化与新生血管的供血及血管的通透性有关[8]。另外,超顺磁性氧化铁微粒以及双靶向氧化铁微粒等能被巨噬细胞吞噬,而作为MRI分子探针来检测斑块内部炎性反应程度及巨噬细胞含量[9]。(4)斑块内出血因出血时间变化,血红蛋白结构和氧化状态不同,MR信号强度亦不相同。研究证实,出血早期,完整红细胞内氧合血红蛋白变为脱氧血红蛋白为顺磁性,在T1WI及3D-TOF呈高信号,T2WI及质子密度加权成像呈等或低信号[3];亚急性期,脱氧血红蛋白变为正铁血红蛋白,随红细胞溶解位于细胞外,在T1WI、T2WI及质子密度加权成像序列呈明显

中国医学装备2018年2月第15卷第2期 China Medical Equipment 2018 February Vol.15 No.2

学术论著 |

一体化PET-MR设备中飞行时间技术和点扩展函数技术对PET图像质量的影响*

董硕① 李东① 吴天棋① 庄静文① 谢峰① 白玫①*

[文章编号] 1672-8270(2018)02-0001-05　　　[中图分类号] R812　[文献标识码] A

[摘要] 目的：研究在一体化PET-MR图像重建中飞行时间(TOF)技术和点扩展函数(PSF)对PET图像质量的影响。方法：依据美国电气制造商协会(NEMA)NU2-2007标准，使用国际电工委员会(IEC)61675-1标准规定的PET图像质量体模，在通用电气公司GE SIGNA型PET-MR及配套AW4.6工作站上完成扫描和图像重建，采用联合使用(TOF+PSF)、单独使用PSF技术(non-TOF+PSF)、单独使用TOF技术(TOF+non-PSF)和两种技术均不使用(non-TOF+non-PSF)4种方法重建PET图像，分析图像的对比度(Q_H和Q_C)、背景变化率(N_j)和信噪比(SNR)。结果：以non-TOF+non-PSF重建结果为参照，单独使用PSF技术、单独使用TOF技术和联合使用TOF+PSF技术重建图像的平均热区对比度(Q_H)分别提高了7.61%、20.94%和40.17%；单独使用TOF技术的图像平均冷区对比度(Q_C)提高了11.29%，联合使用TOF+PSF技术的图像Q_C提高了12.32%；单独使用PSF技术、单独使用TOF技术和联合使用TOF+PSF技术重建图像的平均背景变化率(N_{mean})分别降低了2.28%、21.44%和30.03%；SNR则分别提高了11.52%、44.28%和92.70%。结论：TOF和PSF技术均可提高PET的图像质量，联合使用两种技术对提高重建图像质量效果更为明显。

[关键词] 一体化PET-MR；飞行时间技术；点扩展函数；图像质量

DOI: 10.3969/J.ISSN.1672-8270.2018.02.001
The effects of TOF and PSF on image quality of PET in integrated PET-MR/DONG Shuo, LI Dong, WU Tian-qi, et al//China Medical Equipment,2018,15(2):1-5.

[Abstract] Objective: To research the effects of time of flight (TOF) technique and point spread function (PSF) algorithms on the image quality of PET in the image reconstruction of integrated PET-MR. Methods: The NU 2-2007 protocol of NEMA was followed. The image quality phantom following IEC Standard 61675-1 was adopted in the research. All scan and image reconstruction were performed on PET/MR and matched AW4.6 workstation of GE SIGNA. Different algorithms (TOF+PSF, TOF+non-PSF, non-TOF+PSF, and non-TOF+non-PSF) were applied in image reconstruction of PET. The obtained PET images were quantitatively evaluated and analyzed by following parameters: contrast recovery of hot and cold spheres (Q_H and Q_C), background variability (N_j) and the signal-to-noise ratio (SNR) of hot spheres. Results: For quantitative image quality evaluation, results of (non-TOF+non-PSF) were used as reference. The average Q_H of (non-TOF+PSF), (TOF+non-PSF) and (TOF+PSF) were increased 7.61%, 20.94% and 40.17%, respectively. The average Q_C of TOF alone and (TOF+PSF) were increased 11.29% and 12.32%, respectively. The average N_{mean} of PSF alone, TOF alone and (TOF+PSF) were decreased 2.28%, 21.44% and 30.03%, respectively. And the SNR of PSF alone, TOF alone and (TOF+PSF) were increased 11.52%, 44.28% and 92.70%, respectively. Conclusion: Both TOF and PSF can improve the overall image quality of PET, and it is more obvious when they are used in combination.

[Key words] Integrated PET-MR; Time of flight(TOF); Point spread function(PSF); Image quality

[First-author's address] Department of Medical Engineering, Xuanwu Hospital of Capital Medical University, Beijing 100053, China.

　　一体化PET-MR设备是将正电子发射计算机断层显像(positron-emission tomography, PET)的分子成像功能与磁共振成像(magnetic resonance imaging, MRI)卓越的软组织对比功能结合起来的一种新技术，可以同步进行PET和MR扫描，是一种集结构成像、功能成像和分子成像功能于一体的医学影像设备[1-2]。因此，在基础研究和临床诊断方面都吸引了越来越多的关注。作为目前最先进的医学影像技术之一，一体化PET-MR的图像质量也成为医学影像领域关注的热点。近年来，人们提出了多种能提高PET图像质量的重建算法，其中，飞行时间(time of flight，TOF)技术和点扩展函数(point spread function，PSF)表现优异[3-4]。

　　TOF算法最早提出于20世纪80年代，但是直到近年来该算法才逐渐应用于临床[5-7]。通过TOF算法可以直接确定正电子符合事件发生的位置，在采用TOF技术的PET中，每一个被检测到的光子都会标记其探测时间(或称到达时间)，如果2个光子的探测时间之差小于设定的符合窗，那么这2个光子就会被认为是与同一个湮灭事件相关[10]。该探测时间之间的差值，

*基金项目：国家重点研发计划数字诊疗装备研发专项(2016YFC0103909)"PET-MR在神经系统疾病中的高级临床应用"
①首都医科大学宣武医院医学工程处 北京 100053
*通信作者：jswei65@163.com
作者简介：董硕，女，(1980-)，博士，高级工程师，研究方向：医学图像处理与分析。

第一章 一体化PET/MR科研成果

147 PET/MR

首都医科大学宣武医院一体化 PET/MR 成果集

医学影像学杂志 2018 年第 28 卷第 12 期 J Med Imaging Vol. 28 No. 12 2018

· 短篇论著 ·

护理因素对一体化 TOF PET/MR 图像质量影响的原因分析

Analysis of the effect of nursing factors on integrated TOF PET/MR image quality

马　蕾[1]，卢　洁[1,2]，帅冬梅[1]，宣　萱[1]，马　杰[1]，候亚琴[1]

(1.首都医科大学宣武医院 1.核医学科;2.放射科 北京 100053)

【摘 要】 目的 分析 PET/MR 检查中影响图像质量的护理因素及提出相应的护理预防措施。方法 回顾性分析 2016 年 3~8 月于我院就诊行 PET/MR 检查的患者 72 例，其中男 34 例，女 38 例，平均年龄(58.92±9.12)岁;逐一分析并观察第一患者的图像，筛选出质量不佳的图像，探讨导致图像质量不佳的原因并给出预防措施。结果 72 例行 PET/MR 患者中有 11 例的图像质量不佳，主要原因包括示踪剂皮下渗漏、三通管路内药物剂量高、反复穿刺、污染。结论 护理人员应重视造成成像质量不佳的原因，提高护理技术，保证成像质量。

【关键词】 图像质量;护理因素

中图分类号:R445　文献标识码:A　文章编号:1006-9011(2018)12-2107-02

影像学设备的发展日新月异，一体化 PET/MR 是目前国际最前沿的多模态影像设备，可以同时、同步得到 PET 和 MRI 信息，实现两种成像设备的强强联合与优势互补，为更精准医学提供了崭新的手段[1]。^{18}F-FDG 是 PET 检查最常使用的放射性药物，在组织细胞磷酸化为^{18}F-FDG-6-磷酸，该产物再参与葡萄糖的进一步代谢，由于不能通过细胞膜，从而滞留在细胞内，并在一定时间内保持相对稳定状态。PET 探测器通过采集^{18}F 产生的 γ 光子计数，反映细胞的葡萄糖代谢率，进而反应其代谢程度[2]。然而有时由于护理技术、操作等原因，导致图像质量不佳、伪影重等，无法获取准确的信息，影响医师对病变的准确诊断。本文对 PET/MR 检查患者的图像进行回顾性分析，探讨导致图像出现伪影、质量不佳的护理因素，为今后提高护理技术，保证图像质量提供理论依据。

1 资料与方法

1.1 一般资料

回顾性分析我院 2016 年 3~8 月行一体化 TOF PET/MR 的患者，共 72 例，其中男 34 例，女 38 例，平均年龄(58.92±9.12)岁。72 例患者中，行肿瘤筛查者 19 例，肿瘤-术后检查者 43 例，其它 16 例，包括胸腔积液、硬脊膜动静脉瘘患者及健康体检者。

基金项目:国家科技部十三五重点研发项目资助(编号:2016YFC0103000)

作者简介:马蕾(1975-)，女，北京人，大专学历，初级护师，主要从事核医学护理研究工作

通信作者:卢洁 E-mail:imaginglu@hotmail.com

1.2 检查方法

PET/MR 机型为 GE 公司 SIGNA 一体化 TOF-PET-MRI。显像剂^{18}F-FDG 为我院核医学科放射性药物实验室制备，经伦理委员会论证审批通过。行 PET/MR 检查前所有患者均签署知情同意书。

1.3 护理方法

全部患者需禁食 6h 以上，血糖控制 <10mmol/L 以内。排除有检查禁忌症的患者，如:装有心脏起搏器、人工心脏瓣膜、电子耳蜗植入、心脏监护装置和呼吸机的危重患者等。检查前嘱患者取下所有含磁性物品，并选择合适的血管为患者留置静脉针。护士穿防护设备，根据患者体重将^{18}F-FDG(0.1mci/kg)分装后进行静脉注射。根据图像采集方式(静态/动态)，采取高活室窗口注射给药或床旁弹丸注射给药。1)静态采集，高活室窗口注射给药:患者将其手臂置于防护窗口处，确认留置针在血管后，立即注射^{18}F-FDG;为保证有效的注射剂量，防止示踪剂残留在针头处，注射后用 5ml 生理盐水冲封管路;注射完毕后，拔除留置针，记录注射器及留置针内显像剂残余量;注射^{18}F-FDG 后患者在候诊室视听封闭安静休息 40min，待示踪剂在体内达到峰值后进行 PET/MR 检查;2)动态采集，床旁弹丸注射给药:协助技师在检查室内给患者摆位后，护士在高活室准备好无菌巾、药物及冲管盐水，接到技师电话通知进入检查室，在留置管侧的手臂下垫治疗巾，以免药液溅落污染机器，弹丸注射给药同时、同步开始扫描，注射完毕后冲封管路，夹闭留置针，护士返回高活室测量注射器余量。

中国医学影像技术 2017 年第 33 卷第 5 期　Chin J Med Imaging Technol，2017，Vol 33，No 5　　　　　　　　　　　　　　・791・

❖规范与标准

Guidelines for hybrid PET/MR in brain imaging（2017 Edition）

LU Jie[1]，ZHANG Miao[1]，FANG Jiliang[2]，AI Lin[3]，LAN Xiaoli[4]，

LI Biao[5]，ZUO Changjing[6]，LI Yaming[7*]，

Chinese Medical Association Nuclear Medicine Branch PET/MR

Brain Functional Imaging Working Group Expert Group

（1. *Department of Nuclear Medicine，Xuanwu Hospital，Capital Medical University，Beijing* 100053，*China*；

2. *Department of Radiology，Guang'anmen Hospital，China Academy of Chinese Medical Sciences，*

Beijing 100053，*China*；3. *Department of Nuclear Medicine，Beijing Tiantan Hospital，Capital*

Medical University，Beijing 100050，*China*；4. *Department of Nuclear Medicine，Union*

Hospital，Tongji Medical College，Huazhong University of Science and Technology，

Wuhan 430022，*China*；5. *Department of Nuclear Medicine，Ruijin Hospital，*

School of Medicine，Shanghai Jiao Tong University，Shanghai 200025，*China*；

6. *Department of Nuclear Medicine，Changhai Hospital，Second Military*

Medical University，Shanghai 200433，*China*；7. *Departmem of Nuclear*

Medicine，the First Hospital of China Medical University，

Shenyang 110001，*China*）

［**Abstract**］　The hybrid PET/MR has been gradually applied in clinical practice. However，the hybrid PET/MR is a complex advanced technique，and it brings to the new challenges，especially regarding the workflow and scan protocols. The guidelines for hybrid PET/MR in brain imaging include information related to the indications and contraindications，preparation before examination，procedures of examination（PET imaging，conventional MRI brain imaging and special MRI imaging for brain disease），application of radiopharmaceutical and MRI contrast-enhanced agent. The purpose of the guidelines is to offer a framework that would be practical and helpful for clinical PET/MR brain imaging. In PET tracers，the guidelines only limit to the ^{18}F-FDG.

［**Key words**］　Brain；Positron-emission tomography；Magnetic resonance imaging

DOI：10.13929/j.1003-3289.201702019

一体化 PET/MR 颅脑成像检查规范（2017 版）

卢　洁[1]，张　苗[1]，方继良[2]，艾　林[3]，兰晓莉[4]，李　彪[5]，左长京[6]，李亚明[7*]，

中华医学会核医学分会 PET/MR 脑功能成像工作委员会专家组

（1. 首都医科大学宣武医院核医学科，北京　100053；2. 中国中医科学院广安门医院放射科，北京　100053；

3. 首都医科大学附属北京天坛医院核医学科，北京　100050；4. 华中科技大学同济医学院附属

协和医院核医学科，湖北 武汉　430022；5. 上海交通大学医学院附属瑞金医院核医学科，

上海　200025；6. 第二军医大学附属长海医院核医学科，上海　200433；

7. 中国医科大学附属第一医院核医学科，辽宁 沈阳　110001）

［摘　要］　一体化 PET/MR 已经逐渐在临床应用，其检查流程的规范化是需要迫切解决的重大任务。一体化 PET/MR

［第一作者］卢洁（1975—），女，河北邢台人，博士，主任医师、教授。研究方向：脑功能与分子影像学。E-mail：imaginglu@hotmail.com

［通信作者］李亚明，中国医科大学附属第一医院核医学科，110001。E-mail：ymli2001@163.com

［收稿日期］2017-02-07　　［修回日期］2017-03-29

❖规范与标准

Guidelines for nursing in hybrid PET/MR imaging
(2017 Edition)

HAN Binru[1], SHUAI Dongmei[1], FANG Jiliang[2], AI Lin[3], LAN Xiaoli[4], LI Biao[5],

ZUO Changjing[6], LU Jie[1], LI Yaming[7*], Chinese Medical Association Nuclear

Medicine Branch PET/MR Brain Functional Imaging Working Group Expert Group

(1. Department of Nuclear Medicine, Xuanwu Hospital, Capital Medical University, Beijing 100053, China;

2. Department of Radiology, Guanganmen Hospital, China Academy of Chinese Medical Sciences,

Beijing 100053, China; 3. Department of Nuclear Medicine, Beijing Tiantan Hospital, Capital

Medical University, Beijing 100050, China; 4. Department of Nuclear Medicine,

Union Hospital, Tongji Medical College, Huazhong University of Science and Technology,

Wuhan 430022, China; 5. Department of Nuclear Medicine, Ruijin Hospital, School of

Medicine, Shanghai Jiao Tong University, Shanghai 200025, China; 6. Department of

Nuclear Medicine, Changhai Hospital, Second Military Medical University,

Shanghai 200433, China; 7. Departmem of Nuclear Medicine, the First

Hospital of China Medical University, Shenyang 110001, China)

[Abstract]　The guidelines for standard nursing in the PET/MR imaging examination included preparation of examination, injecting drug, observing during scanning, post scanning care, management of adverse reaction of contrast agent and radiation protection. The purpose of these guidelines could were to provide the practical and effective management for nursing care in PET/MR imaging, and offer a framework for nurses that could provide useful and helpful in clinical practice and research.

[Key words]　Nursing; Positron-emission tomography; Magnetic resonance imaging
DOI: 10.13929/j.1003-3289.201702020

一体化 PET/MR 检查临床护理操作规范(2017 版)

韩斌如[1],帅冬梅[1],方继良[2],艾　林[3],兰晓莉[4],李　彪[5],左长京[6],卢　洁[1],李亚明[7*],

中华医学会核医学分会 PET/MR 脑功能成像工作委员会专家组

(1.首都医科大学宣武医院核医学科,北京　100053;2.中国中医科学院广安门医院放射科,

北京　100053;3.首都医科大学附属北京天坛医院核医学科,北京　100050;

4.华中科技大学同济医学院附属协和医院核医学科,湖北 武汉　430022;

5.上海交通大学医学院附属瑞金医院,上海　200025;6.第二军医大学

附属长海医院核医学科,上海　200433;7.中国医科大学附属

第一医院核医学科,辽宁 沈阳　110001)

[摘　要]　一体化 PET/MR 检查护理规范是关于 PET/MR 检查过程中对于护理人员的工作要求,包括检查前准备、注射药物护理、检查时护理、检查后护理、对比剂不良反应处理和个人辐射防护。旨在为核医学科护士在临床 PET/MR 检

[第一作者]韩斌如(1965—),女,北京人,硕士,主任护师、教授。研究方向:临床护理。E-mail: hanbinru8723@163.com
[通信作者]李亚明,中国医科大学附属第一医院核医学科,110001. E-mail: ymli2001@163.com
[收稿日期] 2017-02-07　　[修回日期] 2017-03-29

• 1620 •　　　　中国医学影像技术 2017 年第 33 卷第 11 期　Chin J Med Imaging Technol, 2017, Vol 33, No 11

❖ 中枢神经影像学

Hybrid PET/MR analysis of neural mechanism for default mode network

WANG Jingjuan[1], CUI Bixiao[1], YANG Hongwei[1], MA Jie[1],
LIANG Zhigang[1], LU Jie[1,2]*

(1. Department of Nuclear Medicine, 2. Department of Radiology, Xuanwu Hospital,
Capital Medical University, Beijing 100053, China)

[Abstract]　Objective　To investigate the relationship between spatial distribution of default mode network and glucose uptake. Methods　Nine healthy subjects were scanned with hybrid PET/MR. Resting state MRI (rs-fMRI) and PET data were obtained. Spatial distribution analysis was performed between default mode network and glucose uptake. The relationship between the functional connectivity of default mode network and the distribution of glucose uptake were further analyzed. Results　The similar spatial distribution pattern was found between default mode network and glucose uptake. Correlation between functional connectivity and glucose uptake in the default mode network showed that the best correlation coefficient between the values of functional connectivity and relative glucose uptake (rGU) was achieved in the right posterior cingulate cortex (r_s=0.833, P<0.001). Conclusion　Hybrid PET/MR is very important to investigate neural mechanism of default mode network.

[Key words]　Positron-emission tomography; Magnetic resonance imaging; Default mode network; Functional connection; Glucose uptake

DOI: 10.13929/j.1003-3289.201705124

一体化 PET/MR 分析脑默认网络工作机制

王静娟[1]，崔碧霄[1]，杨宏伟[1]，马　杰[1]，梁志刚[1]，卢　洁[1,2]*

(1.首都医科大学宣武医院核医学科,2.放射科,北京　100053)

[摘　要]　目的　利用一体化 PET/MR 探讨脑默认网络功能连接和葡萄糖代谢的空间相关性。方法　对 9 名健康人行一体化 PET/MR 脑成像,获得同步的静息态 MR 脑功能成像(fMRI)和 PET 图像。分析静息态脑默认网络脑区连接与葡萄糖摄取分布的相关性。结果　基于静息态 fMRI 的脑默认网络与 PET 图像高代谢区域有很好的空间分布相似性。相关性分析显示,右侧后扣带区域内脑功能连接值与相对葡萄糖摄取(rGU)值的相关性最显著(r_s=0.833,P<0.001)。结论　一体化 PET/MR 可为研究脑默认网络的神经生理机制提供新的手段。

[关键词]　正电子发射型体层摄影术;磁共振成像;脑默认网络;功能连接;葡萄糖摄取

[中图分类号]　R741.04;R817　[文献标识码]　A　　[文章编号]　1003-3289(2017)11-1620-04

　　关于人脑 PET 的研究[1-3]发现,人脑有些区域在

[基金项目]　国家自然科学基金(81671662,81522021)、十三五国家重点研发项目(2016YFC0103000)。
[第一作者]　王静娟(1987—),女,河南濮阳人,博士,技师。研究方向:医学影像技术与应用。E-mail:1127809851@qq.com
[通信作者]　卢洁,首都医科大学宣武医院核医学科,放射科,100053。E-mail:imaginglu@hotmail.com
[收稿日期]　2017-05-22　　[修回日期]　2017-08-29

静息状态较任务状态消耗能量更高,主要包括内侧前额叶、后扣带回、顶下小叶、内侧颞叶,这些脑区为脑默认网络组成部分,对维持人脑的基础功能具有重要作用。通过静息态脑功能 MRI(resting state functional MRI, rs-fMRI)种子点功能连接分析可显示正常人的脑默认网络。此外,临床研究[4]发现,阿尔茨海默病、帕金森综合征、癫痫、抑郁症、精神分裂症、自闭症患者

左侧边栏：首都医科大学宣武医院一体化 PET/MR 成果集

医学影像学杂志 2017 年第 27 卷第 9 期　　J Med Imaging Vol. 27 No. 9 2017

·综　　述·

一体化 PET/MR 在脑功能方面的研究进展

王静娟　综述，卢　洁　审校

（首都医科大学宣武医院核医学科　北京　100053）

【摘　要】　影像学是无创研究脑功能的重要途径。随着影像学技术的快速发展，从单模态磁共振成像、正电子发射断层成像，到多模态成像 PET/CT、PET/MR，多模态已经成为影像学发展的里程碑。目前最先进的多模态成像设备一体化 PET/MR 可以同时得到 PET 成像和 MRI 多序列成像，将两种成像技术结合，为进一步深入研究脑功能提供了可能。本文对目前脑功能方面的研究做一综述。

【关键词】　多模态成像技术；一体化 PET/MR；脑功能

中图分类号：R445.2；R742　　　　文献标识码：A　　　　文章编号：1006-9011（2017）09-1798-02

Progress of hybrid PET/MR in brain function study

WANG Jingjuan, LU Jie

Department of Nuclear Medicine, Xuanwu Hospital Capital Medical University, Beijing 100053, P. R. China

【Abstract】　Imaging is the important way to noninvasively explore brain function. With the rapid development of imaging technology, from single modality imaging magnetic resonance imaging, positron emission tomography to multimodality imaging PET/CT, PET/MR, multimodality imaging has been a milestone of medical imaging. As a novel multimodality imaging equipment, hybrid PET/MR could simultaneously gain PET and multiple sequence MR imaging, which provides the possibility to further explore brain function. The current studies of brain function are reviewed.

【Key words】　Multimodality imaging; Hybrid PET/MR; Brain function

脑功能研究一直是大家关注的热点，影像学是认识脑功能，探索脑功能的重要手段。近年来影像学设备快速发展，研究脑功能的设备主要有磁共振成像（magnetic resonance imaging，MRI）、正电子发射断层成像（positron emission tomography，PET）、PET/CT、以及目前最先进的一体化 PET/MR，为我们进一步深入探究脑机制提供了可能。一体化 PET/MR 能够同时提供 PET 脑代谢和 MRI 脑功能成像信息，逐渐在脑功能研究方面崭露头角。本文重点综述一体化 PET/MR 脑功能的研究进展。

1　功能核磁成像在脑功能方面的研究

MRI 是无创研究脑功能的影像手段，血氧水平依赖功能磁共振成像（blood oxygenation level dependent functional magnetic resonance imaging，BOLD-fMRI）可以无创动态地研究人脑功能活动，其基本原理是利用神经活动时氧合血红蛋白浓度增加导致 MRI 信号差异，从而间接反映脑内神经活动[1]。目前 fMRI 已经广泛应用于脑疾病、神经科学的研究。fMRI 分为任务态和静息态两种模式，任务态通过被试执行特定实验任务研究脑功能的定位，理解特定脑区的功能；静息态通过研究脑区间的功能连接，探索不同的脑功能网络，理解脑工作机制。静息态 fMRI 与任务态 fMRI 比较，具有简便易行，被试只需静卧，容易配合；研究者容易操作和控制扫描等优点，尤其适用于患者的研究。静息态 fMRI 数据分析的常用方法包括：局部一致性、低频波动、独立成分分析、种子点分析、因果模型分析、功能网络等[2,3]。目前，任务状和静息态 fMRI 都已经广泛应用于阿尔茨海默病（Alzheimer's disease，AD）、脑梗死、癫痫等疾病脑功能异常机制的研究[4-8]。

2　PET 成像技术在脑功能方面的研究

PET 是将标记了正电子核素的放射性药物注入被试体内，基于符合判选原理探测正电子核素湮灭后产生的符合光子数据，进而重建反映放射性药物活度分布的图像。通过使用特异性示踪剂测量和显示放射性药物在人体内的分布情况，从而确定体内某种代谢水平和生理功能，达到对疾病的早期诊断，具有很高的灵敏度和准确性。PET 检查分为静态扫描和动态扫描，静态扫描结果是三维灰度图像，显示一段时间的累积效应，研究放射性药物注入体内一段时间后脑内的分布情况，如 ^{18}F-FDG 显示脑内葡萄糖的代谢情况；由于放射性药物的浓度随时间变化，药物时间活度曲线需要若干时间段，每个时间段的扫描产生一帧图像，即动态 PET 扫描，如

基金项目：国家自然科学基金项目（编号：81522021，81671662）

作者简介：王静娟（1987-），女，河南濮阳人，中国科学院高能物理研究所，技师，主要从事影像数据处理工作

通信作者：卢洁　医学博士，博士生导师，主任医师　E-mail：imaginglu@otmoil.com

中国医学影像技术 2017 年第 33 卷第 8 期　Chin J Med Imaging Technol,2017,Vol 33,No 8　　　　　　　　　　　　　·5·

❖ 综述

Progresses of hybrid PET/MR in quantificative evaluation of cerebral blood flow

SHAN Yi, LU Jie*, LI Kun-cheng

(Department of Radiology, Xuanwu Hospital of Capital Medical University, Beijing Key Laboratory of Magnetic Resonance Imaging and Brain Informatics, Beijing 100053, China)

[Abstract]　The hybrid PET/MR has a unique advantage of simultaneous scanning of both PET and MRI images, which has been gradually applied in clinical practice,. In the clinical studies of severe brain diseases (such as cerebrovascular disease, brain tumor and epilepsy), accurate quantification of cerebral blood flow (CBF) can help to understand the etiology, pathogenesis, and to make early diagnosis as well as therapeutic solutions. The hybrid PET/MR can implement a noninvasive, convenient and accurate method of arterial input function for quantification of CBF. The application of the hybrid PET/MR in quantification of cerebral blood flow were reviewed in this article.

[Key words]　Magnetic resonance imaging; Positron-emission tomography; Cerebral blood flow

DOI:10.13929/j.1003-3289.201702090

一体化 PET/MR 评估脑血流量的研究进展

单　艺,卢　洁*,李坤成

(首都医科大学宣武医院放射科 北京磁共振成像脑信息学北京市重点实验室,北京　100053)

[摘　要]　一体化 PET/MR 技术具有一次扫描可同时获得 PET 和 MRI 图像的独特优势,目前已逐步应用于临床。准确定量分析脑血流量(CBF)对研究脑血管病、脑肿瘤、癫痫等脑部重大疾病的发病机制及临床转归具有重要价值。一体化 PET/MR 可实现无创、简便、准确获得动脉输入函数,从而精准定量 CBF。本文对一体化 PET/MR 评估 CBF 的研究进展进行综述。

[关键词]　磁共振成像;正电子发射体层摄影术;脑血流

[中图分类号]　R445.2;R817.4　[文献标识码]　A　[文章编号]　1003-3289(2017)08-0000-04

脑血流量(cerebral blood flow,CBF)对维持脑组织功能和代谢水平起决定性作用,精准定量 CBF 对脑部重大疾病的早期诊断、评估病情、制定诊疗方案及评价疗效具有重要价值。一体化 PET/MR 具有同步扫描的独特优势,一次扫描可同时获得 PET 和 MRI 图像,并可实现图像的精确配准、融合,为定量评估 CBF 提供了新方法。本文对一体化 PET/MR 评估 CBF 的研究进展进行综述。

1　CBF 的概念及其临床意义

1.1　CBF 的概念
CBF 指每 100 g 脑组织单位时间内通过的血流量,是脑灌注成像最常用的参数之一。脑灌注成像可评价血流通过毛细血管网、将携带的氧气及营养物质输送至脑组织并加以利用的过程,反映特定脑区的血流动力学状态及功能。CBF 的升高或降低直接反映脑组织功能代谢水平。

1.2　定量 CBF 的临床意义
脑部重大疾病如缺血性脑卒中、阿尔茨海默病(Alzheimer disease,AD)、癫痫、脑肿瘤等,均可因局部血脑屏障被破坏等病理生理

[基金项目]国家自然科学基金面上项目(81671662)、国家重点研发计划项目(2016YFC0103001)、北京市医院管理局重点医学专业发展计划(ZYLX201609)。

[第一作者]单艺(1990—),女,北京人,硕士,医师。研究方向:脑血管病的磁共振诊断。E-mail:shanyiedu@hotmail.com

[通信作者]卢洁,首都医科大学宣武医院放射科 北京磁共振成像脑信息学北京市重点实验室,100053。E-mail:imaginglu@hotmail.com

[收稿日期]2016-02-22　　[修回日期]2017-06-10

首都医科大学宣武医院一体化 PET/MR 成果集

· 564 ·　　　　　　　　　　　　实用肿瘤学杂志　2017 年第 31 卷第 6 期总第 152 期

PET/MRI 在高级别脑胶质瘤放射治疗中的应用

赵永瑞　**综述**　徐建堃　**审校**

【摘要】　脑胶质瘤是最常见的原发性神经系统肿瘤,其中高级别胶质瘤生长迅速,常呈浸润性生长,且治疗后易复发,死亡率和致残率都很高。手术切除仍是高级别胶质瘤的首选治疗方法,术后放射治疗则是其重要的辅助治疗手段之一。目前放射治疗多以 MRI 图像指导靶区的勾画,但 MRI 在肿瘤显像方面仍存在局限性。随着多种放射性示踪剂的研究及应用,PET 能够通过肿瘤组织的代谢变化来反映肿瘤的浸润范围,还有助于鉴别放射性坏死与肿瘤复发。PET/MRI 的联合应用在高级别脑胶质瘤的放射治疗中具有很好的应用前景。

【关键词】　高级别脑胶质瘤;正电子发射断层显像术;磁共振显像;放射治疗

【中图分类号】　R739.41　【文献标识码】　A

doi:10.11904/j.issn.1002 - 3070.2017.06.016

The application of PET/MRI in high – grade glioma by radiotherapy

ZHAO Yongrui,*XU Jiankun*

Department of Radiation Oncology,Xuanwu Hospital,Capital Medical University,Beijing 100053,China

【Abstract】　Brain glioma is the most common primary nervous system tumors,in which high – grade glioma grows rapidly,often infiltrates growth,and easy recurrence after treatment. Its mortality and morbidity are still high. Surgical resection is the preferred treatment for high – grade glioma. Postoperative radiotherapy is one of the important adjuvant therapy. At present,tumor radiotherapy was guided the sketch of the target area by MRI images,but MRI imaging has limitations. With the development and application of a variety of radioactive tracers,PET reflects the extent of tumor infiltration through the metabolic changes of tumor tissue,and also helps to identify radioactive necrosis and tumor recurrence. The combination of PET/MRI has a good prospect in the radiotherapy of high – grade glioma.

【Key words】　High – grade glioma;Positron emission tomography;Magnetic resonance imaging;Radiotherapy

　　脑胶质瘤是颅内最常见的原发性神经系统肿瘤,约占颅内肿瘤的 46%。世界卫生组织(WHO)根据肿瘤生物学行为及病理表现将其分为 Ⅰ ~ Ⅳ级,其中 Ⅲ、Ⅳ 级为高级别脑胶质瘤,主要包括间变性星形细胞瘤、间变性少突胶质细胞瘤、间变性少突星形胶质细胞瘤和胶质母细胞瘤等,占到颅内胶质瘤的 60% 以上[1],具有弥漫性浸润性生长特性。立体定向活检研究表明在肿瘤周围脑组织区域内仍伴有肿瘤组织浸润,这些区域使用增强 CT 或 MRI 等检查手段与正常脑组织无法区分。因此,对高级别胶质细胞瘤而言,很难做到真正意义上的生物学全切除,其标准治疗原则为最大安全程度的切除辅助放、化疗。

　　然而当前高级别胶质瘤的治疗效果并不满意,WHO Ⅲ/Ⅳ 级胶质瘤患者的中位生存期分别为 2 ~ 5 年和 12 ~ 15 个月[2],为进一步提高局部控制率和生存率就需要明确划定高复发风险区域并尽可能减少正常脑组织的照射。在放疗计划制定中早已将 CT 与 MRI 图像融合,MRI 主要偏向于解剖结构,为肿瘤提供了很好的形态学诊断,在脑胶质瘤分级、手术定位和术后放疗靶区勾画中有着重要的作用。但是,越来越多的研究发现,MRI 在肿瘤显像方面仍存在局限性,如不能准确地反映术后残留肿瘤的位置和范围、不能辨别肿瘤复发进展与治疗后改变等方面。PET 利用组织代谢原理进行功能显像,通过肿瘤组织的代谢变化来反映肿瘤的浸润

作者单位:首都医科大学宣武医院(北京　100053)

作者简介:赵永瑞,男,(1989 -),硕士,住院医师,从事肿瘤放疗工作的研究。

通讯作者:徐建堃,E - mail:xjk_7563@163.com

中国医学影像技术 2017 年第 33 卷第 9 期　Chin J Med Imaging Technol，2017，Vol 33，No 9　　　　　　　　　　　　　• 1401 •

❖影像技术学

Comparision of SUV$_{max}$ of TOF-PET/MR and TOF-PET/CT in body malignant tumor

SONG Tianbin[1]，LU Jie[1,2*]，CUI Bixiao[1]，MA Jie[1]，
YANG Hongwei[1]，MA Lei[1]，LIANG Zhigang[1]
(1. Department of Nuclear Medicine，2. Department of Radiology，Xuanwu Hospital，
Capital Medical University，Beijing 100053，China)

[Abstract]　Objective　To explore the consistency of time-of-flight (TOF) technology of PET/MRI and PET/CT for max standardized uptake value (SUV$_{max}$) of body malignant tumors. Methods　A retrospective analysis of TOF-PET/CT and TOF-PET/MR imaging data about twenty patients with body malignant tumors was performed. Patients were divided into two groups (each $n=10$), including PET/CT first and sequentially PET/MR group and PET/MR first and sequentially PET/CT group. Bland-Altman figure was used to evaluate consistency of SUV$_{max}$ of malignant lesions between TOF-PET/CT and TOF-PET/MR. Multi-way ANOVA was used to analysis effect of machine type and exam order on SUV$_{max}$ of malignant lesions in TOF-PET/CT and TOF-PET/MR. Results　SUV$_{max}$ of malignant lesions in TOF-PET/CT and TOF-PET/MR had good consistency in two groups (PET/CT first and sequentially PET/MR group: Mean difference was 3.06, 95%CI was [−7.5, 13.6]; PET/MR first and sequentially PET/CT group: Mean difference was 3.0, 95%CI was [−2.4, 8.3]). SUV$_{max}$ was not influenced by machine type ($F=0.005$, $P=0.95$), but exam order ($F=46.00$, $P<0.001$). Conclusion　PET/MR and PET/CT with TOF technology have comparative diagnostic value in SUV$_{max}$ of body malignant lesions. SUV$_{max}$ of body malignant lesions increases in delay time, which is not related to machine type, but exam time.
[Key words]　Time-of-flight; Positron-emission tomography, emission-computed; Magnetic resonance imaging; Tomography, X-ray computed; Fluorodeoxyglucose; Standardized uptake value
DOI:10.13929/j.1003-3289.201705157

TOF-PET/MR 和 TOF-PET/CT 在体部
恶性肿瘤 SUV$_{max}$ 值的比较

宋天彬[1]，卢　洁[1,2*]，崔碧霄[1]，马　杰[1]，杨宏伟[1]，马　蕾[1]，梁志刚[1]
(1.首都医科大学宣武医院核医学科，2.放射科，北京　100053)

[摘　要]　目的　探讨时间飞行(TOF)技术 PET/CT 和 PET/MR 检查体部恶性病变 SUV$_{max}$ 值的一致性。方法　回顾性分析接受 TOF-PET/CT 和 TOF-PET/MR 检查的体部恶性肿瘤患者 20 例，分为先 PET/CT 后 PET/MR 组和先 PET/MR 后 PET/CT 组，每组 10 例。采用 Bland-Altman 图评价两次检查病灶 SUV$_{max}$ 值的一致性，采用多因素方差分析评价扫描顺序和机器类型对病灶的 SUV$_{max}$ 测量值的影响。结果　TOF-PET/CT 与 TOF-PET/MR 检查病灶的 SUV$_{max}$ 值有较好的一致性[先 PET/CT 后 PET/MR 组：均值差为 3.06，95%CI(−7.5,13.6)，先 PET/MR 后 PET/CT 组：均值差 3.0，95%CI(−2.4,8.3)]。扫描顺序对于恶性病灶的 SUV$_{max}$ 有影响($F=46.00$,$P<0.001$)，而机器类型对恶性病灶的 SUV$_{max}$ 值无影响($F=0.005$,$P=0.95$)。结论　TOF-PET/MR 和 TOF-PET/CT 在体部恶性病变 SUV$_{max}$ 值测量方面具有相当的诊断价值，且延迟显像 SUV$_{max}$ 的增加与采集时间有关，而与检查机器类型无关。

[第一作者]宋天彬(1984—)，男，山西阳泉人，硕士，医师。研究方向：PET/MR 在体部肿瘤中的临床应用。E-mail：songtb_1984@163.com
[通信作者]卢洁，首都医科大学宣武医院核医学科，100053；首都医科大学宣武医院放射科，100053。E-mail：imaginglu@hotmail.com

[收稿日期]2017-05-29　　[修回日期]2017-07-25

第一章 一体化 PET/MR 科研成果

首都医科大学宣武医院一体化PET/MR成果集

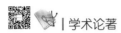 | 学术论著

中国医学装备2017年11月第14卷第11期 China Medical Equipment 2017 November Vol.14 No.11

不同重建条件对一体化PET-MR 图像空间分辨率影响的研究*

庄静文① 谢峰① 吴天棋① 白玫①*

[文章编号] 1672-8270(2017)11-0012-04　　[中图分类号] R812　[文献标识码] A

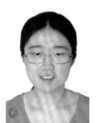

[摘要] 目的：通过模型实验研究，对比不同重建条件对一体化PET-MR图像空间分辨率的影响。方法：参考美国电器制造商协会(NEMA)标准制备点源，使用美国GE公司的Signa PET-MR设备进行扫描，选择不同PET图像重建条件重建图像，读取图像中点源的半高宽(FWHM)，对比飞行时间技术(TOF)、点扩散函数(PSF)、迭代次数以及衰减校正(AC)对于图像空间分辨率的影响。结果：使用PSF技术重建图像，电源FWHM在3.40 mm与4.31 mm之间，而未使用PSF技术重建的图像点源FWHM在4.56 mm与5.83 mm之间，故使用PSF可减小重建图像中点源的FWHM，而TOF和AC对点源FWHM影响不大。结论：PSF和迭代次数可以有效提高图像空间分辨率，TOF和AC对于图像空间分辨率影响不大。在临床使用PET-MR对病灶扫描时应将患者置于孔径中心，在对小病灶的诊断中，PSF技术的使用必不可少，且可根据实际情况适当增加迭代次数。

[关键词] 一体化PET-MR；重建方法；空间分辨率
DOI: 10.3969/J.ISSN.1672-8270.2017.11.004

Research on influence of different reconstruction condition for the spatial resolution of integrative PET-MR image/ZHUANG Jing-wen, XIE Feng, WU Tian-qi, et al//China Medical Equipment,2017,14(11):12-15.
[Abstract] Objective: To compare the influence of different reconstruction condition for the spatial resolution of integrative PET-MR image through experiment research of model. Methods: The standard of NEMA was referred to produce point source, and the signa PET-MR of GE was used to implement scan. Different image reconstruction condition of PET were used to reconstruct image, and then the FWHM of point source were obtained. The influences of TOF, PSF, iterations and AC for spatial resolution of image were compared. Results: The point source FWHM was between 3.40~4.31mm when PSF technique was used to reconstruct image, while it was 4.56~5.83mm without PSF technique. Therefore, PSF could reduce FWHM in reconstructed image. Besides, there were few influences of TOF and AC for FWHM. Conclusion: PSF and iterations could effectively enhance spatial resolution of image, while there were few the influences of TOF and AC for FWHM. In the scan for lesions by using PET-MR, patients should be placed on centre of aperture. And in the diagnosis for small lesion, the using of PSF technique is necessary, and the iteration should properly be increased as the actual situation.
[Key words] Integrative PET-MR; Reconstruction method; Spatial resolution
[First-author's address] Department of Medical Engineering, Xuanwu Hospital of Capital Medical University, Beijing 100053, China.

作者简介

庄静文，女，(1990—)，硕士，助理工程师。首都医科大学宣武医院医学工程处，研究方向：医学影像设备图像质量。

近年来，多模式成像技术进展飞速，正电子发射计算机断层摄影术(positron emission tomography，PET)具有高灵敏度和精准定量的特点，但PET图像却不能清晰显示脏器的解剖结构，因此无法准确对病灶进行定位[1]。核磁共振(magnetic resonance，MR)技术可提供清晰的软组织解剖结构和准确的病灶位置，弥补了PET图像的不足。一体化PET-MR是将PET和MR两种技术有机结合起来的最先进的分子成像设备，由于其具有同时进行PET和MR成像的功能，并且降低了两者硬件之间的相互影响，已经被应用于临床前期研究和临床诊断中[2-3]。作为当今多模式分子显像技术[4]的前沿，PET-MR图像性能和质量已成为行业内关注的焦点，因此很多重建技术应运而生，并被应用于一体化PET-MR图像的重建以提高设备性能和图像质量。

衰减校正(attenuation correction，AC)使重建后的图像具有精准定量化功能，目前一体化PET-MR系统中应用于PET图像的AC方法是采用MR图像信息(即MRAC)，并使用图像分割技术获得脏器不同组织的成分，然后对PET图像进行AC[4]。飞行时间技术(time-of-flight，TOF)产生于20世纪80年代初期，是PET图像重建中应用十分广泛的一种技术，通过测量湮灭光子到达探测器的飞行时间，从而确定放射性核素分布的一种方法，TOF在提高图像信噪比、降低

*基金项目：国家重点研发计划数字诊疗装备研发专项课题(2016YFC0103909) "PET/MR在神经系统疾病中的高级临床应用"
①首都医科大学宣武医院医学工程处 北京 100053
*通讯作者：jswei65@163.com

·802· 中华核医学与分子影像杂志 2017 年 12 月第 37 卷第 12 期 Chin J Nucl Med Mol Imaging, Dec. 2017, Vol. 37, No. 12

·综述·

PET/fMRI 对异常脑活动的精准定位：研究进展与展望

臧玉峰 冯逢 霍力 李彪 兰晓莉 卢洁 田嘉禾 赵周社 Huang Yiyun
311121 杭州师范大学心理科学研究院认知与脑疾病研究中心、浙江省认知障碍评估技术研究重点实验室(臧玉峰);100730 中国医学科学院、北京协和医学院北京协和医院放射科(冯逢),核医学科(霍力);200025 上海交通大学医学院附属瑞金医院核医学科(李彪);430022 武汉,华中科技大学同济医学院附属协和医院核医学科、湖北省分子影像重点实验室(兰晓莉);100053 北京,首都医科大学宣武医院核医学科(卢洁);100853 北京,解放军总医院核医学科(田嘉禾);100176 北京,GE 药业(中国)(赵周社);美国耶鲁大学 PET 中心(Huang Yiyun)
通信作者:臧玉峰, Email: zangyf@ gmail.com
DOI:10.3760/cma.j.issn.2095-2848.2017.12.014

【摘要】 许多脑疾病无明显病灶,其病因可能是源于脑活动或脑区连通性的异常。目前常用的脑成像诊断技术很难对其异常脑活动进行精准定位。新近发展起来的 PET/MR 一体同步显像技术或能弥补此缺陷。该设备已经用于临床诊断,但主要还是利用了 PET 功能影像与 MRI 结构影像的结合,远远没有发挥其"功能-功能"结合的诸多优势。目前,国际上 PET/fMRI 的研究尚处于起步阶段。初步研究表明,PET 与 fMRI 常用功能指标之间的相关性并不高,提示 2 种功能指标可能揭示了不同的生理、病理机制。目前,我国大型研究型医院已经安装了至少 5 台一体化 PET/MR 设备。相对来说,我国的优势在于病源充足,PET 影像发展迅速,且在 fMRI 的计算方法学方面有较高的国际地位。PET/fMRI 的研究通常需要多学科的合作,包括核医学、放射学、化学、医用物理学、影像计算方法学、认知神经科学等等,我国医院的科研管理体制还需要改进,以满足这种多学科高度交叉合作的需求。利用自身优势,改进自身科研管理体制,再加上多中心合作,相信我国在 PET/fMRI 的研究方面能够很快达到国际一流水平,并取得既有科学价值、又有临床价值的科研成果。
【关键词】 脑疾病;诊断;正电子发射断层显像术;磁共振成像;发展趋势
基金项目:国家自然科学基金(81520108016,31471084,81661148045,81671662,81271544)

PET/fMRI for precise localization of abnormal brain activity: a mini review *Zang Yufeng, Feng Feng, Huo Li, Li Biao, Lan Xiaoli, Lu Jie, Tian Jiahe, Zhao Zhoushe, Huang Yiyun*
Center for Cognition and Brain Disorders, Institutes of Psychological Sciences, Hangzhou Normal University, Zhejiang Key Laboratory for Research in Assessment of Cognitive Impairments, Hangzhou 311121, China (Zang YF); Department of Radiology, Peking Union Medical College Hospital, Peking Union Medical College, Chinese Academy of Medical Sciences, Beijing 100730, China (Feng F); Department of Nuclear Medicine, Peking Union Medical College Hospital, Peking Union Medical College, Chinese Academy of Medical Sciences, Beijing 100730, China (Huo L); Department of Nuclear Medicine, Ruijin Hospital, Shanghai Jiao Tong University School of Medicine, Shanghai 200025, China (Li B); Department of Nuclear Medicine, Union Hospital, Tongji Medical College, Huazhong University of Science and Technology, Wuhan 430022, China (Lan XL); Department of Nuclear Medicine, Xuanwu Hospital, Capital Medical University, Beijing 100053, China (Lu J); Department of Nuclear Medicine, General Hospital of PLA, Beijing 100853, China (Tian JH); MR Modality, GE Healthcare China, Beijing 100176, China (Zhao ZS); PET Center, Yale University (Huang YY)
Corresponding author: Zang Yufeng, Email: zangyf@ gmail.com
【Abstract】 Many brain disorders do not show visible lesions and most likely are resulted from abnormalities in regional brain activity or connectivity. Conventional diagnostic neuroimaging techniques are not capable of precisely localizing the abnormal brain activity, but the recently developed integrated PET/MR technology may have the potential to bridge this gap. Integrated PET/MR has been used in clinical practice. However, its primary application is still a combination of functional PET imaging and structural MRI. Simultaneous PET/fMRI, a "functional+functional" imaging technique, holds the advantages of high spatial and temporal resolution, high sensitivity and specificity, and non-invasiveness. Globally, simultaneous PET/fMRI research is still in its beginning stage, and a few initial PET/fMRI studies have shown that voxel-wise correlation between PET and fMRI metrics was not very high, indicating that they may reflect very different as-

中华核医学与分子影像杂志 2016 年 12 月第 36 卷第 6 期　Chin J Nucl Med Mol Imaging, Dec. 2016, Vol. 36, No. 6　　　　　· 547 ·

三维定位与分析。在前期成像技术研究的基础上,结合核素放射激发荧光断层成像的信号特点,构建一种核素放射激发荧光断层成像的新算法,实现由二维透射平面累加成像跨越到三维空间定位定量成像,达到肿瘤细胞的定位、定量及分析。激发产生的荧光属于电磁波的一种,其在生物组织中的传输过程可以用辐射传输方程精确描述。然而,辐射传输方程是一个复杂的积分-微分方程,对于复杂的生物体目前并不能求解。为了克服这个难题,考虑到光在生物组织表现出高散射的特性,将辐射传输方程简化为易于求解的扩散方程,然后使用有限元方法进行离散,最终将光在生物组织的传输转换为线性方程组进行求解。这不仅简化了求解过程,提高了重建速度,更便于设计更加有效的优化求解算法。在线性方程组求解的过程中,考虑到切伦科夫光谱范围广(从蓝紫光谱段到近红外光谱段)、信号弱等特点,利用 CT、PET 等其他显像技术获取结构数据和功能数据等先验信息,提出了一种快速、准确的混合谱核素放射性激发荧光光源重建方法,实现荧光信号的准确定位。该方法在重建精度方面可实现对小于 2 mm 肿瘤的早期检测,同时与多光谱重建算法相比,可极大缩短数据采集时间和重建时间。在获取了肿瘤空间位置分布后,更需通过定量指标判断肿瘤代谢与生长过程。核素放射激发荧光断层成像的定量问题是要建立核素放射激发荧光信号与肿瘤生物学参数信息间的定量关系。研究将依次探索稀土纳米探针的荧光功率与肿瘤摄取的放射性核素计量间、肿瘤摄取核素计量与肿瘤细胞数目间、肿瘤细胞数目与肿瘤状态间的关系,并通过定量研究实现肿瘤组织的早期检测与恶化程度预测,进而为肿瘤治疗方案的设计提供充分信息。

目前此成像研究仍处于前期预临床探究阶段,主要针对小动物开展在体研究。本研究团队为中科院分子影像重点实验室,在探针制备、细胞培养、动物模型构建方面积累一定,并长期与国内各大医院开展积极合作与交流,这对核素放射激发荧光断层成像新技术的预临床研究提供了很大的帮助。

四、预期效益

研究成果可为肿瘤早期诊断探索提供更为精准的定量成像新模式,具有广阔的生物医学应用空间,如抗肿瘤药物疗效评价、早期检测、手术导航等。核素放射激发荧光断层成像新方法是光学分子影像的一次理论突破,也是新一代医学影像手段的重要探究,可实现微小肿瘤的早期精准检测与定位,为肿瘤切除制定更加合理科学的方案。

利益冲突　无

本文直接使用的缩略语:CLI(Cerenkov luminescence imaging),切伦科夫光学成像;CR(Cerenkov radiation),切伦科夫辐射;FDG(fluorodeoxyglucose),脱氧葡萄糖;MTT(3-(4,5-dimethylthiazol-2-yl)-2,5-diphenyltetrazolium bromide),四甲基偶氮唑蓝

(收稿日期:2016-09-20)

·新技术介绍·

一体化 TOF PET/MR 影像技术实现精准定量脑血流量

卢洁　刘振宇　李亚明

100053　北京,首都医科大学宣武医院核医学科(卢洁);100190　北京,中国科学院自动化研究所分子影像重点实验室(刘振宇);110001　沈阳,中国医科大学附属第一医院核医学科(李亚明)

通信作者:卢洁,Email:imaginglu@hotmail.com

基金项目:2016 年国家科技部十三五重点研发计划数字诊疗装备专项(2016YFC0103001)

DOI:10.3760/cma.j.issn.2095-2848.2016.06.016

Study of quantitative cerebral blood flow using integrated TOF PET/MR　*Lu Jie, Liu Zhenyu, Li Yaming Department of Nuclear Medicine, Xuanwu Hospital Affiliated to Captial Medical University, Beijing 100053, China (Lu J); Key Laboratory of Molecular Imaging of Chinese Academy of Sciences, Institute of Automation, Chinese Academy of Sciences, Beijing 100190, China (Liu ZY); Department of Nuclear Medicine, the First Hospital of China Medical University, Shenyang 110001, China (Li YM)*

Corresponding author: Lu Jie, Email: imaginglu@hotmail.com

Fund program: The National Key Research and Development Program of China (2016YFC0103001)

脑血流量对维持正常脑功能起决定作用。脑部疾病(如脑血管病、痴呆等)导致脑血流异常,从而出现各种功能障碍。因此,准确定量脑血流量,对脑疾病的早期诊治有重要价值。"一体化 TOF PET/MR 脑血流定量方法研究及在脑疾病的应用"获 2016 年国家科技部十三五重点研发计划数字诊疗装备专项(2016YFC0103001)经费支持,此项目有望在实现无创精准定量脑血流量方面有重大突破。

一、背景

目前影像学检查中只有 PET 是定量脑血流量的准确方法,但由于传统 PET 方法需连续多次采集患者动脉血,因此无法在临床普及。图像衍生动脉输入函数(imaged-derived arterial input function, IDAIF)法不需采血,但需 PET 和 MRI 图像配准获得动脉输入函数,图像后处理复杂,且易导致配准误差。随着影像学仪器硬件的发展,一体化 PET/MR 仪出现,为研究脑血流量提供了新方法。一体化 PET/MR 具有同步扫描的独特优势,一次扫描可同时获得 PET 和 MRI 图像,MRI 高分辨率解剖图像能够很好地显示颈内动脉,PET 和 MRI 2 种图像精确配准融合,无需后处理就可简便、准确获

第一章 一体化PET/MR科研成果

护理园地

一体化PET/MRI检查的护理配合

帅冬梅,卢 洁*,梁志刚,宣 萱,马 蕾

(北京宣武医院 核医学科,北京 100053)

近年来,临床PET和MRI一体化机器备受关注,一次检查能提供解剖和代谢等综合信息,MRI不仅能提供很好的软组织对比度、降低电离辐射,而且提供多种MRI技术,如功能、波谱和扩散张量成像,在神经系统疾病、肿瘤、心血管和儿科等疾病诊断、疗效评估以及指导个体化治疗均具有重要价值[1]。2015年我院对中国首台GE公司一体化TOF-PET-MRI进行临床研究,对于这一国际最前沿的成像检查,需要护士既具备PET检查的护理知识,又要掌握MRI检查的护理技能,检查过程中对患者的护理直接影响图像采集的成功与否,现将护理体会报告如下。

1 资料与方法

1.1 一般资料

2015年7~10月我科40例患者静脉注射18F-FDG行一体化PET/MRI检查,其中男24例、女16例;年龄21~82岁。临床诊断脑血管病12例、肿瘤20例,其余8例为硬脊膜动静脉瘘、炎性病变、肿瘤筛查。40例患者中17例行MRI增强检查。

1.2 显像设备与方法

PET/MRI机型为GE公司SIGNA一体化TOF-PET-MRI。18F-FDG由本科放射性药物实验室自行制备,经物理学、化学、生物学检测,各项指标合格,放射化学纯度>96%,显像剂通过伦理委员会论证和审批。参照我科检查规程[2,3],分别对脑部疾患、肿瘤及其他疾病患者静脉注射18F-FDG 1mci/kg进行成像。所有患者或患者家属在检查前均签署了知情同意书。40例患者中17例行局部MRI增强检查。

2 护理

2.1 检查前准备

护士检查前向患者及家属告知该检查的目的、意义、方法等,由于注射的18F-FDG示踪剂具有一定放射性,MRI增强检查的对比剂有过敏风险,而且检查时间较长,患者及家属难免产生焦虑不安、恐惧等心理,尤其对肿瘤患者护理人员更应认真倾听他们的需求,了解其心理状况,耐心回答受检者和家属提出的每一个问题,详细讲解检查流程和注意事项,以便能够更好的配合检查。

患者检查前需禁食水4~6h,监测血糖在4~10mmol/L,血糖低的患者给予25g葡萄糖口服;血糖高的患者需提前给予皮下胰岛素或口服降糖药治疗,以使血糖在正常水平,保证检查的准确性。由于MRI采用的是强磁场,因此需要排除有检查禁忌证的患者,如:装有心脏起搏器、人工心脏瓣膜、电子耳蜗植入、心脏监护装置和呼吸机的危重患者等。患者更换检查服,避免衣服有金属物品。禁止将手机、手表、磁卡、钥匙、发卡、项链、假肢和人工关节等金属带进扫描间。有假牙的患者 检查前去除假牙。盆腔检查患者,金属节育环需取出后方可检查。了解患者手部血液循环情况,选择血管明显、弹性好、无皮肤损伤及结痂的手背部静脉血管,常规消毒后进行留置针穿刺,穿刺成功将美敷贴妥善固定穿刺针,防止针尖移动,减少针尖对血管的刺激,并给予生理盐水4ml进行封管。用药准备 我科取得第四类《放射性药品使用许可证》,参照文献和我科放射性药物实验室生产规范[3,4],自行制备18F-FDG显像剂,通过医院伦理委员会论证审批,并在北京市食品药品监督管理局备案。患者准备完毕,护士穿铅衣、戴铅帽、铅围脖、铅镜、手套等防护设备,药物到达后根据患者体重将18F-FDG(1mci/kg)进行药物分装,应用活度计测量准确的活度,进行静脉注射,完毕后给予生理盐水4ml经行封管。MRI对比剂为Gd-DTPA,剂量为0.1mmol/kg,进行静脉注射。

2.2 检查中的护理

2.2.1 注射药物的护理

检查过程中注意周围环境温度、患者肢体循环、患者是否保暖,以保证其血流通畅。只注射18F-FDG的患者留一条静脉通路,在建立好的静脉通路上给予生理盐水4ml冲管,确定静脉通畅后常规速度注入示踪剂,注射完毕后再快速注入生理盐水4ml冲洗管道,防止示踪剂残留在针头处,保证有效的注射剂量,拔除留置针,并将留置针及注射完毕的注射器放入活度计中测量残余量,准确记录给药时间、部位及注射剂量。本组17例患者中7例MRI增强检查患者应用与18F-FDG一条静脉通路,均在留置针处有不同程度的示踪剂浓聚现象,因此其余10例MRI增强患者均留建立两条静脉通路,在留置针数料外标注1、2号,1号为18F-FDG通路,2号为MRI对比剂通路。18F-FDG与MRI对比剂不用同一条通路静脉通路给药,从而解决了示踪剂浓聚问题,保证影像的准确性。患者交谈及运动都会影响检查的准确性,且示踪剂18F-FDG需在体内停留45min才能达到峰值进行检查,所以注射后告知患者需关闭灯光进行视听封闭留在候诊室安静休息等待检查。

MRI增强检查使用高压注射器,按无菌操作将药物抽吸到双筒高压注射器针筒中,生理盐水冲洗静脉通道的用量为50~100ml,常规消毒预留留置针静脉通路进行连接,

(下转第260页)

* 本文通讯作者。

收稿日期:2016-02-26 修回日期:2016-03-26

2015 年 1 月至 2022 年 12 月，获批 PET/MR 相关科研项目 28 项，其中科技部重点研发项目 4 项，国家自然科学基金重点项目 1 项、面上项目 4 项、青年基金项目 6 项、省部级项目 13 项。

1. 项目名称：基于国产 PET/MR 的脑重大疾病诊疗解决方案研究

项目负责人： 卢洁

项目来源： "十四五" 科技部重点研发项目

项目编号： 2022YFC2406900

研究年限： 2022.11—2025.10

资助金额： 中央财政经费 1000 万元，自筹 3000 万元。

项目简介： 我国脑重大疾病发病率居世界首位，给社会和家庭造成沉重负担，其临床诊治复杂，早筛早诊是临床防治关键。影像学检查是诊断脑疾病的重要手段，一体化 PET/MR 是目前医学影像领域最前沿的设备，可同步获取病灶的高清结构、功能、分子多模态信息，对脑疾病早期精准个体化诊断和微创或无创治疗精准定位靶点具有重要价值。由于国产 PET/MR 临床应用尚处于起步阶段，亟须开展其在脑疾病诊疗的临床应用研究，本项注重目培养复合型医师、技术员等人才，对助力国产设备达到国际领先水平具有重大意义。项目分为 6 个课题：①研究脑疾病早期诊断特异性 PET 示踪剂及其临床应用；②制定脑重大疾病 PET/MR 成像规范化流程；③构建脑重大疾病 PET/MR 图像处理及定量阈值；④ PET/MR 在脑重大疾病精准诊断及靶点定位的临床研究；⑤基于 PET/MR 对脑重大疾病无创 / 微创治疗的临床效果进行评价；⑥建立国产 PET/MR 及相关产品在脑疾病应用的评价体系。最终实现国产 PET/MR 脑疾病早期精准诊疗，推动其临床应用，提高国际竞争力，实现替代国外产品的突破，为我国政府制定脑疾病防控政策提供重要依据。

2. 项目名称：脑血流联合脑代谢早期诊断阿尔茨海默病的一体化 PET/MR 研究

项目负责人： 闫少珍

项目来源： 北京市医院管理中心青年人才培养 "青苗" 计划

项目编号： QMS20220820

研究年限： 2023.01—2024.12

资助金额： 6 万元

项目简介： 阿尔茨海默病是老年痴呆最常见的类型（占 50% ~ 75%），轻度认知障碍是阿尔茨海默病的临床前期阶段，每年有 10% ~ 15% 的轻度认知障碍患者进展为阿尔茨海默病。目前全世界尚无阿尔茨海默病的确切治愈方法，但早期诊断可减少约 30%、延缓约 5 年发病，因此早筛、早诊、早干预是临床防治的关键。本项目旨在探讨阿尔茨海默病、轻度认知障碍和认知正常老年人的脑血流灌注及葡萄糖代谢改变模式，评估 ASL 与 ^{18}F-FDG PET 联合早期诊断阿尔茨海默病价值，为早期诊断阿尔茨海默病提供影像学依据，延缓阿尔茨海默病病程进展，减轻中国老龄化社会压力。

3. 项目名称：基于人工智能的多模态跨尺度影像评估颈动脉粥样硬化斑块易损性研究

项目负责人：卢洁

项目来源：国家自然科学基金重点项目

项目编号：82130058

研究年限：2022.01—2026.12

资助金额：290 万元

项目简介：本项目拟联合应用一体化 PET/MR 及 IVOCT 成像对颈动脉粥样硬化斑块易损性进行研究，研发多模态、跨尺度影像数据的新型人工智能融合分析方法，提取易损斑块的宏观、微观结构及代谢特征，构建智能化斑块分类决策模型，并通过纵向随访验证模型的准确性，阐明颈动脉粥样硬化斑块跨尺度影像学特征及其内在联系，揭示斑块易损性的病理生理机制，实现对缺血性脑血管病的早期预警，指导临床个体化精准诊疗。

4. 项目名称：阿尔茨海默病海马功能和代谢网络关系机制的一体化 PET/MR 研究

项目负责人：闫少珍

项目来源：国家自然科学基金青年项目

项目编号：82102010

研究年限：2022.01—2024.12

资助金额：30 万元

项目简介：阿尔茨海默病以进行性认知功能障碍为早期临床特征，海马是阿尔茨海默病最早受累的脑区之一，且与记忆功能障碍密切相关，早期评估海马功能及与认知功能障碍的动态变化关系有望进一步揭示阿尔茨海默病病理生理机制并有助于早期诊断阿尔茨海默病。无创影像学技术为检测海马功能损伤提供了重要手段，高分辨结构 MRI 可精准定量海马体积，静息态功能 MRI 能提供海马功能网络变化情况，^{18}F-FDG PET 可定量监测海马代谢信息，一体化 PET/MR 具有同步扫描的独特优势，可将 MRI 及 PET 图像精准融合，一次扫描便可提取阿尔茨海默病同一生理状态下海马结构、功能网络和代谢特征，是综合、精准获取脑影像数据的强有力手段。因此，本项目采用一体化 ^{18}F-FDG PET/MR 探究阿尔茨海默病海马结构、功能网络和代谢网络损伤特征及其内在联系，并纵向随访，观察阿尔茨海默病海马功能网络与代谢网络动态演变特征及其与神经认知功能的相关性，以期发现海马功能损伤与疾病发展动态变化之间的关系，阐明阿尔茨海默病海马损伤机制，获得早期精准诊断的神经影像学标记，从而为阿尔茨海默病早期预警和干预提供新思路。

5. 项目名称：基于 ^{18}F-NaF PET/MR 评价颅内动脉粥样硬化斑块微钙化及其稳定性的机制研究

项目负责人：吴芳

项目来源：国家自然科学基金青年项目

项目编号：82102008

研究年限：2022.01—2024.12

资助金额：30 万元

项目简介：脑卒中是我国居民的第一位死亡原因，发病率呈逐年上升趋势。颅内动脉粥样硬化是导致我国缺血性脑卒中的常见病因，易损斑块破裂导致血栓形成是缺血性脑卒中的主要原因。早期精确无创性识别易损斑块，对脑卒中高危人群筛查、病因探查、疗效监测及预防再发具有十分重要的意义。斑块内微钙化可以增加纤维帽表面的机械压力，增加斑块破裂风险，是易损斑块的重要组成部分。通过对颅内动脉易损斑块内微钙化进行在体评价，实现易损斑块的早期诊断，可为早期临床干预和预后评估提供重要的依据。因此，颅内动脉粥样硬化斑块微钙化评价将成为重要的新导向。一体化 PET/MR 实现了 PET 和 MR 两种不同设备在相同空间内对各自数据的同时采集，既提供了高分辨率 MR 精细的解剖结构及斑块特征，又提供了 PET 系统的斑块内微钙化定量化信息，使颅内动脉粥样硬化斑块的组织学评估和分子显像成为可能。申请人前期研究发现了颅内动脉斑块 MRI 易损特征，在前期研究基础上，本项目围绕微钙化在颅内动脉粥样硬化斑块破裂中的作用机制及演变规律等关键科学问题，拟进一步应用一体化 PET/MR，探索微钙化与斑块 MRI 特征相关性及与临床症状相关性，并动态观察其演变规律。

6. 项目名称：基于多模态特征结构化技术的急性心肌梗死后心肌重构预警模型研究

项目负责人：刘志

项目来源：国家自然科学基金面上项目

项目编号：62172288

研究年限：2022.01—2025.12

资助金额：60 万元

项目简介：急性心肌梗死是威胁人类生命最主要的疾病之一，现有心肌梗死预后预测量表多通过 6～8 个临床文本指标预测死亡、复发心肌梗死、心力衰竭的发生率，采集数据较为单一。心肌重构作为心肌梗死后早期即可开始并持续进展的不良病理改变，是后期心力衰竭及死亡的主要病理机制。然而目前尚没有心肌重构的定量预警模型，临床缺乏早期干预的指导，这一需求亟待解决。本团队前期研究发现利用心脏 MRI 可以准确量化心肌梗死后水肿心肌内的坏死区域和可恢复心肌。本项目拟采用机器学习算法，结合可变形卷积网络、胶囊网络构建新型神经网络架构，实现 MRI、超声等多模态临床影像数据结构化特征提取；结合前期已建立的 3000 名心肌梗死患者数据库构建多模态特征矩阵，使用多种分类器如支持向量机、随机森林等进行心肌重构定量预测，评估不同分类器效果，预期通过本项目建立符合国人特点的急性心肌梗死后心肌重构定量预警模型，并使用库外同类型数据进行验证，建立高效鲁棒性预警模型。

7. 项目名称：PET/MR 同步测定脑梗死患者运动功能预后的多模态脑机制研究

项目负责人：单艺

项目来源：北京市自然科学基金青年项目

项目编号：7224334

研究年限：2022.01—2023.12

资助金额：10 万元

项目简介：脑梗死是常见病、多发病，致残率很高，3/4 以上患者遗留不同程度的运动功能障碍。人脑运动网络的代偿与重塑，对脑梗死患者运动功能恢复起着决定性作用。利用无创影像学手段精准评估患者运动网络的完整性，是目前国内外研究关注的热点。高分辨脑结构 MRI 可提供运动皮层的形态学特征，静息态 fMRI 可确定运动脑区间的相互关联，^{18}F-FDG PET 可提供脑网络能量代谢的定量指标。不同模态获得的影像学特征彼此互补，但其内在联系及在损伤状态下的代偿重塑模式尚不清楚。本项目将应用一体化 PET/MR 同步获取同一生理和心理状态下脑结构、功能及代谢的同步信息，对脑梗死伴运动障碍患者的多模态影像学特征及临床评分进行纵向随访，综合分析患者运动网络完整性的损伤程度及演变，并与运动功能进行相关性分析，探讨早期精准评价脑梗死患者运动功能预后的客观指标。

8. 项目名称：阿尔茨海默病基底前脑结构与功能早期改变的一体化 PET/MR 研究

项目负责人：闫少珍

项目来源：北京市医管中心培育计划项目

项目编号：PX2022036

研究年限：2022.01—2024.12

资助金额：15 万元

项目简介：基底前脑胆碱能神经元病变、损伤、丢失是阿尔茨海默病早期重要病理表现之一，这些病理变化导致海马等脑区失去胆碱能神经元支配，从而影响认知功能。检测阿尔茨海默病基底前脑损伤有助于理解阿尔茨海默病的病理生理机制，更有助于早期诊断阿尔茨海默病。研究提示基底前脑萎缩是阿尔茨海默病早期重要的影像学表现，并且基底前脑进行性萎缩会伴随认知功能障碍逐渐加重，最终可发展为痴呆。因此，研究阿尔茨海默病和轻度认知障碍患者基底前脑结构、功能网络和代谢特征及其内在联系，是揭示阿尔茨海默病基底前脑损伤机制的基础，有望为阿尔茨海默病早期预警提供精准神经影像指标。本项目利用一体化 PET/MR 同步获得高分辨 T$_1$WI 结构像、静息态 fMRI（功能）和 ^{18}F-FDG PET（葡萄糖代谢）信息，综合分析阿尔茨海默病和轻度认知障碍基底前脑结构、功能网络和代谢特征及其内在联系，并与神经认知功能评分相结合，从而建立阿尔茨海默病早期精准诊断神经影像标记，揭示阿尔茨海默病基底前脑损伤病理生理机制，对阿尔茨海默病早期预警、及时干预、改善预后具有重要意义。

9. 项目名称：基于机器学习的 PET/MR 多模态影像在阿尔茨海默病早期精准诊断研究

项目负责人：闫少珍，刘勇

项目来源：北京市科技新星计划交叉合作课题

项目编号：20220484177

研究年限：2022.12—2024.12

资助金额：50 万元

项目简介：本项目基于机器学习算法对多模态影像数据综合分析，利用阿尔茨海默病和轻度认知障碍的结构 MRI、fMRI、tau PET 数据，获得能够识别早期阿尔茨海默病的最优诊断模型，并与基因和神经认知功能评分相结合，拟解决目前阿尔茨海默病早期影像评估存在的关键问题：①多模态影像数据量大，后处理流程复杂，医师单纯主观、半定量评估难以完成；②由于目前国际上尚缺乏 tau PET 诊断阿尔茨海默病统一的诊断规范标准，不同医师之间的结果一致性差，临床应用困难。本项目拟建立阿尔茨海默病早期精准诊断神经影像模型，协助阿尔茨海默病高危患者早期预警。

10. 项目名称：基于 PET/MR 评价颈动脉粥样硬化斑块炎症及其稳定性的影像学特征研究

项目负责人：卢洁

项目来源：国家自然科学基金面上项目

项目编号：81974261

研究年限：2021.01—2023.12

资助金额：55 万元

项目简介：本项目利用一体化 PET/MR 对颈动脉粥样硬化斑块稳定性进行研究，同步获得精确配准融合的斑块高分辨 MRI 结构、DCE-MRI 新生血管和 ^{18}F-FDG PET 巨噬细胞炎症代谢的影像数据，分析斑块成分、Ktrans 值、Vp 值、TBR 值的相关性，通过长期随访，观察斑块动态演变情况，探究斑块影像学特征与组织病理、临床指标的相关性，阐明斑块易损性的影像学特征，揭示炎症与斑块稳定性的病理生理机制，从而为缺血性脑卒中进行早期预警。

11. 项目名称：基于 [^{18}F]–PBR06 靶向示踪 TSPO 的 PET/MR 多模态分子显像探讨神经精神狼疮前期神经炎症特征与作用研究

项目负责人：苏丽

项目来源：国家自然科学基金青年项目

项目编号：82001733

研究年限：2021.01—2023.12

资助金额：24 万元

项目简介：本项目利用 [^{18}F]-PBR06 靶向示踪 TSPO 的 PET/MR 多模态分子显像技术对神经精神狼疮患者脑内小胶质细胞活化为主的炎症进行研究，同步获得精确配准融合的脑高分辨 MRI 结构、灌注序列和 [^{18}F]-PBR06 PET 脑代谢的影像数据，评估患者认知、情感水平，测定患者外周血炎症因子水平，分析神经精神狼疮患者脑内小胶质细胞活化与脑结构、灌注及代谢影像学特征、高级脑功能、系统性炎症水平的相关性，通过长期随访，观察脑内小胶质细胞活化的动态演变情况，探究神经精神狼疮患者脑内小胶质细胞活化性神经炎症与脑结构功能、临床指标的相关性，阐明该炎症的影像学特征，揭示该炎症与系统性炎症、脑结构功能的病理生理机制，从而为神经精神狼疮进行早期预警，协助判断疾病预后。

12. 项目名称：基于 PET/MR 肌萎缩侧索硬化患者锥体外系相关脑功能及脑网络研究

项目负责人：朱文佳

项目来源：国家自然科学基金青年项目

项目编号：82001352

研究年限：2021.01—2023.12

资助金额：24 万元

项目简介：基于 VMAT2-PET/MR 技术，观察肌萎缩侧索硬化患者多巴胺能神经元受累情况，同时采集 rs-fMRI 相关核磁数据，将黑质功能连接网络、红核功能连接网络及小脑齿状核功能连接网络作为主要关注方向，构建肌萎缩侧索硬化患者锥体外系相关的脑功能连接网络。

13. 项目名称：基于人工智能的结构 MRI 和 ^{18}F-florbetapir PET 阿尔茨海默病影像早期诊断研究

项目负责人：闫少珍

项目来源：北京市科技新星计划交叉合作课题

项目编号：2021B00001609

研究年限：2021.12—2024.12

资助金额：36 万元

项目简介：阿尔茨海默病是老年痴呆最常见的类型，占 50%～75%，我国阿尔茨海默病患病率高且预后差，给社会和家庭带来沉重经济负担。阿尔茨海默病的病程不可逆，尚未发现有效的治疗痴呆的方法，临床上致力于尽可能早诊断出阿尔茨海默病，试图延缓其进展。因此，早期精准诊断干预，以期延缓病程进展，是全世界亟待解决的关键问题。神经影像学技术是无创活体监测阿尔茨海默病脑组织改变的重要手段，高分辨磁共振成像（high-resolution magnetic resonance imaging，HR-MRI）能够定量显示脑结构改变。^{18}F-AV-1451 用于对脑内沉积的神经元纤维缠结进行活体成像。目前阿尔茨海默病早期影像困难，国际上尚缺乏 tau PET 诊断阿尔茨海默病统一的诊断规范标准，不同医师之间的结果一致性差，临床应用困难。因此，本项目利用人工智能技术对多模态影像数据综合分析，提取脑结构、脑内 tau 蛋白聚集特征，构建阿尔茨海默病的早期诊断模型，可实现阿尔茨海默病高危患者的早期预警，帮助指导临床个体化精准诊断和治疗。

14. 项目名称：阿尔茨海默病影像早期诊断标志物的应用开发研究

项目负责人：卢洁

项目来源：北京市科委

项目编号：Z201100005520018

研究年限：2020.03—2024.03

资助金额：150 万元

项目简介：探索并建立阿尔茨海默病的早期诊断模型，从而实现早期干预，以延缓或逆转病程，是目前阿尔茨海默病诊疗领域亟待解决的核心关键问题。近年来新发展的一体化 PET/MR 是国际最前沿的成像设备，具有同步扫描的独特优势，一次扫描同时获得 PET 和 MRI 图像，两种图像的精确配准融合，有望精准定位脑代谢及脑结构异常改变，为临床早期诊断提供有力手段。本项目拟针对目前阿尔茨海默病早期诊断影像学标志物不明确的关键科学问题，运用多模态分子影像学手段（一体化 PET/MR）结合体液生物学及遗传学特征，确定各类影像学、生物学及遗传学标志物在阿尔茨海默病进展过程中的内在动态变化机制，同时定量多模态影像学特征在阿尔茨海默病病理进展过程中的临界阈值，建立阿尔茨海默病的早期影像学诊断模型，为阿尔茨海默病的早期诊断奠定理论及技术基础，并在相关医院推广应用。

15. 项目名称：基于分子成像和计算流体力学技术的颈动脉粥样硬化性狭窄新型评价体系的研发

项目负责人：王亚冰

项目来源：北京市科技计划项目

项目编号：Z201100005520020

研究年限：2020.03—2024.03

资助金额：121 万元

项目简介：本研究针对颈动脉狭窄发生脑卒中的机制，从颈动脉斑块的结构、斑块代谢和血流动力学多个层面，对尚未达到手术干预标准的颈动脉粥样硬化性狭窄患者进行长期随访。通过完整、动态的评价，从病变的发生发展过程中获取不同阶段、多个层面的指标，结合随访期间缺血事件和狭窄程度变化的发生情况，初步建立颈动脉粥样硬化性狭窄病变进展影响因素的综合评价体系。

16. 项目名称：遗忘型轻度认知障碍 PET/MR 脑代谢与脑网络动态变化及关联机制研究

项目负责人：赵志莲

项目来源：国家自然科学基金青年项目

项目编号：81801677

研究年限：2019.01—2021.12

资助金额：20 万元

项目简介：遗忘型轻度认知障碍是阿尔茨海默病临床前期，由于阿尔茨海默病无有效治疗手段，将阿尔茨海默病影像诊断标志物的研究窗口前移到遗忘型轻度认知障碍阶段可能会对阿尔茨海默病诊治产生重大突破。PET 和 MRI 是评价遗忘型轻度认知障碍的有力手段，PET 能够提供脑代谢信息，fMRI 能够提供脑功能信息，联合应用能够更好地评价遗忘型轻度认知障碍的脑改变，由于脑代谢及功能情况受生理、新陈代谢、环境影响，因此本项目利用目前国际最前沿的一体化 PET/MR，进行脑代谢和 fMRI 的同步扫描，分析遗忘型轻度认知障碍患者静息态 fMRI 各功能指标（ALFF、fALFF、ReHo、DC、ICA 网络）、PET 葡萄糖代谢的动态变化及其相关性，并进行纵向随访，揭示遗忘型轻度认知障碍患者脑功能改变与临床认知改变的关系，阐明遗忘型轻度认知障碍患者认知功能障碍与临床转归脑机制，对于早期诊断遗忘型轻度认知障碍，改善预后，具有重要的科学和临床意义。

17. 项目名称：基于多模态影像探究头颈动脉粥样硬化斑块易损机制的人工智能研究

项目负责人：卢洁

项目来源：北京市自然科学基金重点项目

项目编号：Z190014

研究年限：2019.10—2023.10

资助金额：300 万元

项目简介：头颈动脉粥样硬化斑块破裂是导致缺血性脑卒中的主要原因，探索斑块进展的病理生理机制，早期客观、精准判断斑块易损性，是目前国际研究的热点。研究发现头颈动脉粥样硬化斑块的位置、形态、成分等解剖结构及斑块所处的血流动力学环境与判断其易损性密切相关，但目前缺乏结合形态、功能学信息的多模态、定量检测斑块易损性模式，且由于头颈动脉血管图像数据量巨大、后处理流程复杂，需采用基于人工智能的大数据研究方法论，快速、准确地提取并融合易损斑块的多模态影像学特征，构建评估斑块易损性的智能风险预测模型。本项目拟针对目前易损斑块难以检测及准确评估的关键难点，应用基于生理结构分区的新型深度学习算法对多模态影像学数据进行分割、建模，融合斑块多成分流固耦合分析模型，提取头颈动脉粥样硬化斑块的形态学及功能学信息，构建评估斑块易损性的智能风险预测模型，阐明易损斑块进展的病理生理机制，为早期评估患者预后提供精准的客观依据，对缺血性脑卒中的筛查、预警具有重要价值。

18. 项目名称：帕金森病患者脑中神经炎症进展的 18KDa 转位蛋白靶向 PET 显像研究

项目负责人： 乔洪文

项目来源： 国家自然科学基金青年项目

项目编号： 81701726

研究年限： 2018.01—2020.12

资助金额： 20 万元

项目简介： 帕金森病患者脑中存在以小胶质细胞激活为特征的神经炎症反应，但是神经炎症随病情的进展情况尚不明确。TSPO 靶向 PET 显像能够反映脑中小胶质细胞激活情况，定量检测神经炎症。本项目将开发神经炎症显像剂 [^{18}F] PBR06，然后通过 UPDRS、MMSE 量表和 VMAT2 靶向多巴胺能神经元完整性 PET 检查筛选正常人和不同程度的帕金森病患者，进行 [^{18}F] PBR06 PET/MR 显像研究，并对帕金森病患者进行 24 个月跟踪随访。通过横向比较不同程度帕金森病患者量表评分、VMAT2 显像和神经炎症显像结果，分析病情及脑中多巴胺神经元缺失与神经炎症的相关性；通过纵向比较帕金森病患者不同时期评分和 PET 显像结果，分析病情进展、多巴胺能神经元损伤与神经炎症的相关性。本项目能够阐明帕金森病发病中神经炎症的进展情况，提供定量检测神经炎症的 PET 影像学新方法，从而提高疾病的诊疗水平，鉴于我国帕金森病的高发病率和巨大的患者人群，本研究具有重大应用和科研价值。

19. 项目名称：利用 PET/MR 探讨肠道微生物对阿尔茨海默病老年斑形成效应的机制

项目负责人： 王红星

项目来源： 国家自然科学基金面上项目

项目编号： 81771862

研究年限： 2018.01—2021.12

资助金额： 55 万元

项目简介： 本项目首先探讨阿尔茨海默病患者肠道微生物组的变化特征，从阿尔茨海默病患者和健康对照者获得潜在的致病菌和益生菌，并分析外周血中 sST2、IL-33 及 Aβ42 的变化。利用分子影像学活体分析致病菌和益生菌对老年斑形成（Aβ）的效应，并比较致病菌组、益生菌组和空白对照组外周血和大脑内的 Aβ42 水平，以及小鼠大脑额叶和海马区域老年斑的面积。进一步比较致病菌组、益生菌组和空白对照组等 3 组肠道上皮 IL-33、血 IL-33、脑组织 IL-33 的差异，探讨从人体获得的致病菌和益生菌是否影响肠壁 IL-33 的生成。在新冠肺炎疫情条件下，增加了阿尔茨海默病前期出现的失眠和抑郁等脑功能症状的非药物干预方法相关研究，并获得了显著结果。

20. 项目名称：散发性肌萎缩侧索硬化患者多模态神经影像学研究

项目负责人： 朱文佳

项目来源： 首都卫生发展科研专项

项目编号： 2018-4-2015

研究年限：2018.01—2021.12

资助金额：20 万元

项目简介：基于 rs-fMRI 技术，研究肌萎缩侧索硬化患者脑结构及脑功能特点，包括灰质体积、厚度与灰质结构脑网络、脑白质结构连接与网络模型构建、脑功能连接与网络模型构建等，寻找肌萎缩侧索硬化患者影像学标志物。

21. 项目名称：一体化 PET/MRI 在子宫内膜癌诊断及术前精准分期中的应用效果

项目负责人：王世军

项目来源：首都卫生发展科研专项

项目编号：2018-2-2013

研究年限：2018.01—2020.12

资助金额：52 万元

项目简介：子宫内膜癌（endometrial cancer，EC）是原发于子宫内膜的上皮恶性肿瘤，近年来发病率有明显上升趋势。子宫内膜癌的治疗主要是全面分期手术（全子宫 + 双附件 + 盆腔及腹主动脉旁淋巴结切除术）。早期低危型子宫内膜癌（G1 级和 G2 级、子宫肌层受侵深度＜50%、原发肿瘤直径＜2 cm）患者的淋巴结转移率多低于 4%，淋巴结切除对于低危型子宫内膜癌患者预后没有明确的获益，反而可能带来更大的创伤。术前准确评估子宫内膜癌的分期及是否存在高危因素，对实施个体化的手术范围起到决定性作用。经阴道超声、MRI、PET 等影像学检查尚无法准确判断肌层浸润深度、淋巴结是否转移及宫外病变等情况。一体化 PET/MR 结合了 MRI 对软组织分辨好和 PET 对肿瘤转移灶识别强的优点，具备更精确的术前评估能力。目前没有一体化 PET/MR 在子宫内膜癌诊断及术前分期的研究报道。本项目旨在评价一体化 PET/MR 在子宫内膜癌术前分期中的效果，以建立一体化 PET/MR 用于子宫内膜癌术前精准分期的诊断流程及规范。

22. 项目名称：脑梗死后交叉性小脑失联络相关运动功能预后脑机制的 PET/MR 研究

项目负责人：卢洁

项目来源：国家自然科学基金面上项目

项目编号：81671662

研究年限：2017.01—2020.12

资助金额：58 万元

项目简介：脑梗死是致残率最高的疾病之一，探索脑梗死后神经功能的脑重塑机制，是国内外研究所面临的重大问题。研究发现幕上脑梗死后 50% ~ 70% 伴有交叉性小脑失联络征（crossed cerebellar diaschisis，CCD），且交叉性小脑失联络征与患者预后密切相关，但交叉性小脑失联络征发生的脑机制及运动功能预后的代偿机制尚不清楚。脑梗死病灶导致皮层 – 桥脑 – 小脑通路损伤，可能是交叉性小脑失联络征的主要原因。PET 和 MRI 是评价脑梗死后交叉性小脑失联络征的有力手段，PET 能提供脑血流和脑代谢信息，fMRI 能提供脑功能连接情况，DTI 能显示纤维束改变。因此，本项目利用目前国际最前沿的一体化 PET/MR，进行 PET 脑血流代谢和 fMRI、DTI 同步扫描，分析交叉性小脑失联络征患者脑血流、代谢连接、功能连接和白质纤维束的变化情况及其相关性，并长期纵向随访，揭示影像学改变与临床运动功能预后的关系，阐明脑梗死后交叉性小脑失联络征患者运动功能障碍及预后脑机制，对降低患者致残率，指导临床康复治疗有重要意义。

23. 项目名称：一体化 TOF-PET-MR 探讨心力衰竭后认知功能障碍患者的脑结构和脑代谢成像横断面研究

项目负责人：王静娟

项目来源：教育部开放课题

项目编号：2016-ZDSYSKFJJ-12

研究年限：2017.12—2019.12

资助金额：8 万元

项目简介：慢性充血性心力衰竭在临床上常伴有认知功能障碍，但其产生的神经机制很大程度上是未知的。基于研究基础，心力衰竭大鼠存在明显的认知功能障碍，大脑皮层及海马中能量代谢，特别是葡萄糖代谢的相关基因明显下调，海马神经元明显固缩、坏死，提出心力衰竭后认知功能障碍，是由于脑灌注不足和葡萄糖代谢障碍，导致与认知相关的脑区灰质缺失（神经元坏死），最终出现认知功能损害的科学假说。结合首都医科大学宣武医院在神经疾病设备和技术的领先优势，本项目选择心力衰竭兼有认知障碍者、心力衰竭不伴有认知障碍者及非心力衰竭无认知障碍者三组，进行一体化 TOF-PET-MRI 检测，分析静息态和任务态大脑不同区域的解剖结构、功能成像、代谢成像及脑血流的变化；收集心血管危险因素和测定与认知相关的神经递质，以期阐明心力衰竭后认知功能障碍发病的神经机制和中医"心主神明"的科学内涵。本项目具有原始创新性，对中西医结合防治心血管疾病引起的认知功能障碍具有重要的学术意义和临床意义。

24. 项目名称：一体化 PET/MR 在子宫内膜癌术前精准分期诊断中的可行性研究

项目负责人：王世军

项目来源：首都市民健康培育项目

项目编号：Z17110000041702

研究年限：2017.03—2020.05

资助金额：15 万元

项目简介：子宫内膜癌的死亡率从 40 岁开始迅速上升，80 岁达高峰。我国目前正处于老龄化社会，在这种形势下，该疾病的研究是合适且急迫的。一体化 PET/MR 扫描仪是一项高效、准确的分子影像设备，本项目可以验证该技术在子宫内膜癌诊断中的可行性。该技术在临床上的成功应用可以显著提高子宫内膜癌的诊断准确性，并可以辅助提高疗效和患者的生活质量。一体化 PET/MR 用于子宫内膜癌术前精准分期诊断，目前尚无研究，通过本项目可以深化我国对该技术的认知水平，有利于占领领先地位，有巨大的社会效益。一体化 PET/MR 技术经推广使用后可省略多种术前检查步骤，可节省大量医疗资源，为病患节约了医疗成本。子宫内膜癌患者通过一体化 PET/MR 进行术前精准分期，可以缩小早期低危型子宫内膜癌的手术范围，实现个体化治疗，可以降低分期手术淋巴结切除引起的近期、远期并发症发生率，提高患者的生活质量，缩短住院天数，节省医疗资源。

25. 项目名称：一体化 PET/MR 脑血流定量方法研究及在脑疾病应用

项目负责人：卢洁

项目来源："十三五"科技部重点研发项目

项目编号：2016YFC0103000

研究年限：2016.07—2018.12

资助金额：230 万元

项目简介：CBF 对维持脑组织功能和代谢水平起决定作用，脑疾病会导致脑血流异常改变，因此精准定量 CBF，对研究疾病发病机制、早期诊断和治疗有重要价值。目前 PET 是定量测量脑血流的准确方法，但由于传统采血法患者难以接受，无法临床普及应用；图像衍生动脉输入函数法虽不需采血，但需要通过 PET 和 MR 图像配准获得动脉输入函数，后处理复杂，可能出现配准误差。最新一体化 TOF-PET-MRI 技术具有同步扫描的独特优势，一次扫描同时获得 PET 和 MR 图像，两种图像的精确配准融合，可以无创、简便、准确地获得动脉输入函数，为绝对定量 CBF 研究提供新方法。本项目应用一体化 TOF-PET-MRI，建立动态 ^{18}F-FDG 首过 CBF 新算法模型，解决目前难以无创、精准测量 CBF 的难题；应用灵长类动物大脑中动脉闭塞模型，验证 CBF 新算法的准确性和可重复性；通过一体化 TOF-PET-MRI 脑血流测量新算法在缺血性脑血管病、阿尔茨海默病的临床应用研究，发现早期诊断、预后判断及疗效评价的 CBF 指标，为疾病早期诊断和预后判断等提供新方法。本项目对推动神经科学、影像科学和其他临床学科的交叉结合，促进基础研究向临床应用转化，降低患者致残率和致死率具有重要价值。

26. 项目名称：一体化 TOF-PET-MRI 脑血流定量方法研究及在脑疾病的应用——脑血流定量在脑重大疾病的临床应用研究（子课题）

项目负责人：张苗

项目来源："十三五"科技部重点研发项目子课题

项目编号：2016YFC0103004

研究年限：2016.07—2018.12

资助金额：170 万元（子课题金额）

项目简介：CBF 对维持正常脑组织功能和代谢水平起决定作用。目前磁共振评价 CBF 的主要方法有 PWI 和 ASL。PWI 检查无射线辐射，但仍有对比剂过敏风险，容易受机器磁场强、后处理算法等因素影响；ASL 技术完全无创，无须注入对比剂，但信噪比和空间分辨率低，检查时间长，尚未进入临床应用。目前，影像学检查只有 PET 是定量测量 CBF 的"金标准"，但传统 PET 扫描需要在连续动脉采血并离心处理后测定血浆中放射性比活度，属于有创操作；常用的示踪剂 ^{15}O-H$_2$O 代谢速度快，半衰期极短，对于没有安装回旋加速器的机构，无法进行临床常规应用。一体化 TOF-PET-MRI 一次扫描可以同时获得 PET 和 MRI 图像，能够自动进行两种图像的精确配准融合，实现无创、精准定量 CBF；示踪剂 ^{18}F-FDG 的半衰期时间长，可以在成像早期测量 CBF，注射 1 小时后检测脑神经元代谢，达到注射一次示踪剂同时获得脑血流和代谢信息的效果。本项目将一体化 TOF-PET-MRI 动态 ^{18}F-FDG 首过 CBF 成像应用于脑重大疾病（缺血性脑血管病、阿尔茨海默病）的临床研究，分析脑疾病引起的 CBF 异常改变特性，以及疾病过程中 CBF 的动态变化模式，发现早期诊断、预后判断及疗效评价的 CBF 指标。

27. 项目名称：一体化全身正电子发射 / 磁共振成像装备（PET/MR）研制 –PET/MR 在神经系统疾病中的高级临床应用

项目负责人：赵国光

项目来源："十三五"科技部重点研发项目子课题

项目编号：2016YFC0103909

研究年限：2016.07—2020.12

资助金额：50 万元

项目简介：针对本项目研发 PET/MR 系统分辨率高、梯度强度大的特点，本项目将优化 PET/MR 序列参数，建立神经系统疾病的 PET/MR 优化检查方案；研发面向神经系统疾病的数据分析平台。建立神经系统疾病的 PET/MR 优化检查方案，明确 PET/MR 用于神经系统疾病诊断的准确性、特异度和敏感度。研究开发面向神经系统疾病诊断的 PET/MR 定量化数据分析平台。

28. 项目名称：阿尔茨海默病早期诊断的 PET/MR 多模态影像标志物研究

项目负责人：梁志刚

项目来源：首都临床特色应用研究

项目编号：Z161100000516086

研究年限：2016.06—2021.03

资助金额：24 万元

项目简介：阿尔茨海默病是一种神经退行性疾病，起病隐袭，以渐进性记忆力丧失为特征，逐渐累及其他认知与非认知功能，最终导致患者丧失生活自理能力。由于对阿尔茨海默病缺乏有效的治疗手段，目前尚无特效治疗方案，因此能够早期诊断阿尔茨海默病并开始干预是延缓疾病进展的希望所在。寻找能够早期识别阿尔茨海默病的神经影像学生物标志物，是目前国内外研究关注的热点。结构 MRI 可提供皮层的形态学特征，DTI 可确定脑内微观结构的改变，^{18}F-FDG PET 可提供脑区能量代谢的定量指标。不同模态获得的影像学特征互补，从多个角度提供信息。本项目将应用一体化 PET/MR 同步获取脑结构、完整性及代谢的同步信息对阿尔茨海默病进行早期诊断。

1.2022 年度华夏医学科学技术奖一等奖

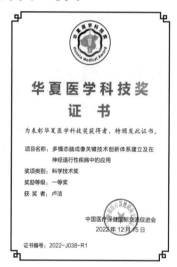

项目名称：多模态脑成像关键技术创新体系建立及在神经退行性疾病中的应用

完成人：卢洁，韩璎，左传涛，崔孟超，吴涛，张敏鸣，舒妮，霍力，闫少珍，胡凌志，吴平，齐志刚，袁健闵，张占军，陈彪

完成单位：首都医科大学宣武医院，复旦大学附属华山医院，北京师范大学，浙江大学医学院附属第二医院，中国医学科学院北京协和医院，上海联影医疗科技股份有限公司

项目简介：神经变性病主要包括阿尔茨海默病和帕金森病，严重危害中老年人健康，我国患病人数居全球首位，早期诊断困难，约 60% 的患者就诊时已为中晚期，因此早期精准诊断是临床诊治的关键。该项目聚焦多模态成像技术创新体系建立及在神经退行性疾病中的应用，经过 10 年科技攻关，取得了系列创新性成果，具有国际领先水平。主要创新点：①针对脑亚区高分辨率精细成像进行新线圈研究，发明了国际首个 32 通道 PET/MR 头线圈，研发射频单元高密度相控阵排列模式，与原有线圈的并行排列模式比较，脑亚区信噪比提高 50% 以上，图像分辨率由 3 mm 提高至 1.4 mm，各项性能指标达到业内最高水平，解决精准诊断阿尔茨海默病和帕金森病特异性脑亚区的高清成像难题；②针对新型高特异性病理靶向分子探针进行研究，研发新型柔性结构高亲和力分子探针，创新应用双膦化合物修饰，打破现有探针的刚性结构，研发与致病蛋白结合位点最佳匹配的分子探针，使脑内特异性摄取较现有探针提高 1 倍，克服了目前已有示踪剂的缺点，在现有同类探针中摄取率最高，为阿尔茨海默病和帕金森病提供特异诊断的原创性药物；③针对阿尔茨海默病和帕金森病多模态图像融合分析技术的难题，研发人工智能神经网络算法，实时融合多参数时空动态信息，提取阿尔茨海默病和帕金森病多模态影像标志物，进行了多中心研究，揭示了阿尔茨海默病和帕金森病的多模态影像动态演变模式，将诊断提前至临床前无症状期，阿尔茨海默病的早诊率由 70% 提高至 87%，帕金森病的早诊率由 75% 提高至 94%，将诊断时间平均提前 4～5 年，实现早期诊断关口前移；④揭示了阿尔茨海默病和帕金森病发病新机制，发现阿尔茨海默病风险基

因 *APOEε4* 和性别交互作用影响脑内 tau 蛋白沉积，阐明了女性高患病率的病理生理机制，指导高危人群筛查。发现帕金森病患者脑内铁沉积增多可导致黑质-纹状体-运动皮层功能连接损伤和神经受体降低，阐明了患者运动功能障碍的脑机制，为临床神经调控治疗提供新靶点。牵头成立中国阿尔茨海默病临床前期联盟和中国帕金森联盟，在 *Brain*、*Radiology*、*EJNMMI* 等国际权威期刊发表 SCI 收录论文 258 篇，其中 2 篇入选全球前 1% ESI 高被引论文、2 篇被世界学术组织 F1000 推荐，参与制定国际临床标准 4 项，牵头制定国内诊断标准及共识 14 项。授权国家专利 30 项，国际专利 5 项，主编/译专著 20 部。成果进行了转化，直接经济效益 3500 万元。项目建立和推广应用神经退行性疾病早期预警影像诊断体系，助力临床医师早期客观诊断，延缓患者病程进展，应对人口老龄化，整体提升研究领域全球竞争力。

2. 其他奖项

（1）国家科技部中青年科技创新领军人才（卢洁）

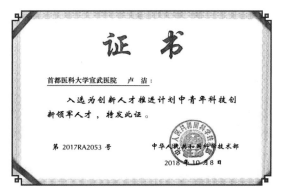

（2）中国产学研合作创新奖（卢洁）

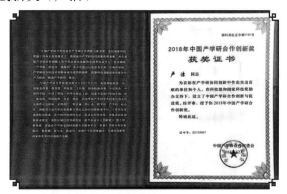

（3）茅以升科学技术奖——北京青年科技奖（卢洁）

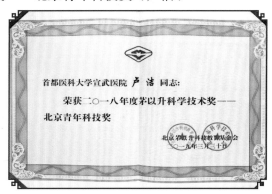

（4）首都青年医学创新与转化大赛一等奖（卢洁）

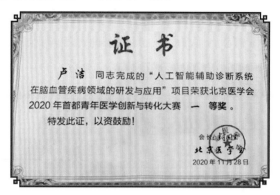

（5）北京医学会优秀中青年医师（卢洁）

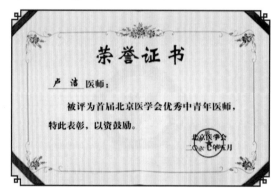

（6）北京医师协会北京优秀医师奖（卢洁）

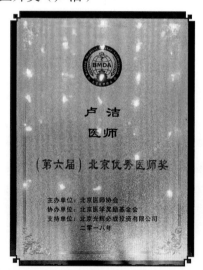

（7）首都医科大学宣武医院优秀导师管理奖（卢洁）

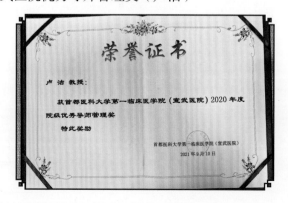

（8）首都医科大学宣武医院校级优秀博士论文指导奖（卢洁）

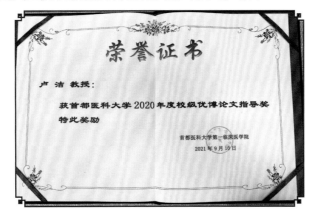

（9）中华医学会核医学分会新锐技师奖（王静娟）

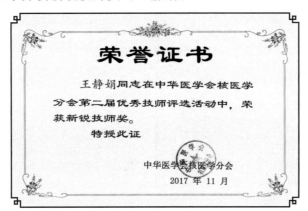

（10）中华医学会核医学分会新锐技师奖（杨宏伟）

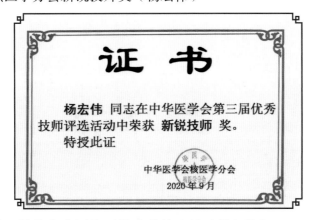

（11）中华医学会核医学分会全国核医学十佳护士长（帅冬梅）

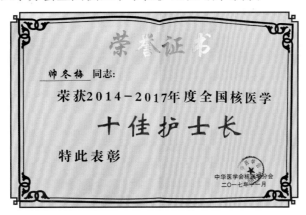

（12）首都医科大学优秀博士学位论文（闫少珍）

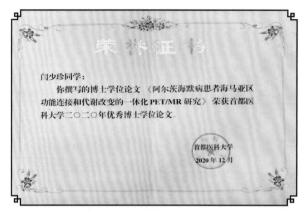

（13）首都医科大学优秀博士学位论文（崔碧霄）

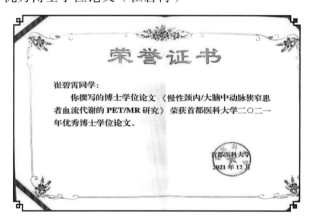

第五节　专著

1.PET/MRI 方法和临床应用（译著）

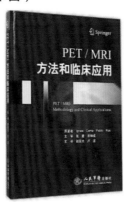

人民军医出版社，2015 年

原著者： Ignasi・Carrio，Pablo・Ros

主　审： 张　建，李坤成

主　译： 赵国光，卢　洁

简介及内容提要： 在 2015 年，国内尚无 PET/MRI 的相关专著，因此我们翻阅了欧洲核医学杂志总编、西班牙巴塞罗那自治大学 Ignasi・Carrio 教授等主编的 *PET/MRI: Methodology and Clinical Applications*，阅读后收获颇丰，萌生了翻译此书的想法，希望将它介绍给国内的同行。本书共 11 章，在介绍 PET/MRI 系统设计的基础上，详细阐述了 PET/MRI 的工作流程和临床实践，PET/MRI 在乳腺癌、淋巴瘤、肝、结直肠癌、颅脑、心脏的临床应用，并对 PET/MRI 系统的风险与安全，以及医疗费用等方面进行了科学评价。本书能够使广大同行了解 PET/MRI 的检查方法、临床应用及其科研价值，便于放射科、核医学科、临床各科室的医师和研究生，以及相关研究人员学习和使用。

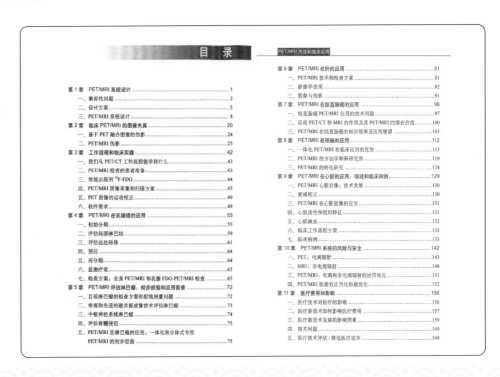

2. 一体化 PET/MR 操作规范和临床应用

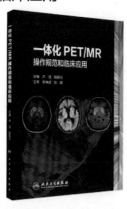

人民卫生出版社，2017 年

主　编：卢　洁，赵国光

主　审：李坤成，张　建

简介及内容提要："未来已经来临，只是尚未流行。"这是 2015 年我们翻译的国内第一部《PET/MR 方法和临床应用》一书中所引用的科幻预言。如今，时间仅过去 1 年多，我们欣喜地看到有关 PET/MR 的科学研究与临床应用得到了迅猛发展，在科研和临床各领域均有广泛应用。全书共分 10 个章节，分别介绍了 PET/MR 成像技术、PET 示踪剂和 MRI 对比剂、一体化 PET/MR 操作流程，以及一体化 PET/MR 在颅脑疾病、肺癌、腹部肿瘤、盆腔肿瘤、淋巴瘤、乳腺癌、心脏疾病等方面的临床应用和研究。其中重点介绍了一体化 PET/MR 在颅脑疾病的应用，这是一体化 PET/MR 的主要优势，尤其与特异性示踪剂相结合，对许多疾病如阿尔茨海默病、帕金森病、肿瘤、癫痫、脑血管病等的病理生理机制、早期诊断和治疗均有重要意义。本书能够帮助国内核医学科、放射科和临床医师了解和认识 PET/MR，促进多学科之间的密切合作。

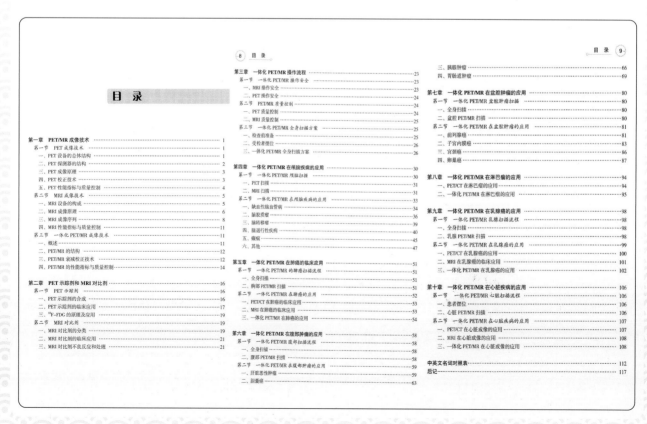

3. 一体化 PET/MR 实操手册

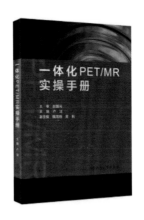

人民卫生出版社，2019 年

主　审：赵国光

主　编：卢　洁

简介及内容提要：2015 年 7 月首都医科大学宣武医院成为国内首台一体化 TOF PET/MR 装机用户，3 年来我们核医学科的医师和技术员经历了艰辛的学习过程，从完全陌生到逐渐了解每个线圈、定位、序列。近年来，国内一体化 PET/MR 装机数量逐渐增加，随着一体化 PET/MR 进入临床应用，各医院急需培养相关的使用人员，首都医科大学宣武医院核医学科先后接收了国内多家医院的人员进行培训。由于一体化 PET/MR 操作复杂，涉及 PET 和 MRI 的两种检查原理、操作流程和数据后处理，使用者很难短期内掌握，我们基于自身积累的经验，编写了这部实用操作手册。本手册由首都医科大学宣武医院和空军军医大学唐都医院的医师共同撰写，分别完成 GE Signa TOF PET/MR 和 Siemens Biograph PET/MR 两部分内容，每部分包括一体化 PET/MR 设备简介、各部位操作流程和图像后处理。该手册内容通俗易懂，文字简练，配有大量图解，方便使用者随时翻看参照，快速了解和操作一体化 PET/MR。

4. 一体化 PET/MR 护理实操手册

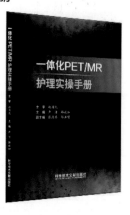

科学技术文献出版社，2020 年

主　审：赵国光

主　编：卢　洁，韩斌如

简介及内容提要：随着实践经验的逐步累积，持续优化及扩展护理人员在一体化 PET/MR 检查中各环节的工作流程及工作范畴，护理质量不断提高，科学化、规范化、标准化的护理工作制度日臻完善。我们利用实践中积累的经验编撰成这本护理实操手册，主要围绕一体化 PET/MR 的设备、检查药物、辐射防护、护理流程及内容、安全管理等方面进行了系统阐述，密切结合理论与实践，在内容设计上纵横交错，兼顾深度及广度，充分考虑内容编排的可读性及可操作性，力求符合一体化 PET/MR 的应用发展趋势及临床实践对护理工作的需求，期冀为从事一线工作的护理人员快速掌握规范护理知识提供参考。

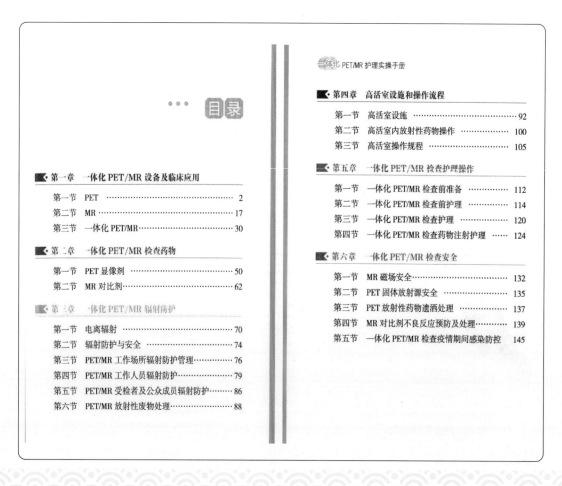

5. 一体化 PET/MR 成像病例图谱

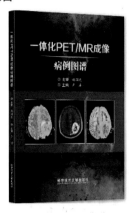

科学技术文献出版社，2020 年

主　审：赵国光

主　编：卢　洁

简介及内容提要：首都医科大学宣武医院自 2015 年装机至今，我们已完成 4000 余例病例采集，我们前期出版的《一体化 PET/MR 操作规范和临床应用》《一体化 PET/MR 实操手册》主要为临床扫描流程和初步临床应用经验。目前国内一体化 PET/MR 虽然已逐渐进入临床应用，但仍处于起步阶段，病例资料积累不足，亟须一本病例分析手册加强对疾病影像征象的认识。本书由经验丰富的 PET/MR 成像临床医师执笔，涵盖缺血性脑血管病、癫痫、神经变性疾病及全身各系统肿瘤共 47 个 PET/MR 成像临床应用中的经典病例。我们将病例的临床特点、一体化 PET/MR 影像表现和病理学特征进行详细分析和对照，重点突出 PET/MR 对于疾病精准诊断的价值。书中病例除涵盖 PET 传统示踪剂及 MRI 常规序列图像外，还展示了 ^{18}F-FET、^{11}C-PIB、^{18}F-AV45 等新示踪剂及 DWI、DTI、ASL、MRS 等新序列图像，方便读者全面、深入地了解疾病的影像表现，满足不同读者的需求。本书内容翔实、临床实用性强，有助于临床及影像医师快速掌握一体化 PET/MR 成像诊断要点及临床应用等知识。

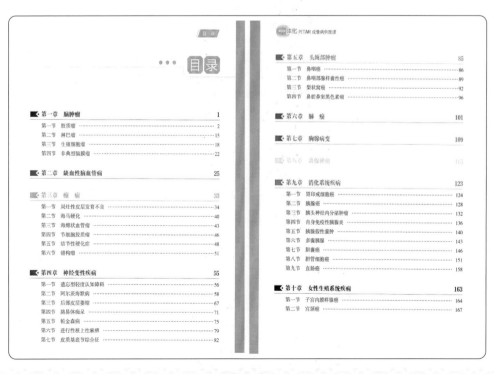

6. PET/MR 脑功能与分子影像：从脑疾病到脑科学

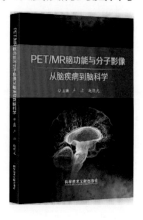

科学技术文献出版社，2021 年

主 编： 卢 洁，赵国光

简介及内容提要： 随着 PET/MR 设备的发展及在我国的推广应用，临床亟须掌握 PET 和 MRI 的复合型人才。我们前期出版的《一体化 PET/MR 操作规范和临床应用》《一体化 PET/MR 实操手册》和《一体化 PET/MR 成像病例图谱》内容主要集中于设备临床操作的规范性，以及临床典型病例表现。本书在前期工作的基础上，汇总了我们团队 PET/MR 脑疾病和脑科学方面的经验积累及国内外最新研究进展。全书共 16 章，内容包括设备简介、脑功能成像技术、脑疾病应用、脑科学研究，层层递进。脑功能成像技术围绕 MRI 功能成像、灌注成像及 PET 动态成像原理、数据后处理方法；脑疾病涉及阿尔茨海默病、帕金森病、癫痫、脑肿瘤、脑血管病、脑损伤、抑郁症、精神分裂症、多发性硬化、偏头痛等常见疾病，具有临床实用性及科研指导性。本书适合神经影像科、神经内科、神经外科及脑科学领域相关专业的医师阅读，可帮助其掌握一体化 PET/MR 影像诊断要领及开展相关科研公众，同时适用于脑科学研究工作者。

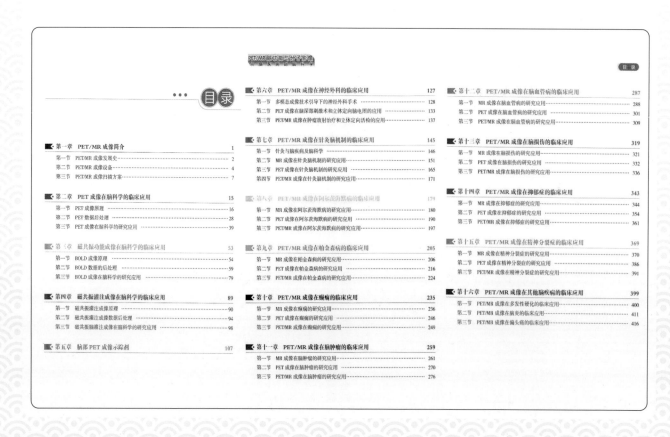

7. 下咽癌 PET/CT 和 PET/MRI 病例荟萃

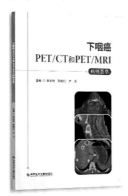

科学技术文献出版社，2022 年

主　编： 鲜军舫，陈晓红，卢　洁

简介及内容提要： 下咽癌是原发于下咽部恶性肿瘤的统称，绝大多数（95%）为鳞状细胞癌，发病率低，预后较差。尽管近几年来下咽癌治疗采用多学科团队诊疗模式，但晚期患者的 5 年生存率仍然很低，因此早期发现和准确分期及选择有效的治疗方案是下咽癌诊治的重点和难点。影像学检查是早期发现下咽癌和准确分期的重要方法，为下咽癌治疗决策提供了可靠的客观依据。本书针对临床重点关注的下咽癌诊治问题，详细地总结和分析了下咽癌 PET/CT 与 PET/MRI 的表现及在临床诊治中的价值，具有以下特点。①以临床需求为导向来阐述：20 例下咽癌病例涵盖了不同类型和分期的下咽癌的主要症状、体征、喉镜表现、PET/CT 与 PET/MRI 表现，并针对临床关注点进行解读和分析，更好地理解和掌握下咽癌的诊断和分期，以及各种诊断方法的优缺点。②多模态影像学运用与比较：创新性地将一体化 PET/MRI 用于下咽癌诊断与分期，并与每个病例的 PET/CT 表现进行对比分析，详细阐述了 CT、MRI、PET/CT 及 PET/MRI 在下咽癌诊治和评估中的优缺点与价值。③资料全面：每个病例包括主要症状、体征、喉镜表现与图像、PET/CT、PET/MRI 表现与图像、HE 染色图像及免疫组化结果与图像，资料翔实可靠，图像精美。本书采用要点式书写方式，内容简明扼要、重点突出、可读性强，适用于放射科、核医学科医师和技师，以及耳鼻咽喉头颈外科、肿瘤科和相关学科的医师与相关人员。

1. 一种血管异常图像识别方法、装置、电子设备和存储介质

授权日期：2022 年

授权号：CN 113610841 A

发明人：卢洁，傅璠，单艺

摘　要：本方案公开了一种血管异常图像识别方法、装置、电子设备和存储介质，步骤包括：对待识别的血管图像中的体素点进行标记，获得体素点标记信息，再基于体素点标记信息，确定血管区域中的最大联通域，利用所述最大联通域，识别、待识别血管图像的异常血管图像。通过这种方式能够快速、准确地从正常血管中分离出复杂血管区域，再对复杂血管的真实属性进行识别，从而提高识别的准确度，降低误诊率和漏诊率。

2. 一种医学成像系统

授权日期：2020 年

授权号：CN 210055993 U

发明人：卢洁，赵国光，刘慧，贺强，郑均安

摘　要：本实用新型实施例公开了一种医学成像系统，包括：扫描装置具有扫描腔，用于对受检者执行扫描并获得扫描数据；扫描床可沿扫描腔的轴向移动，用于承载受检者进入扫描腔；光学发射装置设置于扫描腔上，用于向受检者发射结构光信号；光学接收装置设置于扫描腔上用于接收反射结构光信号；光学信号处理装置用于确定受检者的生理信号；图像重建装置用于图像重建得到目标图像。本实用新型实施例可实现在获取扫描数据的过程中同步获取受检者的呼吸和心跳信号，重建出质量高的医学图像，从而简化获取医学图像的扫描准备工作，增加获取医学图像的成功率。

3. 一种头部线圈装置

授权日期：2020 年

授权号：CN 209863823 U

发明人：卢洁，赵国光，史宇航，刘慧

摘　要：本实用新型实施例公开了一种头部线圈装置，该装置包括：头部线圈本体；光学发射单元，设置于所述头部线圈上，用于向受检者的面部发射结构光信号；光学接收单元，设置于所述头部线圈上，并与所述光学发射单元间隔预设距离，用于接收经反射的反射结构光信号并获取所述受检者的面部图像；其中，所述结构光信号、所述反射结构光信号及所述面部图像用于确定所述受检者的面部信息。本实用新型实施例解决了现有头部线圈不能实时监测受检者的眼睛状态和头部运动信息的问题；本实用新型实施例可在获取头部扫描数据的过程中同步监测受检者的眼睛状态和头部运动信息，从而增加获取脑医学图像的成功率。

4. 用于磁共振系统的扫描床及磁共振系统

授权日期：2019 年

授权号：CN 209107354 U

发明人：赵国光，卢洁，沈振华，贺强

摘　要：本实用新型实施例提供了一种用于磁共振系统的扫描床及磁共振系统。该扫描床包括床板、位于床板底部的床板支架，以及与床板支架底端连接的床板基座，床板基座内部的容置腔中设置有无线充电装置和电池，床板基座的侧壁上设置有线圈插槽，线圈插槽中固定有直流针；床板底座的底部设置有供扫描床移动的滑动装置，床板基座与磁共振系统可拆卸连接；无线充电装置可采用外部无线充电设备对电池进行无线充电；电池用于对扫描床的电机及通过直流针对外部待供电设备进行供电。该扫描床减少了与磁共振系统的电源线连接，其可靠性高，操作便利且结构简化，降低了搬运带来的风险，保证了患者生命体征的稳定及患者的生命安全，减少了医疗事故的发生。

5. 一种防辐射注射装置

授权日期：2019 年

授权号：CN 209092511 U

发明人：卢洁，赵澄，崔碧霄，帅冬梅，马杰

摘　要：本实用新型实施例公开了一种防辐射注射装置，包括双头卡扣组件和三通阀组件。双头卡扣组件包括第一卡接部、第二卡接部、第一握持部、第二握持部、弹性卡扣、弹性部件。第一卡接部和第二卡接部为弹性卡环；第一握持部为中空结构，一端为连接端且与第一卡接部连接，另一端为活动端，顶部开设一卡孔；第二握持部为一端开口的中空结构，顶部至少开设两个卡孔，套接在第一握持部外侧，其未开口端与第二卡接部连接；弹性卡扣包括弹性连接部和突起部，突起部设在弹性连接部一端，弹性连接部另一端固定在第一握持部内底面上，突起部可穿过卡孔；弹性部件一端与第一握持部活动端连接，另一端与第二握持部未开口端内壁连接。三通阀组件包括三通阀和注射管。

6. 正电子发射断层成像系统有源模体定位方法

授权日期：2019 年

授权号：CN 106333701 B

发明人：邓子林，卢洁

摘　要：本发明提供了一种利用正电子发射断层成像系统进行有源模体定位方法，包括：使用该有源模体的重建图像；选择重建图像中穿过有源模体部分图像的任一截面，沿任一方向获取该截面的灰度轮廓曲线；根据该灰度轮廓曲线选取阈值，并基于该阈值对该重建图像进行二值化处理；根据二值化处理后的重建图像获取该有源模体的中心位置。本发明不依赖于精确且计算量大的图像重建过程，易于实现且定位精度较高。

7. 确定脑部图像冠状位方向的方法及装置

授权日期：2019 年

授权号：CN 103793905 B

发明人：卢洁，王旭，邓丽芳

摘　要：本发明公开了一种确定脑部图像冠状位方向方法及装置。所述方法包括：根据脑部图像重建中心矢状面图；在所述中心矢状面图中分割出脑干区域；在所述脑干区域中确定脑干后边缘

方向；取所述脑干后边缘方向或平行于所述脑干后边缘的方向为所述冠状位方向。所述装置包括：重建单元，根据脑部图像重建中心矢状面图；分割单元，在所述中心矢状面图中分割出脑干区域；确定方向单元，在所述脑干区域中确定脑干后边缘方向；建立方向单元，取所述脑干后边缘方向或平行于所述脑干后边缘方向为所述冠状位方向。通过本发明确定的脑部图像冠状位方向，与所述脑干后边缘方向平行，能更好地满足脑部成像扫描的需要。

8. 一种磁共振检查用头部固定装置

授权日期：2019 年

授权号：CN208876531 U

类型：实用新型专利

发明人：卢洁，赵澄，张苗

摘　要：本实用新型实施例涉及医学设备技术领域，本专利公开了一种磁共振检查用头部固定装置，该装置在现有的磁共振检查保护垫的头垫部分增加了包围部，在包围部上设置了用于固定被检查者头部位置的头部固定器，头部固定器具有充气部，充气部可通过充气放气调整气囊的膨胀度，使气囊通过合适的压力挤压头部，将头部固定在适于检查的位置，可以更好地适应不同被检查者头部大小；头部固定器上还设有可容纳降噪耳机的凹槽，可通过气囊的压力将降噪耳机固定在贴合被检查者耳部的位置，使其不易滑动，起到正常降噪作用，避免因噪音导致被检查者不适而移动头部位置。本实用新型实施例的优点在于贴合性好，固定效果佳，操作方便，舒适稳定，成本低廉。

9. 磁共振头部扫描的线圈装置及其磁共振系统

授权日期：2019 年

授权号：CN 208795833 U

发明人：侯祥明，卢洁

摘　要：本实用新型实施例涉及医学设备技术领域，特别是涉及一种磁共振头部扫描的线圈装置及其磁共振系统。该磁共振头部扫描的线圈装置包括用以套设于患者头部的可伸缩头套，以及设于所述头套内的线圈；所述线圈能够随头套的变形而变形，头套包括与患者头部适配的套体，套体内具有型腔，套体上设有型腔连通的第一开口，并能够通过第一开口将患者头部套入型腔内；所述套体具有相对设置的两个侧面，每一个侧面上均设有分别与第一开口及型腔相连通的第二开口，患者耳部能够通过所述第二开口伸出至型腔的外部。本实用新型实施例的优点在于：贴合性好、检测信噪比高、成像质量高，另外其操作更加方便，成本更低。

10. DICOM 文件的存取方法及其装置

授权日期：2019 年

授权号：CN 105512246 B

发明人：卢洁，李建功

摘　要：本发明提供了一种 DICOM 文件的存取方法及其装置，包括：输入 DICOM 文件；确定 DICOM 文件的文件索引是否在文件信息表中有相应记录；如有，则在文件索引关系表中创建文件索引链接以将 DICOM 文件的文件索引链接到其上层文件索引；否则，将 DICOM 文件存储在 DICOM 文件数据库中，在文件信息表中创建记录以将所述 DICOM 文件的文件索引链接到所存储的文件存储路径，并在文件索引关系表中创建文件索引链接以将所述 DICOM 文件的文件索引链接到其上层文件索引。本发明提供的方法及其装置有效减小了 DICOM 文件的磁盘占用空间，同时缩短了存取 DICOM 文件的时间。

11. 用于制备放射性药物的一次性辅助装置

授权日期：2019 年

授权号：CN 208414286 U

类型：实用新型专利

发明人：乔洪文，卢洁，陈彪

摘　要：本发明涉及一种用于制备放射性药物的一次性辅助装置及方法，属于放射性药物制备装置技术领域，一次性辅助装置由以下部分组成：依次相连接的三个放射化学反应五联三通阀和产品制剂化五联三通阀，放射化学反应五联三通阀中的第一三通阀的左端通过鲁尔接头及硅胶管连接到供气口，第一三通阀的上端连到靶材料回收口，第二三通阀通过离子交换小柱与装有放射性核素 F-18 溶液的锥形容器相连接，放射化学反应五联三通阀中的第十三三通阀通过鲁尔接头与半制备型 HPLC 进样口相连接。本发明装置适用于放射性药物的半制备型高效液相色谱法纯化，保证试剂全部加入反应瓶中或被抽出，能够确保试剂用量的一致性，有利于放射性药物生产的标准化并且能够减少试剂的用量。

一体化 PET/MR
成果推广

一体化 PET/MR 集合 PET 和 MRI 两种成像方法的优势，对于脑疾病的早期诊断、鉴别诊断、指导临床治疗具有显著优势。基于首都医科大学宣武医院一体化 PET/MR 的研究成果及国内外专家的研究工作，组织相关的学术活动和交流，为推动 PET/MR 的临床应用贡献力量。

PET/MR
第一节　PET/MR 脑功能成像工作委员会

在中华医学会核医学分会李亚明主任委员的建议和支持下，于 2016 年 9 月 2 日成立 PET/MR 脑功能成像工作委员会，由核医学专家、放射学专家、脑功能图像后处理专家、放射性药物专家、防护和质控专家共同组成。首都医科大学宣武医院核医学科卢洁教授担任主任委员，左长京（上海长海医院）、李彪（上海交通大学医学院附属瑞金医院）、兰晓莉（华中科技大学同济医学院附属协和医院）、艾林（首都医科大学附属北京天坛医院）担任副主任委员，委员包括白玫（首都医科大学宣武医院）、崔瑞雪（中国医学科学院北京协和医院）、方继良（中国中医科学院广安门医院）、冯逢（中国医学科学院北京协和医院）、富丽萍（中日友好医院）、耿建华（中国医学科学院肿瘤医院）、胡振华（中国科学院自动化研究所）、贾红梅（北京师范大学）、凌雪英（暨南大学附属第一医院）、刘斌（四川大学华西医院）、刘伟（北京大学人民医院）、乔洪文（首都医科大学宣武医院）、孙洪赞（中国医科大学附属盛京医院）、孙夕林（哈尔滨医科大学第四附属医院）、谭海波（复旦大学附属华山医院）、王亚蓉（西安交通大学第一附属医院）、魏龙晓（空军军医大学唐都医院）、翟士桢（北京大学肿瘤医院）、张苗（首都医科大学宣武医院）、邹启红（北京大学）、左西年（中国科学院心理研究所）。该工作委员会成立会议暨第一次工作会议在北京商务会馆召开，李亚明主任委员介绍了工作委员会的发起背景，卢洁教授介绍了工作委员会的筹备情况，并汇报了未来五年的工作计划，委员们对工作计划展开了热烈讨论，提出了宝贵的意见和建议。李亚明主任委员对 PET/MR 脑功能成像工作委员会的成立表示祝贺并寄予厚望，工作委员会以引领行业发展为己任，为推动核医学和神经科学的飞速发展贡献力量。

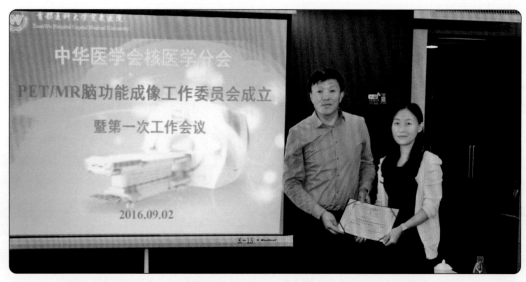

李亚明主任委员为卢洁教授颁发 PET/MR 脑功能成像工作委员会主任委员聘书

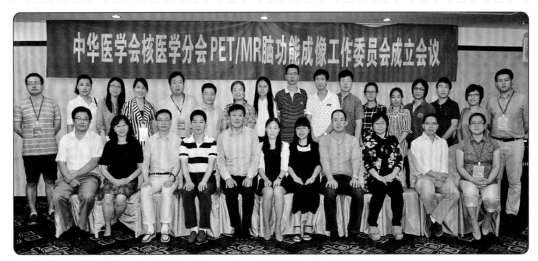

李亚明主任委员与全体委员合影

PET/MR
第二节　全国 PET/MR 脑功能成像学习班

　　首都医科大学宣武医院自 2016 年至 2022 年已连续七年举办全国 PET/MR 脑功能成像学习班，邀请国内外相关领域专家进行专题讲座，与国内外同行增进交流、深入合作，搭建多学科交流平台，分享和推广一体化 PET/MR 在精准医学的研究应用经验，推动 PET/MR 在神经科学领域的发展。

1. 首届全国 PET/MR 脑功能成像学习班

　　首届全国 PET/MR 脑功能成像学习班于 2016 年 9 月 2—4 日在北京举行，首都医科大学宣武医院赵国光院长、首都医科大学王松灵校长、北京市医院管理局边宝生副局长、中华医学会核医学分会李亚明主任委员等出席了开幕式。中国医科大学附属第一医院李亚明教授、中国人民解放军军事医学科学院范明教授和北京大学磁共振成像研究中心高家红教授分别对 PET/MR、脑科学、神经影像的发展作了主旨报告。国内核医学、放射学、神经科学领域专家进行了学术讲座：国家自然科学基金委员会李恩中处长讲解了神经影像学基金申报的注意事项；中国科学院自动化研究所胡振华副研究员介绍了新型核素光学多模融合成像；上海交通大学医学院附属瑞金医院李彪教授分享了 PET/MR 配置申报及运行前准备工作的经验和体会；中国人民解放军总医院徐白萱教授、暨南大学附属第一医院徐浩教授分别介绍了 PET/MR 在神经退行性疾病、癫痫中的应用；中国科学院高能物理研究所单保慈教授、中国科学院心理研究所左西年教授介绍了神经影像数据的后处理；中国医学科学院北京协和医院冯逢教授、首都医科大学宣武医院张苗教授介绍了 MRI 的原理、技术和应用；华中科技大学同济医学院附属协和医院兰晓莉教授、首都医科大学附属北京天坛医院艾林教授、中国医科大学附属盛京医院孙洪赞教授分享了 PET 及 PET/MR 在脑肿瘤中的应用；GE 医疗公司赵周社博士介绍了 PET 的成像原理；中国医学科学院肿瘤医院耿建华教授、首都医科大学宣武医院乔洪文博士分别介绍了 PET/MR 的质量控制和放射性药物；首都医科大学附属北京友谊医院杨吉刚教授分享了 SCI 收录论文写作经验；主办方卢洁教授分享了首都医科大学宣武医院一体化 TOF-PET/MR 的操作流程和在神经系统疾病中的应用体会。学术讲座结束后，学员前往首都医科大学宣武医院现场观摩一体化 TOF-PET/MR 的临床应用及科研应用。

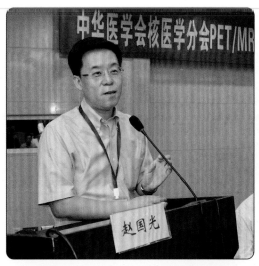

首都医科大学宣武医院赵国光院长致辞

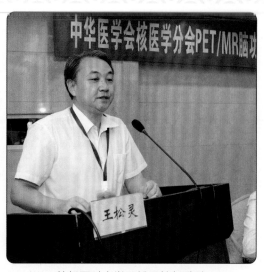

首都医科大学王松灵校长致辞

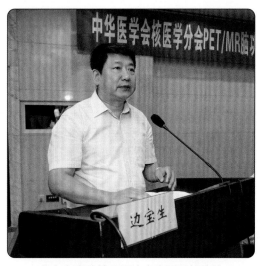

北京市医院管理局边宝生副局长致辞

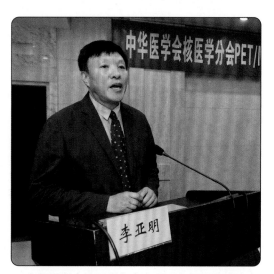

中华医学会核医学分会李亚明主任委员致辞

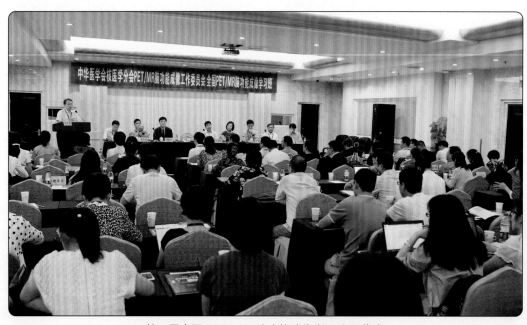

第一届全国PET/MR脑功能成像学习班开幕式

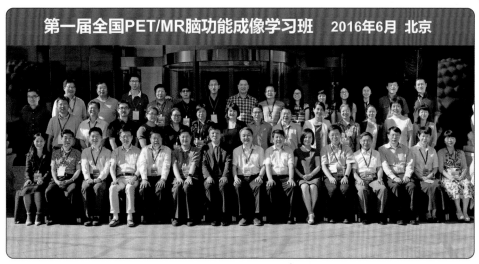

第一届全国 PET/MR 脑功能成像学习班合影

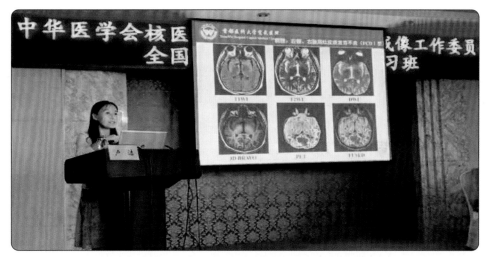

第一届全国 PET/MR 脑功能成像学习班，卢洁教授讲座

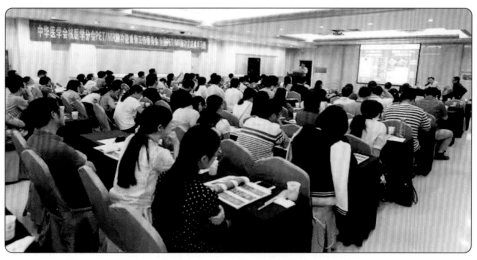

第一届全国 PET/MR 脑功能成像学习班现场

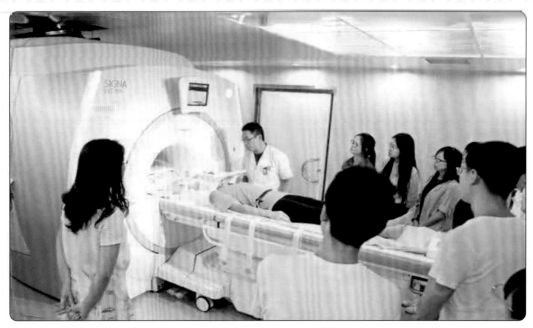

学员现场观摩一体化 PET/MR 扫描

2. 第二届全国 PET/MR 脑功能成像学习班暨《一体化 PET/MR 操作规范和临床应用》新书发布会

第二届全国 PET/MR 脑功能成像学习班于 2017 年 9 月 15—17 日在北京商务会馆举办，核医学、放射学、生物医学工程和神经科学研究领域专家进行了讲座，内容涵盖 PET/MR 在脑功能成像的临床应用、科研进展、发展趋势、课题申报等。2017 年 9 月 15 日上午举行开幕式及 PET/MR 专著《一体化 PET/MR 操作规范和临床应用》新书发布仪式，出席的领导和专家包括首都医科大学宣武医院赵国光院长、中华医学会核医学分会主任委员李亚明教授、中华医学会放射学分会副主任委员暨首都医科大学医学影像学系主任李坤成教授、中国人民解放军军事医学科学院范明教授、北京大学磁共振成像研究中心高家红教授、中华医学会核医学分会副主任委员王铁教授、上海医学会核医学分会副主任委员李彪教授、杭州师范大学认知与脑疾病研究中心臧玉峰教授、中国微循环学会神经变性病专业委员会磁共振学组主任委员韩璎教授等。首都医科大学宣武医院李坤成教授、韩璎教授、吴涛教授、高勇安教授、张苗教授、杨延辉教授、齐志刚教授，中国人民解放军军事医学科学院范明教授，北京大学磁共振成像研究中心高家红教授，中华医学会核医学分会李亚明主任委员，上海交通大学医学院附属瑞金医院李彪教授，中国医学科学院北京协和医院冯逢教授，复旦大学附属华山医院左传涛教授，中国科学院深圳先进技术研究院郑海荣研究员，中国科学院计算机网络信息中心赵地教授，杭州师范大学臧玉峰教授，中国科学院心理研究所左西年教授，中国人民解放军总医院徐白萱教授、马林教授，空军军医大学唐都医院魏龙晓教授，天津医科大学总医院于春水教授，首都医科大学附属北京天坛医院艾林教授，中国医学科学院肿瘤医院耿建华教授，中国中医科学院广安门医院方继良教授，哈尔滨工业大学电子与信息工程学院马婷教授，浙江大学张宏教授，首都医科大学附属北京友谊医院杨吉刚教授分别从国内外脑科学研究进展，PET/MR 发展现状，质量控制，神经系统的 PET 显像剂，神经影像数据处理与分析，PET/MR 在癫痫、帕金森病、阿尔茨海默病、脑肿瘤等神经系统疾病的应用方面介绍了各自的经验和体会。

2017 年 9 月 15 日举办了首都医科大学宣武医院赵国光院长、卢洁教授主编专著《一体化 PET/MR 操作规范和临床应用》的新书发布仪式由北京广播电视台、中国国际广播电台、好医生网、鼎湖影像等多家媒体进行了现场报道。首都医科大学宣武医院作为国内最早对一体化 PET/MR 设备进行验证和评价的单位，对设备质量控制、操作技术规范、示踪剂、全身各系统肿瘤、中枢神经系统重大疾病和心脏病开展了研究，书中介绍了 PET/MR 在脑部疾病中的应用经验，对阿尔茨海默病、帕金森病、癫痫及脑血管病等的病理生理机制、早期诊断和治疗均具有重要的指导意义。

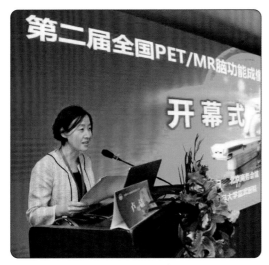

卢洁教授主持开幕式

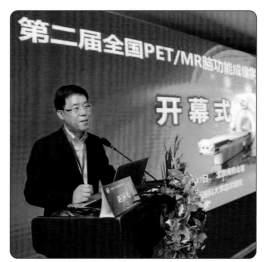

首都医科大学宣武医院赵国光院长致辞

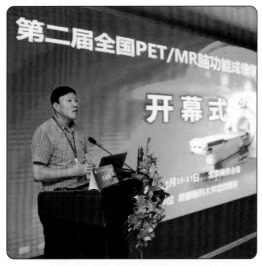

中华医学会核医学分会李亚明主任委员致辞

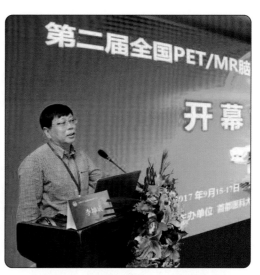

首都医科大学宣武医院李坤成教授致辞

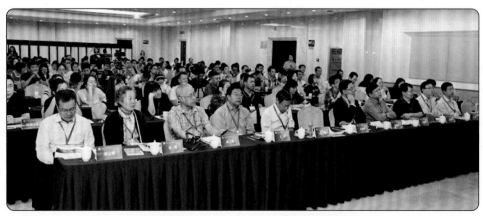

第二届全国 PET/MR 脑功能成像学习班开幕式

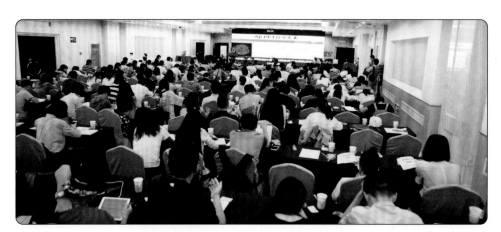

第二届全国 PET/MR 脑功能成像学习班现场

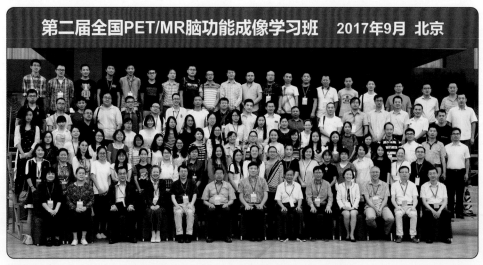

第二届全国 PET/MR 脑功能成像学习班合影

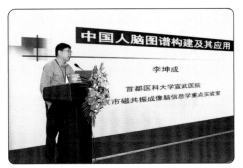
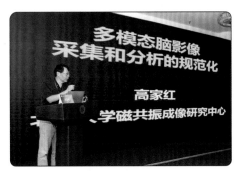

李坤成教授讲座　　　　　　　　　　　　高家红教授讲座

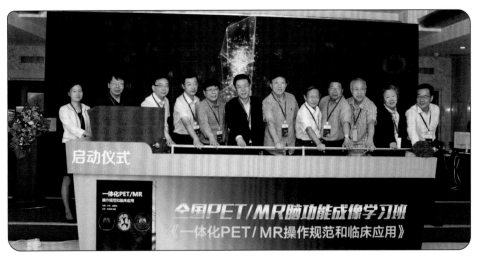

《一体化 PET/MR 操作规范和临床应用》新书发布启动仪式

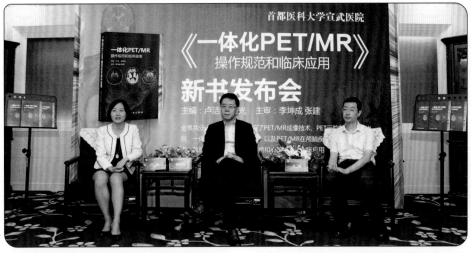

首都医科大学宣武医院赵国光院长（中）、卢洁教授（左一）、吴航处长（右一）
在新书发布会接受媒体采访

3. 第三届全国 PET/MR 脑功能成像学习班

第三届全国 PET/MR 脑功能成像学习班于 2018 年 10 月 20—21 日在北京大方饭店举办，核医学、放射学、生物医学工程、药学、神经科学研究领域专家从 PET/MR 的临床应用、科研进展、优势与面临挑战等方面进行了 30 场讲座。2018 年 10 月 20 日上午举行开幕式，出席的领导和专家包括首都医科大学宣武医院党委书记张国君教授，中华医学会放射学分会主任委员、中国医学科学院北京协和医院放射科主任金征宇教授，北京医学会核医学分会候任主任委员、中国人民解放军总医院第一医学中心核医学科主任徐白萱教授，中国人民解放军空军特色医学中心张挽时教授，中国科学院深圳先进技术研究院副院长郑海荣教授，美国纽约西奈山伊坎医学院 MRI、CT 主任 Lawrence N Tanenbaum 教授，美国耶鲁大学医学院 PET 中心 Yiyun Huang 教授，美国哈佛大学医学院刘河生教授、冉崇昭教授，复旦大学附属华山医院 PET 中心副主任左传涛教授，中国中医科学院广安门医院方继良教授等。中国医学科学院北京协和医院金征宇教授、冯逢教授、朱朝晖教授，中国人民解放军总医院第一医学中心马林教授、徐白萱教授，中国科学院深圳先进技术研究院郑海荣教授，中国科学院自动化研究所田捷教授，天津医科大学总医院于春水教授，河南省人民医院王梅云教授，北京医院陈敏教授，中国科学院化学研究所高明远教授，中国科学院高能物理研究所单保慈教授，空军军医大学唐都医院魏龙晓教授，复旦大学附属华山医院左传涛教授，中国医学科学院肿瘤医院耿建华教授，天津医科大学第二医院张雪宁教授，首都医科大学附属北京友谊医院杨吉刚教授，首都医科大学附属北京天坛医院马军教授、艾林教授，中日友好医院马国林教授，大连大学附属中山医院张清教授，Elsevier 大中华区曹引总经理，美国纽约西奈山伊坎医学院 Lawrence N Tanenbaum 教授，美国耶鲁大学医学院 PET 中心 Yiyun Huang 教授，美国哈佛大学医学院刘河生教授、冉崇昭教授。在此次学习班上首都医科大学宣武医院李坤成教授、韩璎教授、卢洁教授、高勇安教授、殷雅彦博士分别就 PET 原理、心脑疾病的 PET/MR 研究、PET/MR 临床应用中的优势与面临的挑战等内容进行了介绍；首都医科大学宣武医院年轻医师就 PET/MR 在缺血性脑血管病、认知障碍、颈动脉斑块等疾病中的应用进行了经验分享。

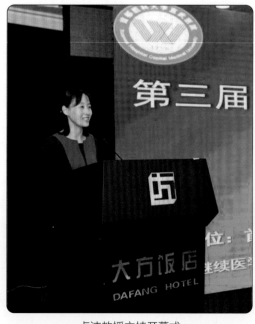

卢洁教授主持开幕式

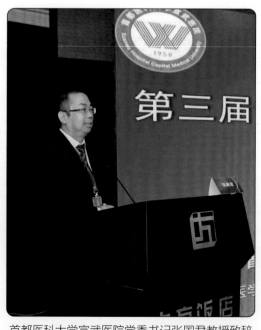

首都医科大学宣武医院党委书记张国君教授致辞

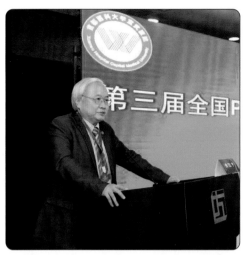
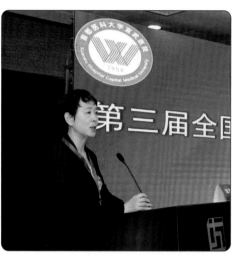

中国医学科学院北京协和医院金征宇教授致辞　　中国人民解放军总医院第一医学中心
　　　　　　　　　　　　　　　　　　　　　　徐白萱教授致辞

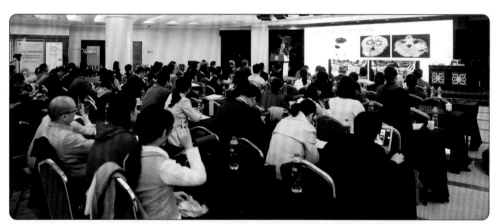

第三届全国 PET/MR 脑功能成像学习班现场

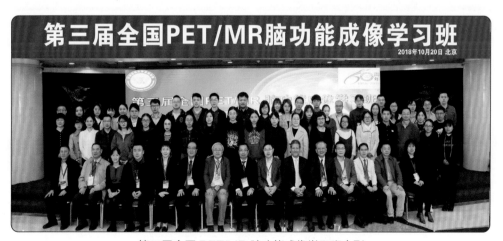

第三届全国 PET/MR 脑功能成像学习班合影

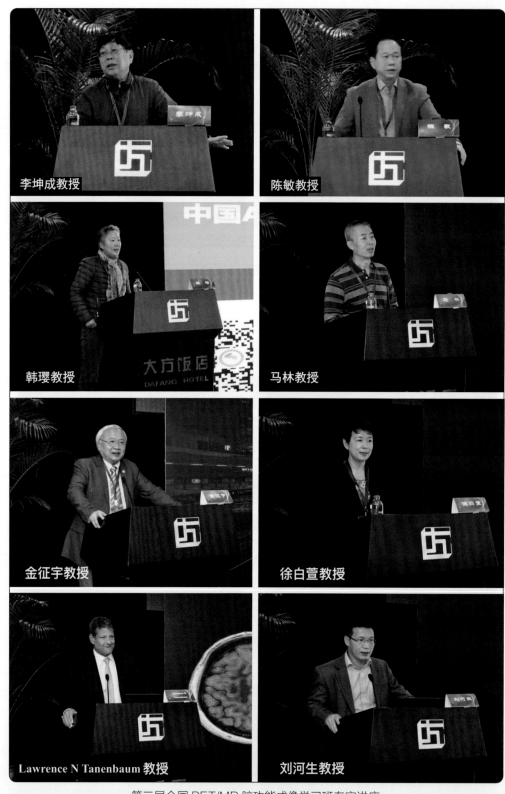

第三届全国 PET/MR 脑功能成像学习班专家讲座

4.第四届全国 PET/MR 脑功能成像学习班暨全国 PET/MR 脑功能成像高阶强化培训班

第四届全国 PET/MR 脑功能成像学习班于 2019 年 10 月 8—12 日在首都医科大学宣武医院新区会议室举办，本次学习班为高阶强化培训班，采用小班教学模式，招收学员 20 余人，分为理论授课 3 天，实践操作 2 天。来自核医学、放射学、生物医学工程、药学、神经科学研究领域的专家进行了讲座，内容涵盖 PET/MR 在脑功能成像中的临床应用、科研进展、发展趋势、文章投稿等。2019 年 10 月 8 日上午举行开幕式，出席的领导和专家包括中国医师协会核医学医师分会会长、北京医学会核医学分会主任委员、首都医科大学附属北京朝阳医院核医学科主任王铁教授，首都医科大学宣武医院赵国光院长等。在本次学习班上中国人民解放军总医院第一医学中心徐白萱教授，中国人民解放军空军特色医学中心张挽时教授，中国医学科学院北京协和医院冯逢教授，首都医科大学附属北京友谊医院杨正汉教授，上海交通大学医学院附属瑞金医院李彪教授，复旦大学附属中山医院石洪成教授，北京师范大学崔孟超教授，中国科学院高能物理研究所单保慈教授，空军军医大学唐都医院魏龙晓教授，复旦大学附属华山医院左传涛教授，首都医科大学附属北京天坛医院艾林教授，《中华放射学杂志》编辑部主任张琳琳，首都医科大学宣武医院唐毅教授、韩璎教授、吴航教授、齐志刚教授、张苗教授、杨延辉教授、赵志莲教授、曹丽珍教授、张海琴教授、苏玉盛教授、尚琨博士、李琼阁博士、李静博士、殷雅彦博士和乔洪文博士，欧洲医学和生物学磁共振学会前主任委员、GE PET/MR 全球培训中心特邀高级顾问、苏黎世大学医学院影像中心主席 Gustav K.von Schulthess 及美国华盛顿大学医学院 Manu S.Goyal 教授分别从 PET/MR 的临床应用、诊断前沿、新技术进展、科研进展、发展趋势、《中华放射学杂志》投稿要求等方面进行了介绍；会后由崔碧霄博士及杨宏伟技师、马杰技师主持一体化 PET/MR 现场观摩和讲解。

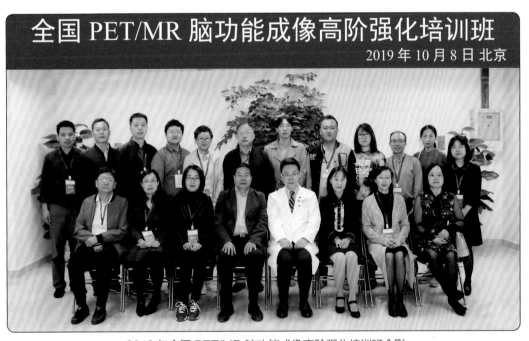

2019 年全国 PET/MR 脑功能成像高阶强化培训班合影

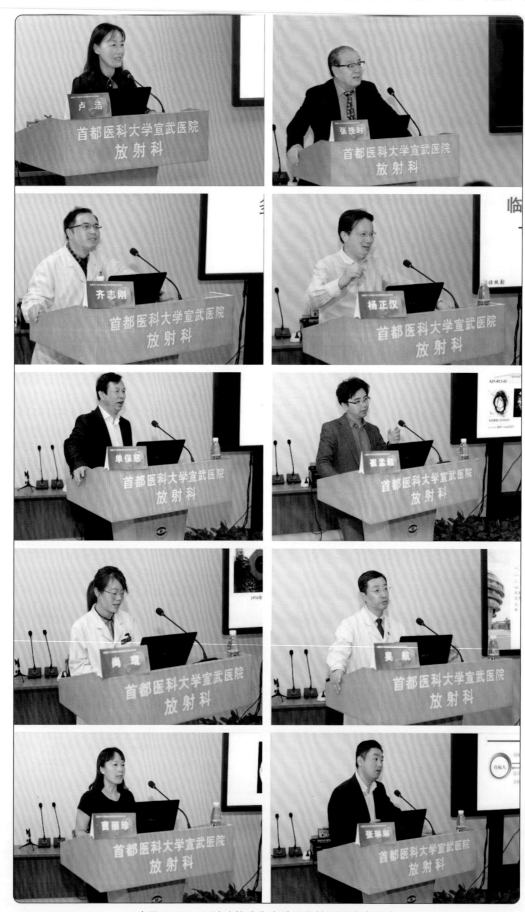

全国 PET/MR 脑功能成像高阶强化培训班专家讲座

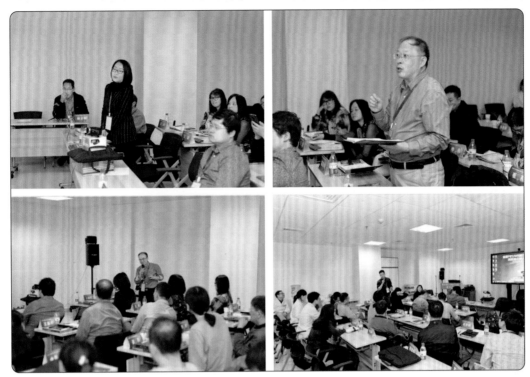
全国 PET/MR 脑功能成像高阶强化培训班现场，学员与专家互动交流

5. 第五届全国 PET/MR 脑功能成像学习班暨《一体化 PET/MR 护理实操手册》新书发布

第五届全国 PET/MR 脑功能成像学习班于 2020 年 10 月 29—31 日在首都医科大学宣武医院新区会议室举办，受新冠肺炎疫情影响本次学习班采用线上线下相结合的方式，由北京专家现场授课，外地专家线上授课。2020 年 10 月 29 日上午举行开幕式及《一体化 PET/MR 护理实操手册》新书发布，出席的领导和专家包括首都医科大学宣武医院院长赵国光教授，北京医学会核医学分会候任主任委员暨中国人民解放军总医院第一医学中心核医学科主任徐白萱教授等。来自核医学、放射学、生物医学工程、药学、神经科学等研究领域的专家，包括北京大学肿瘤医院杨志教授，中国医学科学院北京协和医院霍力教授，北京大学第三医院邬海博教授，中国人民解放军总医院第六医学中心程流泉教授，中国科学院自动化研究所田捷教授、刘勇教授，河南省人民医院王梅云教授，中国科学院高能物理研究所单保慈教授，华中科技大学同济医学院附属协和医院兰晓莉教授，上海交通大学医学院附属瑞金医院李彪教授，复旦大学附属中山医院石洪成教授，中国医科大学附属盛京医院辛军教授，上海市东方医院赵军教授，南京市第一医院王峰教授，复旦大学附属华山医院左传涛教授，中国医学科学院肿瘤医院耿建华教授，首都医科大学附属北京天坛医院艾林教授，首都医科大学附属北京安贞医院张晓丽教授，首都医科大学附属北京友谊医院杨正汉教授，北京师范大学崔孟超教授等在放射性药物研发与制备、PET/MR 在不同疾病的影像表现特点、诊断及鉴别诊断、科研进展等方面进行了介绍。

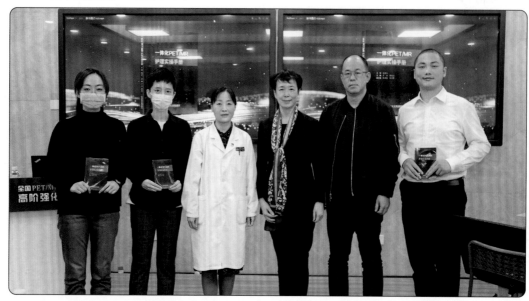

《一体化 PET/MR 护理实操手册》新书发布会，卢洁教授（左三）、徐白萱教授（右三）、
艾林教授（右二）向学员赠书

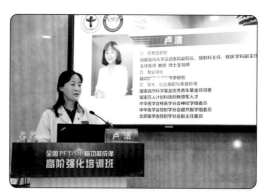

卢洁教授讲座

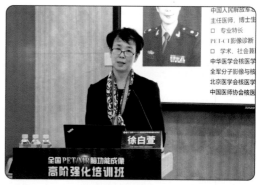

徐白萱教授讲座

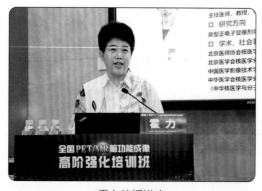

霍力教授讲座

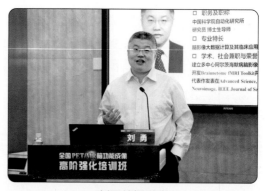

刘勇教授讲座

6. 第六届全国 PET/MR 脑功能成像学习班暨《PET/MR 脑功能与分子影像：从脑疾病到脑科学》新书发布

第六届全国 PET/MR 脑功能成像学习班于 2021 年 9 月 10—12 日采用全部线上授课形式举办。中国医科大学附属第一医院李亚明教授，第四军医大学第一附属医院西京医院汪静教授，中国人民

解放军总医院第一医学中心徐白萱教授，北京大学肿瘤医院杨志教授，复旦大学附属中山医院石洪成教授，华中科技大学同济医学院附属协和医院兰晓莉教授，中国人民解放军空军特色医学中心张挽时教授，浙江大学张宏教授，中国科学院精密测量科学与技术创新研究院周欣教授，中国科学院田捷教授，北京大学陈良怡教授，厦门大学刘刚教授，中国医学科学院北京协和医院冯逢教授、霍力教授，中国人民解放军东部战区总医院张龙江教授，四川大学华西医院吕粟教授，上海大学蒋皆恢教授，首都医科大学附属北京天坛医院艾林教授，上海交通大学医学院附属瑞金医院李彪教授，上海市第六人民医院李跃华教授，中日友好医院谢晟教授，中南大学湘雅二医院刘军教授，暨南大学附属第一医院徐浩教授，上海长海医院左长京教授，复旦大学附属华山医院左传涛教授，上海市东方医院赵军教授，南京市第一医院王峰教授，中国医科大学附属盛京医院孙洪赞教授，首都医科大学附属北京安贞医院张晓丽教授，首都医科大学附属北京友谊医院杨正汉教授等从 MRI 新技术、影像大数据的临床应用、分子影像与病理、临床转化等方面进行了介绍。

2021 年 9 月 10 日首都医科大学宣武医院赵国光院长、卢洁教授主编专著《PET/MR 脑功能与分子影像：从脑疾病到脑科学》一书发布，本书全面总结了首都医科大学宣武医院应用一体化 PET/MR 成像在脑疾病诊疗和研究方面的最新进展，并介绍了国内外脑科学领域的最新成果，包括脑疾病临床应用和脑科学研究现状，有助于广大医学影像专业人员掌握一体化 PET/MR 影像诊断要领，同时本书在脑功能与分子影像的科研工作中也具有重要的参考价值。

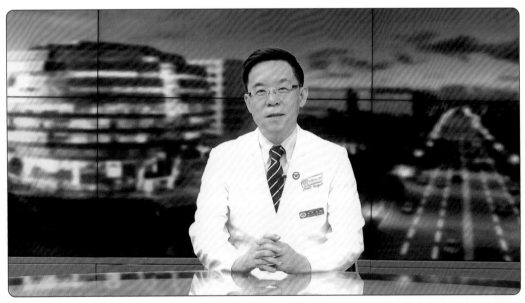

赵国光院长致辞

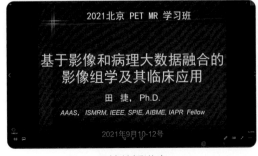

田捷教授讲座

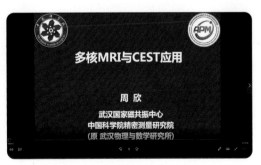

周欣教授讲座

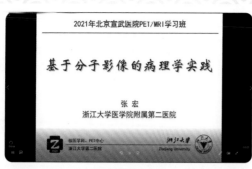
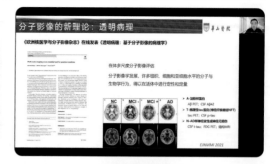

张宏教授讲座　　　　　　　　　　　　左传涛教授讲座

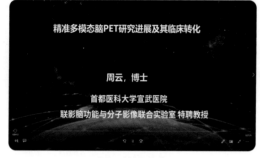
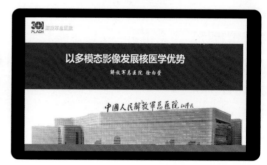

周云教授讲座　　　　　　　　　　　　徐白萱教授讲座

7. 第七届全国 PET/MR 脑功能成像学习班

　　第七届全国 PET/MR 脑功能成像学习班于 2022 年 10 月 14—16 日在线上举办，核医学、放射学、生物医学工程、药学和神经科学等研究领域的专家进行了讲座，主要内容包括 PET/MR 国内外最新应用与实践经验、国际前沿科研成果等。2022 年 10 月 14 日上午举行开幕式，出席的领导和专家包括首都医科大学宣武医院赵国光院长、中国人民解放军总医院第一医学中心徐白萱教授及北京大学肿瘤医院杨志教授等。中国医科大学附属第一医院李亚明教授，中国科学院分子影像重点实验室田捷教授，复旦大学人类表型组研究院田梅教授，厦门大学刘刚教授，苏州大学高明远教授，北京师范大学崔孟超教授，上海大学蒋皆恢教授，复旦大学附属中山医院石洪成教授，北京大学肿瘤医院杨志教授，上海市东方医院赵军教授，南京市第一医院王峰教授，华中科技大学同济医学院附属同济医院朱小华教授、樊卫教授，中山大学附属第一医院张祥松教授，中国人民解放军总医院第一医学中心徐白萱教授，华中科技大学同济医学院附属协和医院兰晓莉教授，中国医学科学院北京协和医院霍力教授，中国医科大学附属盛京医院辛军教授、孙洪赞教授，郑州大学第一附属医院韩星敏教授，首都医科大学附属北京天坛医院艾林教授，浙江大学张宏教授，暨南大学附属第一医院徐浩教授、王璐教授，上海交通大学医学院附属瑞金医院李彪教授，上海长海医院左长京教授，复旦大学附属华山医院左传涛教授，青岛大学附属医院王振光教授，首都医科大学附属北京安贞医院张晓丽教授，中国科学院深圳先进技术研究院郑海荣教授，中国科学院精密测量科学与技术创新研究院周欣教授，北京医院蔡葵教授，上海市第六人民医院李斌教授，上海市第一人民医院王悍教授，首都医科大学附属北京友谊医院杨正汉教授，中国科学院高能物理研究所单保慈教授，中国医学科学院肿瘤医院耿建华教授，美国耶鲁大学医学院 PET 中心 Yiyun Huang 教授，新加坡国立大学陈小元教授，美国威斯康星大学麦迪逊分校蔡伟波教授，维也纳总医院李翔教授，芬兰国家 PET 中心韩春雷教授，昭和大学明石定子教授分别介绍了 PET/MR 脑功能与分子影像的基础原理、扫描流程、图像分析等临床常见问题，以及新型放射性药物的研发与转化、分子影像精准治疗等。

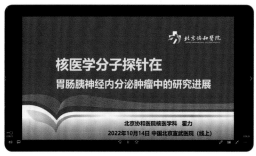

霍力教授讲座

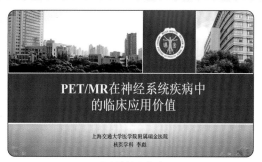

李彪教授讲座

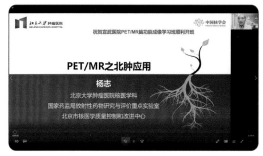

杨志教授讲座

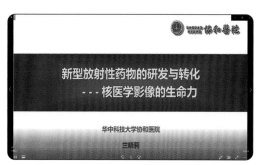

兰晓莉教授讲座

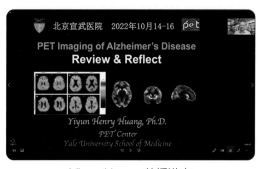

Yiyun Huang 教授讲座

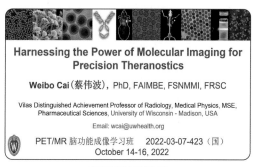

蔡伟波教授讲座

PET/MR
第三节　国内外学术会议交流

　　自 2016 年 1 月至 2022 年 12 月，卢洁教授在国际会议上做特邀报告 3 篇，团队成员有 33 篇研究摘要入选美国核医学与分子影像学会年会（Society of Nuclear Medicine and Molecular Imaging，SNMMI）、北美放射学会（Radiological Society of North America，RSNA）等国际学术会议壁报或口头发言，15 篇研究摘要入选中华医学会核医学分会学术年会、中华医学会全国放射学学术大会、中华医学会全国医学影像技术学学术大会等国内学术会议壁报或口头发言。

1. 特邀报告

[1] Jie Lu. PET/MR imaging：new frontier in Alzheimer's disease. The 10th International Congress on Magnetic Resonance Imaging & 27th Annual Scientific Meeting of KSMRM. 2022，Seoul，Korea.

[2] Jie Lu. PET/MR imaging：new frontier in Alzheimer's disease. The 14th Asian Oceania Congress of Nuclear Medicine and Biology. 2022，Kyoto，Japan.

[3] Jie Lu. Hybrid PET/MR in epilepsy. Joint Annual Meeting ISMRM-ESMRMB，2018，Paris，France.

2. 国际学术会议

[1] Shaozhen Yan. Sex and APOE ε 4 genotype modify early detection of Alzheimer's disease using random forest based on ^{18}F-flortaucipir PET. 2022，SNMMI，poster.

[2] Bixiao Cui，Min Wang，Jie Lu. Quantification of brain glucose metabolism by ^{18}F-FDG PET/MR with image-derived input function in ischemic cerebrovascular disease. 2022，SNMMI，poster.

[3] Bixiao Cui，Hongwei Yang，Jie Ma，et al. Chronic symptomatic unilateral anterior circulation stenosis or occlusion patients：a study of simultaneous cerebral blood flow and metabolism. 2021，SNMMI，poster.

[4] Yue Zhang，Jie Lu，Hongwei Yang，et al. Correlation between inflammation and neovascularization in carotid atherosclerotic plaques based on hybrid ^{18}F-FDG PET/MRI：a pathological validation study. 2020，SNMMI，oral.

[5] Hongwei Yang，Jie Lu，Bixiao Cui，et al. Quantitative performance and optimal regularization parameter in block sequential regularized expectation maximization reconstructions in carotid plaques with ^{18}F-FDG PET /MR. 2020，SNMMI，oral.

[6] Jie Lu. Altered coupling between resting-state glucose metabolism and functional activity in medial temporal lobe epilepsy with hippocampal sclerosis：a hybrid PET/MR study. 2020，SNMMI，oral.

[7] Shuangshuang Song，Jie Lu. Grade and IDH genotype prediction in glioma by a hybird PET/MR with FET-PET and DSC-PWI. 2020，SNMMI，oral.

[8] Kun Shang，Jiehui Jiang，Jie Lu. Functional connectivity of epileptic network in medial temporal lobe epilepsy and the relationship with disease parameters：a hybrid PET/MR study. 2020，SNMMI，poster.

[9] Shaozhen Yan，Chaojie Zheng，Bixiao Cui，et al. Relationship between nucleus basalis of Meynert resting state functional connectivity and brain ^{18}F-FDG metabolism in Alzheimer's disease：a hybrid PET/MR study. 2020，SNMMI，poster.

[10] Yue Zhang.Association between neovascularization and inflammation in carotid atherosclerotic plaques evaluated by hybrid ^{18}F-FDG PET/MRI：a pathological validation study. 2020，RSNA，oral.

[11] Shaozhen Yan. The relationship between connectivity and metabolism of hippocampal cornus ammonis 1（CA1）in Alzheimer's disease using hybrid FDG-PET/MRI. 2019，SNMMI，oral.

[12] Shaozhen Yan，Hongwei Yang，Jie Ma，et al. The alters of functional MRI and PET（18F-FDG and ^{18}F-AV45）in posterior cingulate of Alzheimer's disease using hybird PET/MRI. 2019，SNMMI，poster.

[13] Yue Zhang，Jie Lu，Hongwei Yang，et al. Evaluation of hybrid ^{18}F-FDG PET/MR imaging of vulnerable plaque features in patients with carotid plaques. 2019 SNMMI，oral.

[14] Tianbin Song，Bixiao Cui，Jie Ma，et al. Evaluation of the detection ability of integrated

PET/MR for lymph node metastases in patients with stage I-IIA1 endometrial and cervical cancer. 2019 SNMMI，oral.

[15] Bixiao Cui，Jie Lu，Hongwei Yang，et al. Change of cerebral blood flow and glucose metabolism in patients with ischemic cerebrovascular disease. 2019 SNMMI，poster.

[16] Tianbin Song，mingyang wang，Bixiao Cui，et al. Assessment of infarction and metabolism with integrated TOF- PET/MR in MCAO rats. 2019 SNMMI，poster.

[17] Yue Zhang，Jie Lu. Varying correlation between inflammation and microvascularization in carotid atherosclerotic plaques with hybrid ^{18}F-FDG PET/MR. 2019，RSNA，oral.

[18] Yue Zhang，Jie Lu. Vulnerable plaque features can be detected in carotid plaques with hybrid ^{18}F-FDG PET/MR imaging. 2019，RSNA，oral.

[19] Jingwen Zhuang，Mei Bai. A phantom study on radiotracer dose reduction in integrated PET/MR system. 2019，EANM，poster.

[20] Bixiao Cui，Jie Lu，Jie Ma，et al. Comparison of cerebral blood flow measurement with ^{18}F-FDG positron emission tomography（PET）and arterial spin labeling（ASL）on hybrid PET-MR. 2018，SNMMI，poster.

[21] Tianbin Song，Jie Lu，Bixiao Cui，et al. Preoperative assessment of diagnostic value in staging pancreatic cancer with hybrid TOF-PET/MR imaging versus PET/CT. 2018，SNMMI，poster.

[22] Bixiao Cui，Jie Lu，Kun Shang，et al. The study of correlation between the ^{18}F-FDG PET-IDIF and ASL sequence imaging on hybrid PET-MR. 2017，SNMMI，oral.

[23] Jingjuan Wang，Kun Shang，Bixiao Cui，et al. Disabled effective connectivity from hippocampus to posterior central gyrus in temporal lobe epilepsy with hippocampal sclerosis. 2017，SNMMI，oral.

[24] Tianbin Song，Bixiao Cui，Jie Ma，et al. The effect of examination order of dual-imaging protocol of PET/MR and PET/CT Imaging in ^{18}F-FDG uptake of focal malignat lesion. 2017，SNMMI，poster.

[25] Kun Shang，Jingjuan Wang，Bixiao Cui，et al. Hybrid TOF PET-MRI in localizing seizure focus in patients with MRI negative temporal lobe epilepsy. 2017，SNMMI，poster.

[26] Tao Wan，Bixiao Cui，Yaping Wang，et al. A radiomics approach for automated identification of aggressive tumors on combined PET and multi-parametric MRI. 2017，International Conference on Neural Information Processing，poster.

[27] Shuo Dong，Dong Li，Tianqi Wu，et al.The effect of technology on PET image quality of integrated PET/MR equipment. 2016，SNMMI，oral.

[28] Bixiao Cui，Jie Ma，Kun Shang，et al. Evaluation of neoplastic lesions using TOF and PSF in hybrid PET/MRI. 2016，SNMMI，poster.

[29] Bixiao Cui，Jie Ma，Kun Shang，et al. The effect of time-of-flight（TOF）technique in eliminating "hot trachea" artifacts in hybrid PET/MR scanning. 2016，SNMMI，poster.

[30] Bixiao Cui，Su Yusheng，Ziling Deng，et al. Clinical evaluation of TOF-PET image

reconstruction with small lesion. 2016，SNMMI，poster.

[31] Tianqi Wu，Ping Wu，Jingwen Zhuang，et al. Effect of acquisition time and matrix on the image quality in integarted PET/MR. 2016，SNMMI，poster.

[32] Feng Xie，Jingwen Zhuang，Tianqi Wu，et al. Evaluation of PET spatial resolution on integrated PET/MR. 2016，SNMMI，poster.

[33] Feng Xie，Jingwen Zhuang，Tianqi Wu，et al. Study on Shine-Through artifacts in integrated PET/MR imaging. 2016，SNMMI，poster.

3. 国内学术会议

[1] 崔碧霄. 基于一体化 PET/MR 联合血流、代谢在慢性缺血性脑血管病患者的初步应用. 中华医学会核医学分会 2021 年学术年会，口头发言.

[2] 杨宏伟. BSREM 重建算法在颈动脉斑块 ^{18}F-FDG PET/MR 成像的初步研究. 中华医学会核医学分会 2021 年学术年会，壁报.

[3] 郭坤，王静娟. SPM-PET 结合 MAP 在核磁阴性的难治性癫痫中的定位价值. 中华医学会核医学分会 2021 年学术年会，壁报.

[4] 宋天彬，杨宏伟. 一体化 TOF-PET/MR 检查对肺部小结节（≤ 10 mm）的检出及 ^{18}F-FDG 代谢显示价值的探讨. 中华医学会第 26 次全国放射学学术大会（CCR2019），口头发言.

[5] 杨宏伟. 基于一体化 PET/MR 的 Q. 静态运动校正采集模式对体部病灶成像的影响. 2019 年中华医学会第 27 次全国医学影像技术学学术大会暨山东省第 14 次放射技术学学术大会，口头发言.

[6] 宋天彬，崔碧霄. DWI 序列在一体化 TOF-PET/MR 检查中对体部 ^{18}F-FDG 阳性微小病灶的诊断价值探讨. 中华医学会核医学分会 2018 年学术年会，口头发言.

[7] 杨宏伟. 一体化 TOF-PET/MR 飞行时间技术对图像质量的影响. 中华医学会核医学分会 2018 年学术年会，口头发言.

[8] 崔碧霄. 一体化 PET/MR ^{18}F-FDG PET-IDIF 方法与 ASL 方法测量脑血流量的相关性研究. 中华医学会核医学分会 2017 年学术年会，壁报.

[9] 乔洪文. [^{18}F]Florbetapir 脑部 PET/MR 显像视觉判定准确性分析. 中华医学会核医学分会 2017 年学术年会，壁报.

[10] 宋天彬. DWI 序列在 PET/MR 检查中对体部 ^{18}F-FDG 阳性病灶的应用必要性探讨. 中华医学会核医学分会 2017 年学术年会，壁报.

[11] 尚琨，崔碧霄. 一体化 TOF PET/MR 在 MRI 阴性难治性癫痫中的初步应用. 中华医学会核医学分会 2016 年学术年会，壁报.

[12] 崔碧霄，尚琨，卢洁，等. 一体化 PET/MR 设备 TOF 和 PSF 技术检出肿瘤病灶价值探讨. 中华医学会第 23 次全国放射学学术大会（CCR2016），壁报.

[13] 崔碧霄，卢洁，马杰，等. 一体化 TOF PET/MR 在胰腺疾病中的初步应用. 中华医学会第 23 次全国放射学学术大会（CCR2016），壁报.

[14] 马杰，崔碧霄，卢洁，等. 一体化 TOF PET/MR 的 PET 质量控制. 中华医学会第 23 次全国放射学学术大会（CCR2016），壁报.

[15] 崔碧霄，王鑫，张海琴，等. 一体化 PET/MR 飞行时间技术和点扩散函数技术检测肿瘤病灶价值的探讨. 2015 年第七届全国核医学与分子影像学术会议暨首届全国 PET/MR 学术研讨会会议，壁报.

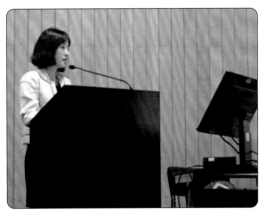

卢洁教授在国际磁共振年会（2018 年，法国）作特邀学术报告

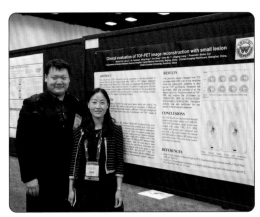

崔碧霄博士与卢洁教授参加美国核医学与分子影像学会年会（2016 年 SNMMI）

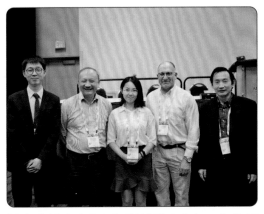

闫少珍博士（中）与张越博士（左一）参加美国核医学与分子影像学会年会（2019 年 SNMMI），与美国耶鲁大学医学院 PET 中心 Yiyun Huang 教授（左二）、耶鲁大学医学院放射与分子影像系 Evan Morris 教授（右二）、美国圣路易斯华盛顿大学周云教授（右一）合影

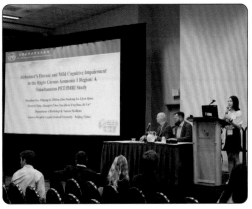

闫少珍博士在美国核医学与分子影像学会年会发言（2019 年 SNMMI）

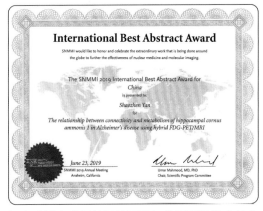

闫少珍博士获得美国核医学与分子影像学会年会国际最佳摘要奖（2019 年 SNMMI）

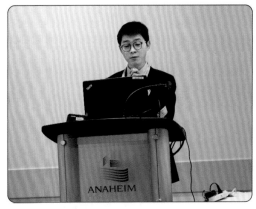

张越博士在美国核医学与分子影像学会年会发言（2019 年 SNMMI）

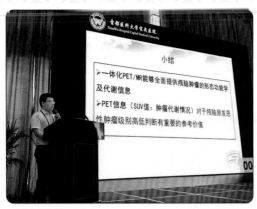

宋天彬博士在中华医学会第 26 次全国放射学学术大会发言（2019 年 CCR）

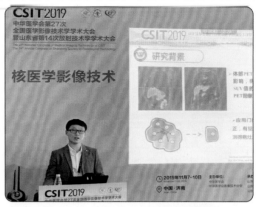

杨宏伟技师在中华医学会第 27 次全国医学影像技术学学术大会发言（2019 年 CSIT）

PET/MR
第四节　国内外推广交流

　　2015 年 7 月，GE 公司全球 PET/MR 培训经理 Julie 女士在首都医科大学宣武医院进行了一周的培训。2018 年 8 月 14 日首都医科大学宣武医院依托首都医科大学核医学系举办了北京国际核医学与分子影像高峰论坛，邀请加利福尼亚大学洛杉矶分校分子与医学药理学系和生物数学系教授 Sung-cheng（Henry）Huang、圣路易斯华盛顿大学放射学和生物医学工程副教授 Yuan-Chuan Tai、约翰斯·霍普金斯大学医学院放射科物理与信息学联合主任 Yun Zhou 和悉尼大学信息技术学院多媒体实验室副主任 Xiuying WANG、美国耶鲁大学生物医学工程和精神病学教授 Evan D. Morris、美国国立卫生研究院国家精神卫生研究所分子成像分部 PET 物理学家 Jeih-San Liow、约翰斯·霍普金斯大学医学院行为药理学系精神病学和行为科学助理教授 Fred Barrett、华盛顿大学多模态临床前成像实验室联合主任 Kooresh Shoghi、约翰斯·霍普金斯大学医学院放射学教授 Benjamin M. W. Tsui 和芬兰图尔库大学医院 Chunlei Han 等专家做专题讲座，北京核医学界同仁参加了本次学术论坛，其对开阔科研思路，加强国际合作具有指导意义。2018 年 8 月 25 日，首都医科大学宣武医院参加由 GE 医疗发起的国内 SIGNA™ PET/MR 精英社群——盖亚俱乐部在上海的成立仪式。2019 年 2 月，卢洁教授率领团队成员前往瑞士苏黎世大学附属医院交流学习，搭建中瑞核医学合作的桥梁。2019 年 3 月 25 日，在首都医科大学宣武医院举办了国际神经影像研讨会，Gary H. Glover（斯坦福大学影像学暨神经科学与生物物理学教授，美国国家工程院院士）、国际人类脑图谱学会主席高家红教授，中国人民解放军空军特色医学中心张挽时教授，GE 医疗集团首席科学家 Dr. R. Scott Hinks 等国内外专家出席了会议；会议期间，首都医科大学宣武医院与 GE 公司签署战略合作协议，成为 GE PET/MR 全球培训中心。2021 年 9 月 28 日，首都医科大学宣武医院与联影医疗技术集团有限公司签署了战略合作协议，成立宣武—联影脑功能与分子影像联合实验室。2015 年 7 月至 2022 年 12 月，全国兄弟医院的医师、护士及技术人员等 30 余人赴首都医科大学宣武医院进修学习，推动了 PET/MR 的临床应用。

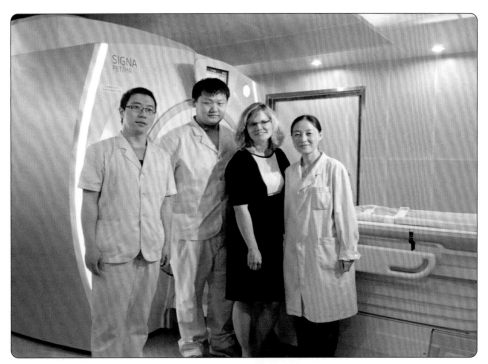

GE 公司培训专员 Julie 与卢洁教授团队合影（2015 年）

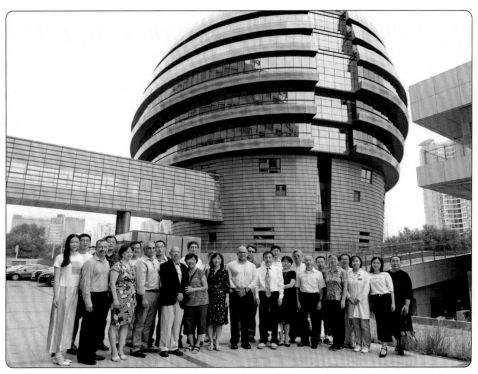

北京国际核医学与分子影像高峰论坛（2018 年）

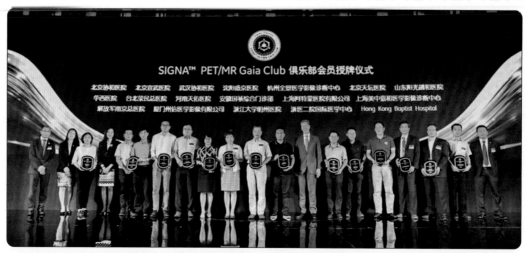

首都医科大学宣武医院参加盖亚俱乐部授牌仪式（2018 年）

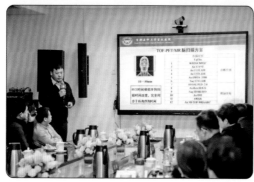

崔碧霄博士在"SIGNA™ PET/MR Gaia Club 系列活动之高级临床科研论坛"做报告（2018 年）

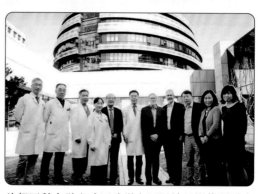

首都医科大学宣武医院举办国际神经影像研讨会（2019 年）

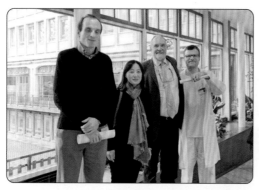

卢洁教授团队在瑞士苏黎世大学附属医院交流学习（2019 年）

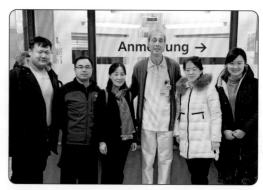

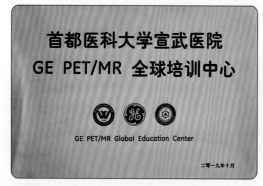

首都医科大学宣武医院 GE PET/MR 全球培训中心成立（2019 年）

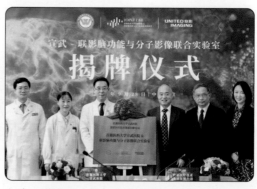

宣武—联影脑功能与分子影像联合实验室签约仪式（2021 年）

姓　名	单位及职务	进修时间
郭　坤	空军军医大学唐都医院 主治医师	2016 年 12 月 15—31 日
张　微	空军军医大学唐都医院 技师	2016 年 12 月 15—31 日
阮伟伟	华中科技大学同济医学院附属协和医院 技师	2017 年 10 月 17—20 日
刘　芳	华中科技大学同济医学院附属协和医院 副主任医师	2017 年 9 月 4—8 日
王　婷	华中科技大学同济医学院附属协和医院 护师	2017 年 9 月 4—8 日
张其锐	中国人民解放军东部战区总医院 硕士研究生	2018 年 1—2 月
权　巍	中国人民解放军东部战区总医院 硕士研究生	2018 年 1—2 月

第二章　一体化 PET/MR 成果推广

姓　名	单位及职务	进修时间
赵　升	云南省肿瘤医院 主治医师	2018 年 1—6 月
李鹏宇	河南省人民医院 技师	2019 年 8 月 5—10 日
周凯悦	大连医科大学附属第二医院 技师	2018 年 9—11 月
杜　彪	郑州大学第一附属医院 主治医师	2019 年 9 月—2020 年 3 月
陈颖琦	中国人民解放军东部战区总医院 主任护师	2020 年 1 月 6—17 日
潘　璟	中国人民解放军东部战区总医院 初级药师	2020 年 1 月 6—17 日
唐春香	中国人民解放军东部战区总医院 主治医师	2020 年 1 月 6—17 日

	姓　名	单位及职务	进修时间
	马　璐	中国人民解放军东部战区总医院 技师	2020 年 1 月 6—17 日
	高珂梦	江苏省人民医院 住院医师	2021 年 4—12 月
	杨　品	兰州大学第二医院 主治医师	2021 年 9 月—2022 年 3 月
	刘　婷	广州中医药大学金沙洲医院 副主任医师	2022 年 9—12 月
	俞美香	延边大学附属医院（延边医院） 主治医师	2022 年 7 月—2023 年 1 月

第二章　一体化 PET/MR 成果推广

PET/MR

第三章

一体化 PET/MR 研究团队

首都医科大学宣武医院是以神经科学和老年医学为重点的三级甲等综合医院，为国家神经疾病医学中心、国家老年疾病临床医学研究中心，是全国大型神经病学诊疗、科研和教学中心。放射与核医学科是国家重点专科，拥有先进影像学设备，包括 2 台一体化 PET/MR、术中 MR 等多台高端影像设备。团队针对脑血管病、阿尔茨海默病、帕金森病、癫痫、脑肿瘤等脑重大疾病开展神经影像学研究，研究成果发表在 *Neuron*、*Nature Communications*、*Brain*、*Radiology*、*EJNMMI* 等国际顶级期刊。目前科室 161 人，包括诊断医师 56 人，其中主任医师 9 人，副主任医师 17 人，主治医师 19 人；技师 73 人，其中副主任技师 2 人，主管技师 7 人；护士 17 人，其中主管护师 9 人。

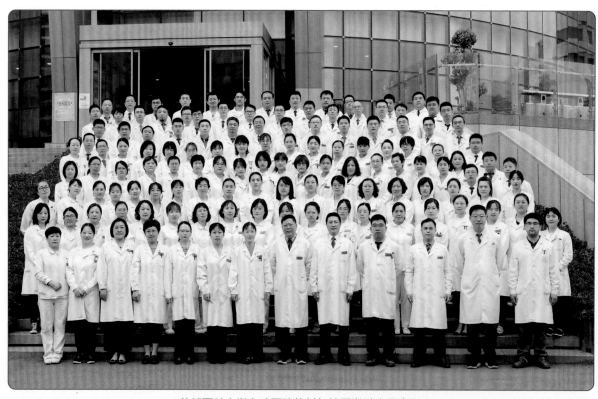

首都医科大学宣武医院放射与核医学科人员合影

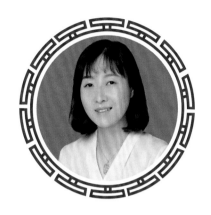

卢 洁

主任医师，教授，博士研究生导师

首都医科大学宣武医院副院长、放射与核医学科主任，国家神经疾病医学中心副主任

神经变性病教育部重点实验室副主任、磁共振成像脑信息学北京市重点实验室主任

学术成果：

以第一作者或通讯作者发表 SCI 收录论文 200 余篇，代表作发表在 *Neuron*、*Nature Communications*、*Radiology*、*Brain*、*Neurology*、*EJNMMI* 等国际权威期刊；主持国家自然科学基金重点项目、国家自然科学基金优秀青年科学基金项目、科技部"十四五"及"十三五"国家重点研发计划、北京自然科学基金重点项目等 19 项课题；主编（译）专著 10 部；授权专利 10 项；专家共识 13 项；获华夏医学科技奖一等奖、北京市留学人员创新创业特别贡献奖、国家"万人计划"科技创新领军人才、茅以升北京青年科技奖、中国产学研合作创新奖、中华医学会放射学分会杰出青年奖、北京医学会首都青年医学创新与转化大赛一等奖等多项学术奖励。

学术兼职：

中华医学会放射学分会全国委员、中国医学影像技术研究会放射学分会副主任委员、北京医学会放射学分会副主任委员、北京医师协会放射医师分会副会长等；担任 *EJNMMI*、*Neuroimage* 等国际期刊编委。

第二节 一体化 PET/MR 研究团队主要成员

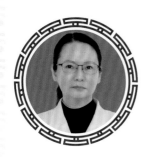

张 春

医学博士，主任医师，教授，硕士研究生导师
首都医科大学宣武医院放射与核医学科副主任

主要研究方向：

肿瘤的放射性核素靶向治疗、神经系统核医学。

学术兼职：

中华医学会核医学分会功能显像学组委员、北京医学会核医学分会委员、中国医学装备协会核医学装备与技术专业委员会常务委员、中国医学影像技术研究会核医学分会委员、北京中西医结合学会核医学专业委员会常务委员。

发表文章：

以第一作者或通讯作者发表 SCI 及核心期刊收录论文 20 余篇。

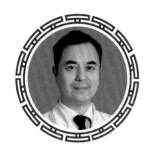

齐志刚

医学博士，主任医师，副教授，硕士研究生导师
首都医科大学宣武医院放射与核医学科主任助理

主要研究方向：

阿尔茨海默病与脑肿瘤的多模态成像研究。

学术兼职：

北京神经内科学会神经影像专业委员会主任委员、阿尔茨海默病防治协会影像专业委员会副主任委员、中华医学会放射学分会神经学组委员、北京医学会放射学分会委员、北京医师协会放射医师分会理事、中国图学学会医学图像与设备专业委员会常务委员、中国神经科学学会神经影像学分会委员。

发表文章：

发表 SCI 收录论文 10 余篇，统计源期刊收录论文 30 余篇。

参加及主持课题：

参与北京市科学技术委员会科技重大专项脑科学研究项目课题、北京市科学技术委员会科技支撑市委市政府重点工作课题；主持国家自然科学基金委员会主任基金项目及科技部重点研发计划数字诊疗装备研发专项课题。

国内外学术会议交流：

多次参加北美放射学会（RSNA）、欧洲放射学大会（ECR）、阿尔茨海默病协会国际会议（AAIC）、国际医学磁共振学会（ISMRM）、中华医学会放射学分会年会、中国医师协会放射医师分会年会等国际国内会议交流；2019 年初赴苏黎世大学医院进行为期 1 个月的一体化 PET/MR 临床应用学习。

参编专著：

参编《一体化 PET/MR 成像病例图谱》《PET/MR 脑功能与分子影像：从脑疾病到脑科学》《一体化 PET/MR 操作规范和临床应用》等专著。

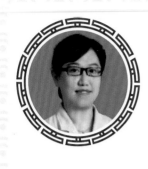

张 苗

医学博士，主任医师，副教授，硕士研究生导师
首都医科大学宣武医院放射与核医学科主任助理

主要研究方向：

脑血管病多模态影像学研究。

学术兼职：

中华医学会放射学分会医学影像人工智能工作组委员、中国医师协会放射医师分会对比剂学组委员、中国医疗保健国际交流促进会影像医学分会委员、中国研究型医院学会超微与分子病理学专业委员会委员、北京神经内科学会神经影像专业委员会常务委员、北京医学会放射学分会神经学组委员、北京女科技工作者协会理事；担任《中国脑血管病杂志》青年编委。

发表文章：

以第一作者发表 SCI 收录论文 3 篇（单篇最高影响因子：29.146），以第一作者发表统计源期刊收录论文 20 余篇。

参加及主持课题：

主持国家自然科学基金青年基金项目和科技部重点研发项目子课题 2 项、北京市科学技术协会"金桥工程种子基金"项目 1 项；参与 10 余项国家及省部级科研课题。

国内外学术会议交流：

多次参加北美放射学会年会（RSNA）、欧洲放射学大会（ECR）、亚洲大洋洲放射学大会（AOCR）、中华医学会放射学分会年会等国际国内会议交流。

参编 / 译专著：

参编 / 译《一体化 PET/MR 操作规范和临床应用》《一体化 PET/MR 成像病例图谱》《一体化 PET/MR 实操手册》《PET/MR 脑功能与分子影像：从脑疾病到脑科学》《PET/MRI 方法和临床应用》等专著。

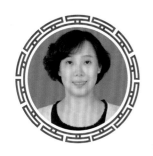

张海琴

医学博士，副主任医师
首都医科大学宣武医院放射与核医学科

主要研究方向：

神经系统疾病和肿瘤的多模态影像诊断。

学术兼职：

北京神经内科学会神经影像专业委员会委员、北京医学会核医学分会新型探针多中心研究学组委员、北京医学会核医学分会肿瘤学组委员、北京医学会核医学分会青年委员会委员、首都医科大学核医学系务委员会委员。

发表文章：

以第一作者或通讯作者发表统计源期刊收录论文 10 余篇。

参加及主持课题：

参与多项国家级及市局级课题，其中 PET/MR 相关项目有"十四五"科技部重点研发项目"基于国产 PET/MR 的脑重大疾病诊疗解决方案研究"、国家自然科学基金青年项目"帕金森病患者脑中神经炎症进展的 18KDa 转位蛋白靶向 PET 显像研究"；主持校级课题"帕金森病患者基底节环路神经连接网络功能代偿及失衡 – 基于一体化 PET/MRI 多模态成像"。

参编 / 译专著：

参编 / 译《一体化 PET/MR 操作规范和临床应用》《一体化 PET/MR 实操手册》《一体化 PET/MR 护理实操手册》《一体化 PET/MR 成像病例图谱》《核医学：核心复习》《比较神经影像学》《神经病学》等专著。

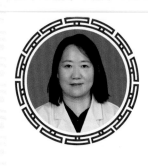

赵志莲

医学博士，副主任医师，副教授，硕士研究生导师
首都医科大学宣武医院放射与核医学科腹部神经医疗组长

主要研究方向：

阿尔茨海默病多模态影像研究。

学术兼职：

北京神经内科学会神经影像专业委员会委员、北京医学会放射学分会头颈学组委员、北京抗癌协会神经肿瘤专业委员会委员、中国研究型医院学会神经再生与修复专业委员会神经影像与神经再生学组委员、中国医师协会放射医师分会教学技术委员会委员、中华医学会放射学分会神经学组 youth club 成员。

发表文章：

以第一作者及并列第一作者发表 SCI 收录论文 5 篇（单篇最高影响因子：5.133）；以第一作者或通讯作者发表统计源期刊收录论文 8 篇。

参加及主持课题：

主持国家自然科学基金青年项目"遗忘型轻度认知障碍 PET/MR 脑代谢与脑网络动态变化及关联机制研究"、院级课题 1 项；参与国家自然科学基金重大项目"癫痫病人脑连接的个体化特征分析"、北京市科委基金项目"轻度认知障碍智能诊断模型研究"。

国内外学术会议交流：

2013、2014 年度北美放射学会（RSNA）2 次口头发言交流。

参编专著：

参编《一体化 PET/MR 成像病例图谱》《PET/MR 脑功能与分子影像：从脑疾病到脑科学》等专著。

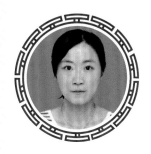

黄 靖

医学博士，副主任医师
首都医科大学宣武医院放射与核医学科

主要研究方向：

多发性硬化的一体化 PET/MR 研究。

学术兼职：

北京医学会放射学分会青年委员、北京神经内科学会神经影像专业委员会委员、中国药物滥用防治协会成瘾医学分会委员、中国生物物理学会表型组学分会委员。

发表文章：

以第一作者及并列第一作者发表中英文文章 20 篇，其中 SCI 收录论文 7 篇（单篇最高影响因子：13.828）。

参加及主持课题：

参与国家自然科学基金面上项目"视神经脊髓炎患者早期认知障碍的脑结构和功能基础及动态演变纵向研究"、国家自然科学基金青年项目"视神经脊髓炎和多发性硬化深部灰质损伤的多模态 MRI 研究"；主持校级及院级课题各 1 项。

国内外学术会议交流：

2014 年北美放射学会（RSNA）1 次壁报交流、1 次口头发言交流，2021 年国际医学磁共振学会（ISMRM）1 次壁报交流，2014、2016—2019 年中华医学放射学年会 4 次壁报交流，1 次口头发言交流。

参编 / 译专著：

参编 / 译《中枢神经系统脱髓鞘疾病影像学》《PET/MR 脑功能与分子影像：从脑疾病到脑科学》《一体化 PET/MR 护理实操手册》《fMRI 基础与临床应用》等专著。

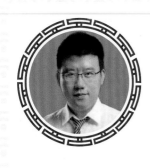

宋天彬

医学博士，副主任医师
首都医科大学宣武医院放射与核医学科核医学组医疗组长

主要研究方向：

帕金森病及体部肿瘤的一体化 PET/MR 研究。

学术兼职：

北京核医学分会辐射防护学组副组长、北京核医学分会继续教育学组委员、北京医学奖励基金会肺癌医学青年专家委员会影像学组委员、中国医师协会放射医师分会呼吸学组委员、中国人体健康科技促进会肿瘤医学影像专业委员会委员、中国生物医学工程学会医学影像工程与技术分会青年委员。

发表文章：

以第一作者及并列第一作者发表 SCI 收录论文 9 篇（单篇最高影响因子：10.057）；以第一作者或通讯作者发表统计源期刊收录论文 8 篇。

参加及主持课题：

参与国家自然科学基金青年项目"帕金森病患者脑中神经炎症进展的 18KDa 转位蛋白靶向 PET 显像研究"、首都卫生发展科研专项课题"一体化 PET/MR 在子宫内膜癌诊断及术前精准分期中的应用效果"；主持院级课题 1 项。

国内外学术会议交流：

2017—2019 年度美国核医学与分子影像学会年会（SNMMI）3 次壁报交流、1 次口头发言交流。2018—2019 年 2 次中华医学核医学年会及 1 次中华医学放射学年会口头发言。

参编 / 译专著：

参编 / 译《一体化 PET/MR 成像病例图谱》《PET/MR 脑功能与分子影像：从脑疾病到脑科学》《下咽癌 PET/CT 和 PET/MRI 病例荟萃》《一体化 PET/MR 护理实操手册》《肿瘤 PET/CT 图谱：胸部肿瘤卷》《核医学：核心复习》《fMRI 基础与临床应用》等专著。

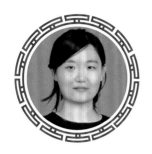

单 艺

医学硕士研究生，在读博士研究生，主治医师
首都医科大学宣武医院放射与核医学科科研秘书、新区医疗组组长

主要研究方向：

脑梗死的多模态脑成像研究。

学术兼职：

中国图学学会医学图像与设备专业委员会委员、中国针灸学会针灸医学影像专业委员会委员、北京医学会放射学分会中医影像学组委员、北京神经内科学会神经影像专业委员会委员。

发表文章：

以第一作者或通讯作者发表 SCI 收录论文 7 篇，统计源期刊收录论文 7 篇。

参加及主持课题：

参与国家自然科学基金重点项目"基于人工智能的多模态跨尺度影像评估颈动脉粥样硬化斑块易损性研究"、北京市自然科学基金重点项目"基于多模态影像探究头颈动脉粥样硬化斑块易损机制的人工智能研究"、国家科技部重点研发计划"一体化 TOF-PET-MRI 脑血流定量方法研究及在脑疾病应用"；主持北京市自然科学基金青年项目"PET/MR 同步测定脑梗死患者运动功能预后的多模态脑机制研究"。

国内外学术会议交流：

2017 年国际医学磁共振学会（ISMRM）壁报交流、2017 年欧洲放射学年会（ECR）口头交流，2019 年 1—2 月于瑞士苏黎世大学医院核医学科进修 PET/MR 诊断。

参编 / 译专著：

参编 / 译《一体化 PET/MR 成像病例图谱》《PET/MR 脑功能与分子影像：从脑疾病到脑科学》《一体化 PET/MR 实操手册》《一体化 PET/MR 操作规范和临床应用》《PET/MRI 方法和临床应用》《fMRI 基础与临床应用》等专著。

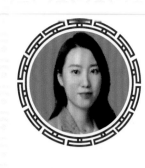

吴 芳

医学硕士研究生，在读博士研究生，主治医师

首都医科大学宣武医院放射与核医学科北区磁共振组组长

主要研究方向：

脑血管病影像学研究。

学术兼职：

中国生物医学工程学会医学影像工程与技术分会青年委员、北京神经内科学会神经影像专业委员会委员；担任 *Frontiers in Neurology* 评审编辑。

发表文章：

以第一作者及并列第一作者发表 SCI 收录论文 7 篇（单篇最高影响因子：10.1）；以第一作者发表统计源期刊收录论文 5 篇。

参加及主持课题：

主持国家自然科学基金青年项目"基于 ^{18}F-NaF PET/MR 评价颅内动脉粥样硬化斑块微钙化及其稳定性的机制研究"、北京市医院管理中心"培育计划"课题"基于多模态磁共振成像的脑小血管病小动脉结构和功能损伤的早期识别研究"、北京市委组织部优秀人才青年骨干个人项目"基于多延迟动脉自旋标记成像技术的烟雾病血流动力学研究"；主持校级及院级课题各 1 项。

国内外学术会议交流：

2018 年国际卒中大会口头发言，2018 年第 104 届北美放射学会（RSNA）口头发言，2019 年国际医学磁共振学会（ISMRM）壁报交流。

参编专著：

参编《肺部高分辨率 CT（第 2 版）》《心血管影像诊断学（第 2 版）》等专著。

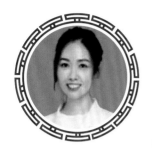

闫少珍

医学博士，住院医师，青年博士研究生导师
首都医科大学宣武医院放射与核医学科

主要研究方向：

神经变性病的一体化 PET/MR 研究。

学术兼职：

中国图学学会医学图像与设备专业委员会委员、北京神经内科学会神经影像专业委员会委员。

发表文章：

以第一作者发表 SCI 收录论文 4 篇（单篇最高影响因子：15.552）；以第一作者发表统计源期刊收录论文 6 篇。

主持课题：

主持国家自然科学青年基金"阿尔茨海默病海马功能和代谢网络关系机制的一体化 PET/MR 研究"、北京市科技新星计划交叉课题"基于机器学习的 PET/MR 多模态影像在阿尔茨海默病早期精准诊断研究"、北京市科技新星"基于人工智能的结构 MRI 和 ^{18}F-florbetapir PET 阿尔茨海默病影像早期诊断研究"、北京市医管中心培育计划"阿尔茨海默病基底前脑结构与功能早期改变的一体化 PET/MR 研究"。

国内外学术交流及获奖：

2019—2010 年美国圣路易斯华盛顿大学访问学者，2019 年美国核医学与分子影像学会年会（SNMMI）国际最佳摘要奖，2020 年 SNMMI 神经科学领域优秀壁报一等奖，2021 年 SNMMI 神经科学领域十佳优秀壁报奖，2021 年北京医学会放射学分会英语演讲比赛二等奖，2020 年首都医科大学优秀博士论文。

参编 / 译专著：

参编 / 译《一体化 PET/MR 成像病例图谱》《PET/MR 脑功能与分子影像：从脑疾病到脑科学》《fMRI 基础与临床应用》等专著。

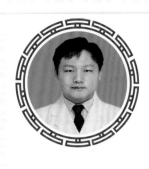

崔碧霄

医学博士，住院医师

首都医科大学宣武医院放射与核医学科

主要研究方向：

神经系统疾病的一体化 PET/MR 研究。

学术兼职：

中国图学学会医学图像与设备专业委员会委员、北京神经内科学会神经影像专业分会委员。

获奖情况：

2021 年首都医科大学优秀博士论文。

发表文章：

共发表文章 30 篇，其中以第一作者及并列第一作者发表 SCI 收录论文 4 篇（单篇最高影响因子：15.717）；以第一作者发表统计源期刊收录论文 4 篇。

参加及主持课题：

参与科技部"十三五""十四五"重点专项各 1 项，国家自然科学基金重点项目 1 项、面上项目 2 项；主持院级课题 1 项。

国内外学术会议交流及获奖：

美国核医学与分子影像学会年会（SNMMI）9 次壁报交流、1 次口头发言交流，中华医学核医学年会 2 次口头发言，中华医学放射学年会 1 次口头发言，2019 年 1—2 月于瑞士苏黎世大学医院核医学科进修 PET/MR 诊断。

参编/译专著：

参编/译《PET/MR 脑功能与分子影像：从脑疾病到脑科学》《一体化 PET/MR 护理实操手册》《下咽癌 PET/CT 和 PET/MRI 病例荟萃》《一体化 PET/MR 成像病例图谱》《一体化 PET/MR 实操手册》《一体化 PET/MR 操作规范和临床应用》《核医学：核心复习》《PET/MRI 方法和临床应用》《fMRI 基础与临床应用》等专著。

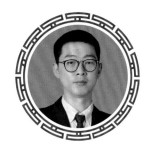

张 越

医学博士，住院医师
首都医科大学宣武医院放射与核医学科

主要研究方向：

颈动脉斑块易损性的一体化 PET/MR 研究。

学术兼职：

北京神经内科学会神经影像专业分会委员、中国图学学会医学图像与设备专业委员会委员。

发表文章：

以第一作者发表 SCI 收录论文及统计源期刊收录论文共 8 篇。

参加及主持课题：

主持首都医科大学临床专科学院（系）培养基金开放课题：基于 PET/MR 评估颈动脉粥样硬化斑块易损性的影像学特征研究；参与国家自然科学基金重点项目：基于人工智能的多模态跨尺度影像评估颈动脉粥样硬化斑块易损性研究；参与国家自然科学基金面上项目：基于 PET/MR 评价颈动脉粥样硬化斑块炎症及其稳定性的影像学特征研究；参与北京市自然科学基金重点项目：基于多模态影像探究头颈动脉粥样硬化斑块易损机制的人工智能研究；主持首都医科大学宣武医院国自然青年培育项目课题 1 项。

国内外学术会议交流：

国际会议：2018—2020 年连续 3 年在北美放射学年会（RSNA）进行口头发言共 4 次；2019、2020 年连续两年在美国核医学年会（SNMMI）进行口头发言共 2 次。

国内会议：2019 年在中华医学会放射学分会学术会议进行口头发言 1 次。

参编 / 译专著：

参编 / 译《PET/MRI 脑功能与分子影像：从脑疾病到脑科学》《一体化 PET/MR 成像病例图谱》《一体化 PET/MR 实操手册》《fMRI 基础与临床应用》等专著。

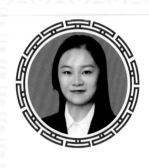

殷雅彦

北京大学医学物理和工程工学博士研究生，助理研究员

首都医科大学宣武医院放射与核医学科博士后

主要研究方向：

脑氧代谢功能磁共振成像技术及临床应用。

学术兼职：

中国图学学会医学影像与设备专业委员会高级委员、北京神经内科学会神经影像专业委员会委员、北京脑网络组与类脑智能学会委员，担任 *Frontiers in Neuroscience* 审稿专家、*Frontiers in Stroke* 审稿专家。

发表文章：

以第一作者及并列第一作者发表 SCI 收录论文 3 篇（单篇最高影响因子：7.4）。

主持课题：

主持国家自然科学基金青年项目、中国博士后基金面上项目、院级青苗培育项目、院级科技培育转化项目。

国内外学术会议交流：

2017 年、2018 年国际医学磁共振学会（ISMRM）口头报告 2 次，2019 年国际人类脑图谱学会（OHBM）大会壁报 1 次，2020 年国际医学磁共振学会（ISMRM）电子壁报 1 次，2019 年青海省医学会放射学分会大会报告 1 次，"一带一路"神经影像高峰论坛大会报告 1 次，2022 年黄河医学影像论坛线上大会报告 1 次。

参编 / 译专著：

参编 / 译《PET/MR 脑功能与分子影像：从脑疾病到脑科学》《fMRI 基础与临床应用》等专著。

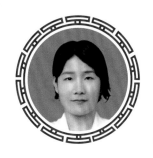

王静娟

中科院高能物理研究所粒子物理与原子核物理工学博士研究生
首都医科大学宣武医院放射与核医学科专职科研人员

主要研究方向：

难治性癫痫术前影像学定位的一体化 PET/MR 研究。

发表文章：

以第一作者及并列第一作者发表 SCI 收录论文 10 篇（单篇最高影响因子：10.057）。

参加及主持课题：

参与国家自然科学基金面上项目、"十三五"课题、北京市科学技术委员会重点项目；主持
首都医科大学培育基金 1 项、中医内科学教育部重点实验室开放基金课题 1 项、院级培育课题 1 项。

国内外学术会议交流及获奖：

2017—2019 年美国核医学与分子影像学会年会（SNMMI）口头发言，2018 年、2019 年中华
医学放射学年会口头发言，中华医学会核医学新锐技师奖。

参编 / 译专著：

参编 / 译《一体化 PET/MR 成像病例图谱》《PET/MR 脑功能与分子影像：从脑疾病到脑科
学》《fMRI 基础与临床应用》等专著。

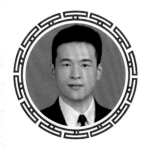

乔洪文

北京师范大学化学学院理学博士研究生、首都医科大学宣武医院神经内科博士后
首都医科大学宣武医院放射与核医学科化学师

主要研究方向：

新型放射性药物开发与转化。

发表文章及专利：

以第一作者及并列第一作者发表 SCI 收录论文 8 篇；申请发明专利 2 项、实用新型专利 1 项。

主持课题：

主持国家自然科学基金青年项目"帕金森病患者脑中神经炎症进展的 18KDa 转位蛋白靶向
PET 显像研究"、院级课题 1 项。

参编专著：

参编《PET/MR 脑功能与分子影像：从脑疾病到脑科学》《一体化 PET/MR 护理实操手册》
等专著。

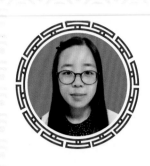

候亚琴

医学硕士研究生，在读博士研究生，主治医师
首都医科大学宣武医院放射与核医学科

主要研究方向：

癫痫一体化 PET/MR 研究。

发表文章：

以第一作者发表 SCI 收录论文 1 篇；以第一作者发表统计源期刊收录论文 6 篇。

参加课题：

参与国家自然科学基金面上项目"耳穴刺激经迷走神经调控脂肪代谢"。

国内外学术会议交流：

2018 年度美国核医学与分子影像学会年会（SNMMI）壁报交流。

参编 / 译专著：

参编 / 译《一体化 PET/MR 成像病例图谱》《PET/MR 脑功能与分子影像：从脑疾病到脑科学》《一体化 PET/MR 护理实操手册》《核医学：核心复习》等专著。

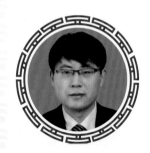

王　臣

医学硕士研究生，在读博士研究生，主治医师
首都医科大学宣武医院放射与核医学科

主要研究方向：

心脑血管系统影像研究。

发表文章：

以第一作者或通讯作者发表统计源期刊收录论文 5 篇。

参加课题：

参与北京市科学技术委员会课题"低剂量心脑联合 CTA 动脉硬化斑块负荷评价在缺血性心脑血管病二级预防中价值的临床研究"。

国内外学术会议交流：

中华医学放射学年会口头发言 1 次。

参编专著：

参编《临床实用影像诊断学》《脑血管病影像评价观点》等专著。

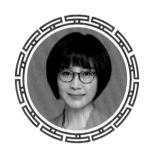

武春雪

医学博士，副主任医师
首都医科大学宣武医院放射与核医学科博士后

主要研究方向：

神经影像、脑血管畸形。

学术兼职：

中华医学会放射学分会磁共振学组委员、中国医师协会放射学分会国际交流学组委员、北京核医学分会继续教育学组委员、北京医学会放射学分会人工智能学组学组秘书、北京医学会放射学分会儿科学组委员、中国抗癌协会神经肿瘤专业委员会中枢神经系统淋巴瘤学组委员。

发表文章：

以第一作者及并列第一作者发表 SCI 收录论文 4 篇；统计源期刊收录论文 10 篇。

参加及主持课题：

参加国家自然科学基金青年项目"基于 QSM 定量成像分析铁沉积影响脑血管畸形出血及癫痫发生风险的机制研究"、国家自然科学基金面上项目"基于深度学习的脑垂体瘤 MRI 医学影像智能识别与诊断"；主持国家自然科学基金青年项目"基于磁共振血流动力学特征构建脑动静脉畸形出血风险预测的机器学习模型"；主持院级课题 1 项。

国内外学术会议交流：

2021 年国际医学磁共振学会（ISMRM）壁报、2019 年国际医学磁共振学会（ISMRM）口头发言。

参编专著：

参编《一体化 PET/MR 成像病例图谱》《一体化 PET/MR 护理实操手册》《PET/MR 脑功能与分子影像：从脑疾病到脑科学》等专著。

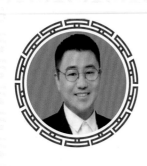

臧振享

德国海德堡大学曼海姆医学院精神病学医学博士研究生

首都医科大学宣武医院放射与核医学科博士后

主要研究方向：

神经影像学方法及其在神经、精神类疾病中的应用。

学术兼职：

担任 *Human Brain Mapping*、*NeuroImage Reports* 审稿专家。

发表文章：

以第一作者及并列第一作者发表 SCI 收录论文 7 篇（单篇最高影响因子：25.911）。

参加课题：

参与国家科技部"十四五"重点研发计划"基于国产 PET/MR 的脑重大疾病诊疗解决方案研究"。

参译专著：

参译《fMRI 基础与临床应用》。

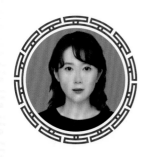

李玮华

英国伦敦帝国理工学院临床医学医学博士

首都医科大学宣武医院放射与核医学科博士后

主要研究方向：

神经退行性疾病的一体化 PET/MR 研究。

发表文章：

以第一作者及并列第一作者发表 SCI 收录论文 4 篇（单篇最高影响因子：10.338）。

国内外学术会议交流：

2015 年 NECTAR 会议口头发言，2017 年第 23 届世界神经病学大会（WCN）口头发言，2017 年、2018 年欧洲神经病学大会口头发言 2 次，2016 年、2017 年国际帕金森氏症和运动障碍大会电子壁报 2 次。

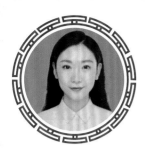

宋双双

医学博士，主治医师
青岛大学附属医院核医学科

主要研究方向：

中枢神经系统肿瘤的 PET/MR 研究。

发表文章：

以第一作者及并列第一作者发表 SCI 收录论文 7 篇（单篇最高影响因子：10.057）；以第一作者发表统计源期刊 8 篇。

参加及主持课题：

主持国家自然科学基金青年项目"基于 PET/MR 影像特征联合影像组学的脑胶质瘤 IDH 基因型预测研究"、山东省医药卫生科技发展计划项目"基于 PET/MRI 影像组学的脑胶质瘤预后与分子标志物 MGMT 相关机制的研究"；主持院级课题 1 项。

国内外学术会议交流：

2020 年美国核医学与分子影像学会年会（SNMMI）口头发言。

参编 / 译专著：

参编 / 译《一体化 PET/MR 成像病例图谱》《PET/MR 脑功能与分子影像：从脑疾病到脑科学》《fMRI 基础与临床应用》等专著。

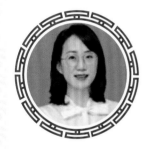

郭 坤

医学博士，主治医师
空军军医大学西京医院核医学科

主要研究方向：

难治性癫痫术前定位与致痫网络机制的 PET/MR 研究。

发表文章：

以第一作者及并列第一作者发表 SCI 收录论文 9 篇，统计源期刊收录论文 9 篇。

参加课题：

参与国家自然科学基金面上项目"STN-DBS 调控运动皮质癫痫的机制研究以及自身免疫性脑炎相关机制研究"。

参编 / 译专著：

参编 / 译《PET/MR 脑功能与分子影像：从脑疾病到脑科学》《一体化 PET/MR 护理实操手册》《一体化 PET/MR 实操手册》《fMRI 基础与临床应用》等专著。

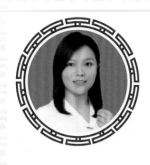

李琼阁

北京航空航天大学生物医学工程工学硕士

首都医科大学宣武医院放射与核医学科技师

主要研究方向：

脑疾病的功能磁共振成像研究。

学术兼职：

北京放射技术学会青年委员、中国图学学会医学图像与设备专业委员会委员、中华医学会影像技术分会委员，担任《广州医科大学学报》中青年委员审稿专家。

发表文章：

以第一作者及并列第一作者发表 SCI 收录论文 2 篇（单篇最高影响因子：5.702）；以第一作者发表统计源期刊收录论文 4 篇。

主持课题：

主持院级课题 1 项。

国内外学术会议交流：

2017—2019 年度美国核医学与分子影像学会年会（SNMMI）壁报交流。

参编专著：

参编《PET/MR 脑功能与分子影像：从脑疾病到脑科学》等专著。

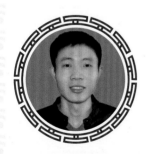

田德峰

首都医科大学生物医学工程工学硕士研究生

首都医科大学宣武医院放射与核医学科技师

主要研究方向：

一体化 PET/MR 图像质量控制及重建算法研究。

发表文章：

以第一作者发表 SCI 收录论文 1 篇；以第一作者发表统计源期刊收录论文 3 篇。

参编专著：

参编《临床工程学》等专著。

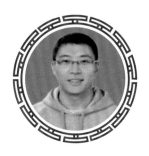

马 杰

本科，技师
首都医科大学宣武医院放射与核医学科

参加课题：

参与课题有"一体化 PET/MR 探讨心力衰竭后认知功能障碍患者的脑结构和脑代谢研究""一体化 PET/MR 脑血流定量新方法的手术评估""一体化 PET/MR 脑胶质瘤的手术评估""一体化 PET/MR 颈动脉斑块的评估""一体化 PET/MR 在子宫内膜癌诊断及术前精准分期中的应用效果"等。

参编专著：

参编《一体化 PET/MR 实操手册》等专著。

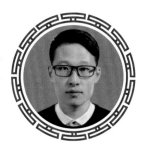

杨宏伟

医学本科，技师
首都医科大学宣武医院放射与核医学科

主要研究方向：

PET/MR 技术及设备质量控制。

发表文章：

以第一作者发表 SCI 收录论文 1 篇，统计源期刊收录论文 1 篇。

参加课题：

参与"阿尔茨海默病影像早期诊断标志物的应用开发研究"。

国内外学术会议交流及获奖：

2020 年美国核医学与分子影像学会年会（SNMMI）口头发言，2018 年、2021 年中华医学会核医学年会壁报交流，全国医学影像技术学大会口头发言，荣获中华医学会核医学分会"新锐技师"奖。

参编专著：

参编《一体化 PET/MR 实操手册》《一体化 PET/MR 护理实操手册》《下咽癌 PET/CT 和 PET/MRI 病例荟萃》等专著。

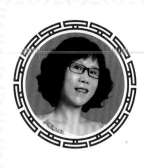

帅冬梅

主管护师

首都医科大学宣武医院放射与核医学科护理组长

主要研究方向：

放药注射及治疗。

学术兼职：

北京医学会核医学分会第十届科普宣传委员。

发表文章：

以第一作者发表统计源期刊收录论文 7 篇。

参加课题：

主持院级护理重点项目课题"一体化 PET-MR 双药物注射检查的护理操作流程研究"。

参编专著：

参编《一体化 PET/MR 护理实操手册》等专著。

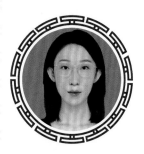

王振明

影像医学与核医学在读博士研究生

主要研究方向：

难治性癫痫术前定位和预后评估的影像学研究。

发表文章：

以第一作者及并列第一作者发表 SCI 收录论文 5 篇（单篇最高影响因子：7.4）；以第一作者发表统计源期刊收录论文 1 篇。

参加课题：

参与国家自然科学基金面上项目"STN-DBS 调控运动皮质癫痫的机制研究以及自身免疫性脑炎相关机制研究"。

参编 / 译专著：

参编 / 译《PET/MR 脑功能与分子影像：从脑疾病到脑科学》《一体化 PET/MR 护理实操手册》《fMRI 基础与临床应用》等专著。

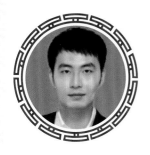

李笑然

影像医学与核医学在读博士研究生

主要研究方向：

恶性脑肿瘤及妇科恶性肿瘤的 PET/MR 相关研究。

发表文章：

以第一作者及并列第一作者发表 SCI 收录论文 3 篇（单篇最高影响因子：7.034）；以第一作者发表统计源期刊收录论文 1 篇。

国内外学术会议交流：

2022 年中华医学会核医学年会口头发言。

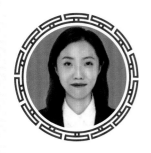

於 帆

影像医学与核医学在读博士研究生

主要研究方向：

颈动脉斑块的一体化 PET/MR 研究。

发表文章：

以第一作者发表 SCI 收录论文 2 篇；统计源期刊收录论文 5 篇。

参加课题：

参与国家自然科学基金重点项目"基于人工智能的多模态跨尺度影像评估颈动脉粥样硬化斑块易损性研究"。

国内外学术会议交流：

2022 年国际医学磁共振学会年会（ISMRM）大会 2 次口头发言，2019 年中华医学会放射学年会口头发言。

参编专著：

参编《PET/MR 脑功能与分子影像：从脑疾病到脑科学》等专著。

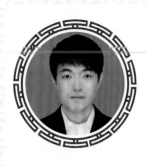

郑 冲

影像医学与核医学在读博士研究生

主要研究方向：

心力衰竭后认知功能障碍的一体化 PET/MR 研究。

发表文章：

以第一作者发表 SCI 收录论文 1 篇；以第一作者发表统计源期刊收录论文 3 篇。

参加课题：

参与国家重点研发计划"基于国产 PET/MR 的脑重大疾病诊疗解决方案研究"、国家自然科学基金面上项目"基于 PET/MR 评价颈动脉粥样硬化斑块炎症及其稳定性的影像学特征"、北京自然科学基金重点项目"基于多模态影像探究头颈动脉粥样硬化斑块易损机制的人工智能研究"。

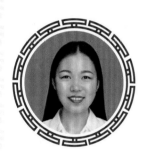

袁 丽

影像医学与核医学在读硕士研究生

主要研究方向：

脑胶质瘤 MRI 研究。

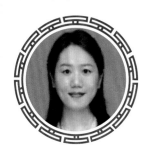

谷珊珊

影像医学与核医学在读博士研究生
民航总医院核医学科主治医师

主要研究方向：

脑卒中神经保护机制 PET/MR 研究。

学术兼职：

北京医学会核医学分会继续教育学组委员、北京医学会核医学分会影像组学学组委员。

发表文章：

以第一作者发表统计源期刊收录论文 6 篇。

参加课题：

参与院级课题 1 项"基于 PET/MR 的缺血性心肌病认知功能障碍机制研究"。

国内外学术会议交流：

2014 年长城国际心脏病学会议及亚太心脏大会壁报交流。

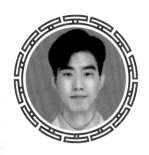

毕　晟

影像医学与核医学，在读硕士研究生

主要研究方向：

神经退行性疾病的一体化 PET/MR 研究。

发表文章：

以第一作者发表统计源期刊收录论文 1 篇。

参加课题：

参与国家自然科学基金青年项目"阿尔茨海默病海马功能和代谢网络关系机制的一体化 PET/MR 研究"。

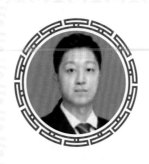

孙赫屿

生物医学工程在读硕士研究生

主要研究方向：

颈动脉粥样硬化斑块的一体化 PET/MR 研究。

参与课题：

参与国家自然科学基金重点项目"基于人工智能的多模态跨尺度影像评估颈动脉粥样硬化斑块易损性研究"。

一体化 PET/MR
企业支持团队

PET/MR
第一节　GE 医疗科研支持团队

2014 年 GE 医疗推出全球首款 SiPM 一体化 TOF PET/MRI-SIGNA™ 全息数字 PET/MR，近年来持续投入大量资源推动产品技术快速迭代创新，组建了目前业内强大的 ONE MI 分子影像临床科研支持团队，与国内顶尖医院开展广泛合作。2015 年亚洲第一台 TOF SIGNA™ 全息数字 PET/MR 落地首都医科大学宣武医院，GE 医疗 ONE MI 临床科研支持团队集 GE 医疗全球研究院、产品研发团队、临床应用团队、科研支持团队等专业力量，携手宣武医院开展从设备创新到临床试验，从技术创新到科研合作，从人才培养到行业普及等一系列医研产学合作。通过结合宣武医院临床优势，共同推动一体化 PET/MR 在癫痫、神经退行性疾病、脑血管疾病、肿瘤等重大疾病临床应用。

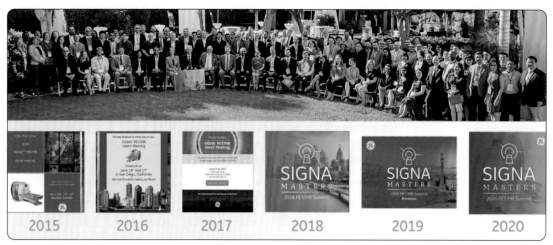

宣武 -GE 医疗 ONE MI PET/MR 合作团队

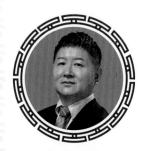

熊　伟

博士　GE PET/MR 临床应用经理

负责并带领 PET/MR 临床应用团队全程参与首都医科大学宣武医院一体化 PET/MR 装机后的所有临床应用相关培训及指导，包括多种序列优化、数据采集方案、临床方向指导等一系列工作，保障首都医科大学宣武医院 PET/MR 正常高效使用及临床科研的顺利开展。

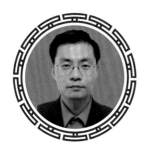

徐家骅

博士　GE ONE MI 高级应用经理

带领 ONE MI 高级应用团队参与并负责首都医科大学宣武医院一体化 PET/MR 科研合作，包括实验设计、实验数据后处理及统计分析、新型药物开发、论文修改等一系列工作，助力宣武医院 PET/MR 临床科研成果的高效产出。

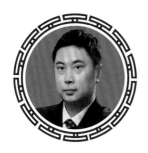

郑志超

博士　GE PET/MR 临床应用专家

全程参与并协助首都医科大学宣武医院一体化 PET/MR 装机后临床应用相关培训及指导，包括临床图像优化、临床数据采集、临床科研可行性讨论等一系列工作，保障首都医科大学宣武医院 PET/MR 正常高效使用及临床科研工作的顺利开展。

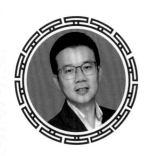

梁洒远

博士　GE PET/MR 产品经理

先后以科研支持及产品经理的身份参与首都医科大学宣武医院一体化 PET/MR 临床科研合作及支持，包括科研方向分享、科研项目支持、成果宣传等系列工作，助力首都医科大学宣武医院 PET/MR 临床科研成果产出及推广。

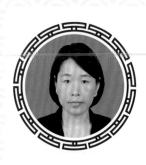

马淑杰

博士　GE PET/MR 临床应用专家

作为 GE 医疗与宣武医院合作的主要联系人，常驻首都医科大学宣武医院确保一体化 PET/MR 日常临床科研工作的顺利开展。

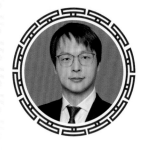

刘华伟

博士　GE PET/MR 高级应用专家

支持首都医科大学宣武医院一体化 PET/MR 科研合作，包括实验设计、科研序列使用、论文修改等工作，助力宣武医院 PET/MR 科研项目开展及文章发表。

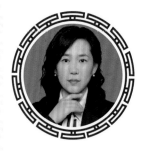

李　红

博士　GE PET/MR 高级应用专家

支持首都医科大学宣武医院一体化 PET/MR 科研合作，包括科研方向可行性、科研项目管理、数据后处理等工作，助力首都医科大学宣武医院 PET/MR 科研项目开展及文章发表。

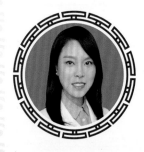

孙牧川

博士　GE PET/MR 临床应用专家

支持宣武医院一体化 PET/MR 临床科研工作开展，包括临床应用支持、科研项目支持等工作，助力首都医科大学宣武医院 PET/MR 科研项目开展及文章发表。

第二节　联影医疗科研支持团队

　　上海联影医疗科技股份有限公司将 PET/MR 作为最为重要的多模态分子影像产品之一，坚持凝聚全球的技术专家，与中国的放射学、核医学专家共同推进临床诊断和科研探索。业界首台"时空一体"超清 TOF PET/MR 于 2019 年 1 月在首都医科大学宣武医院正式投入临床科研使用，围绕神经疾病精准诊疗与脑科学前瞻探索，双方成立了宣武 – 联影脑功能与分子影像联合实验室，将持续推动神经和老年疾病的早期诊断、精准治疗、新型探针与新药研发等，进行全方位的联动创新，共同探索 PET/MR 的临床与科研价值。

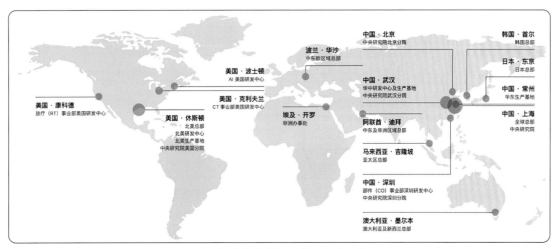

联影打造全球创新研发、生产网络

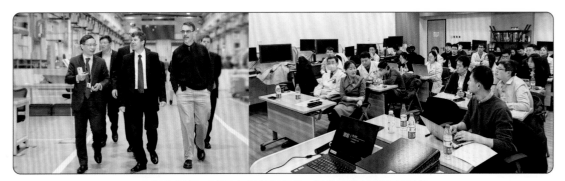

定制化创新，灵活响应客户需求，提供高端科研定制服务

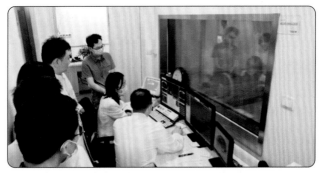

宣武 – 联影医疗 PET/MR 合作团队

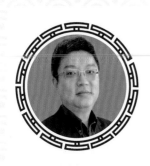

李　峥

博士

博士毕业于北京航空航天大学电子信息工程学院，现任北京联影智能影像技术研究院运营院长，联影智能医疗科技（北京）有限公司联席总经理，长期从事医疗影像人工智能等领域的研究。

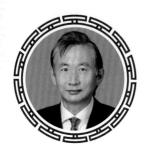

周　云

博士

联影医疗分子医学与药理学中心主任，上海科技大学生物医学工程学院特聘教授，加利福尼亚大学洛杉矶分校生物医学物理学博士。曾任职于约翰斯·霍普金斯大学医学院放射系和圣路易斯华盛顿大学放射系，研究方向包括基于多模态 PET 的定量分析基础理论及其在神经、心脏、肿瘤及药物评估等领域的应用。

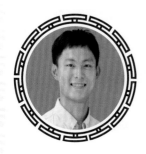

袁健闵

博士

毕业于英国剑桥大学临床医学院，博士后工作于美国斯坦福大学临床医学院。从事 PET/MR 序列开发、图像采集和重建、人工智能算法研究。主要研究方向为心血管成像、血管壁斑块成像、肿瘤、儿科影像，曾作为首位华人获得欧洲医学和生物学磁共振学会年会（ESMRMB）青年科学家奖。发表 SCI 收录论文近 30 篇，其中作为第一作者 8 篇。获专利 1 项。长期担任 *MRM*、*JMRI*、*MRI*、*MAGMA* 等杂志审稿人。目前作为联影中央研究院科研合作专家，主持上海市扬帆科研项目 1 项，参与国家自然科学基金委员会面上课题 2 项、上海市启明星科研计划 1 项、北京市自然科学基金项目 2 项。

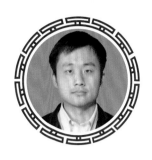

胡凌志

博士

美国华盛顿大学医学物理博士，联影研究院研发总监。发表 SCI 期刊收录论文 20 余篇，国际会议论文 30 余篇，美国专利 13 余项，担任 *Journal of Magnetic Resonance Imaging*、*Molecular Imaging and Biology*，*Magnetic Resonance in Medicine* 等 10 余部 SCI 收录期刊审稿人。主持科技部"十三五"重点研发项目"一体化 PET/MR 装备研制"，主持上海市经信委"嵌入式乳腺 PET/MR"项目，参与自然科学基金委员会"多核一体化同步成像仪"重大仪器研发项目。

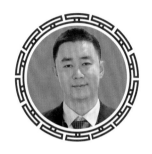

曹拓宇

博士

毕业于美国纽约州立大学，在医学影像领域有 10 余年的工程及研发经验。发表期刊、会议论文 20 余篇，授权 / 申请 10 项国内、国际专利。在上海联影作为 PET/MR 项目的系统负责人，领导了 PET/MR 的系统集成、测试、算法和高级应用开发工作。此外，作为项目负责人领导了嵌入式 PET/MR 项目的研发工作，领导团队克服了多个电磁兼容、可靠性、算法等技术难题，整机性能已经通过了上海市的项目验收。目前作为项目负责人承担上海市科学技术委员会"产学研医合作领域项目"1 项。

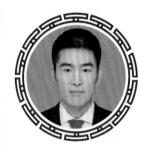

杨　阳

博士

毕业于北京大学物理学院。从事 MRI 的序列开发、数据采集和图像分析 6 年。主要研究方向为 PET/MR 的序列开发及其临床应用、PET/MR 在神经影像方面的应用、脑氧摄取分数对比度的应用及睡眠状态下的白质脑功能研究等。在 *NeuroImage* 上发表学术论文 1 篇、国际会议摘要数篇。

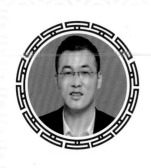

孙红岩

博士

加拿大曼尼托巴大学医学物理专业博士，美国医学物理学家协会（AAPM）会员，加拿大医学物理学家组织（COMP）会员，加拿大辐射防护协会（CRPA）会员，美国电气与电子工程师协会（IEEE）会员。加拿大辐射防护协会（CRPA）Anthony J. MacKay 奖获得者。主要研究方向：医学影像、剂量学、放射治疗学、医学物理学等。现任联影中央研究资深科研合作专家。

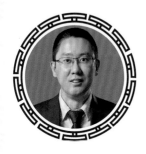

胡战利

博士

联影研究院双聘教授，中国科学院深圳先进技术研究院研究员、博士研究生导师、国家自然科学基金优秀青年基金获得者、"广东特支计划"青年拔尖人才，研究领域为医学 PET 与 CT 成像、临床图像人工智能分析。一直致力于医学成像方法研发，突破现有医学成像技术在空间分辨率、时间分辨率和辐射剂量等方面的极限。在实现学术前沿突破的同时参与了我国多项高端医疗装备和科研仪器的自主研发。因在高端医学仪器关键技术实现和研究方面的创新性成果获得"中国科学院科技促进发展奖"。近年来以第一作者或通讯作者在 *PMB*、*Medical Physics*、*IEEE TCI*、*IEEE TRPMS*、*Neurocomputing* 等本领域权威期刊发表 SCI 收录论文 20 余篇；作为第一发明人授权的 9 项发明专利技术和 2 个软件著作权已转让企业。先后主持国家自然科学基金面上项目 / 优秀青年基金项目、广东省国际合作项目和企业横向项目等。

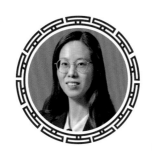

张 娜

博士

联影研究院双聘教授，中科院深圳先进院副研究员、博士研究生导师。先后入选深圳市"孔雀计划"海外高层次人才和深圳市后备级高层次人才。研究领域为快速高分辨 MRI 及在脑血管病精准诊疗中的应用。曾赴美国加州国际心脑血管顶级实验室（Cedars-Sinai 医疗中心）交流学习。发表本领域 SCI 收录的权威期刊和会议论文共计 50 余篇。多次获邀在国际医学磁共振大会上做报告介绍最新研究成果，并获得大会颁发的 Summa Cum Laude、Magna Cum Laude 等奖项。先后授权美国 / 中国发明专利 10 余项，并实现转化。参与研发的"脑血管磁共振计算成像技术及应用"获得 2018 年中国电子学会科技进步一等奖。主持国家自然科学基金、广东省自然科学基金、深圳市基础研究等多项课题；同时作为核心骨干先后参与国家重大科研仪器研制项目、科技部数字诊疗装备研发项目、国家自然科学基金重点项目等。

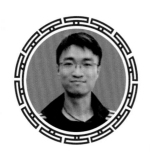

郑超杰

博士

上海联影分子医学与药理学研究中心高级算法工程师，澳大利亚悉尼大学软件工程学士、计算机科学硕士和博士研究生，美国圣路易斯华盛顿大学医学院博士后。主要研究方向是医学图像处理、机器学习与影像组学分析、PET 定量分析与参数成像。在研究期间提出了基于机器学习的肿瘤和肝脏图像分割方法，由拓扑树引导的图像配准方法，参与了乳腺癌预后、白血病复发预测的 PET/CT 影像组学分析，多模态 PET 脑影像在阿尔茨海默病上的定量分析，基于机器学习的双示踪剂信号分离技术，新型 PET 示踪剂在肺部、心脏部位的定量分析与参数成像等项目。

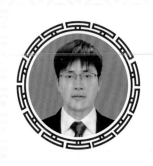

李学飞

博士

上海联影分子医学与药理学研究中心分子探针开发高级专家，武汉大学药学院博士，曾任上海合全药业高级研究员。并先后在英国卡迪夫大学生物化学系、美国圣路易斯华盛顿大学医学院放射化学系从事博士后研究。在药物合成工艺路线开发、多肽药物筛选与结构优化、肿瘤 PET 显影剂上有丰富研发经验，相关研究成果以第一作者或共同作者发表多篇论文，获批国际专利 3 项。此外还筹建过药物化学实验室，具有研发团队管理经验。目前担任国际学术期刊 *PLoS One*、*Tetrahedron Letters* 审稿人。

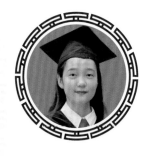

葛 琪

博士

毕业于中山大学医学统计系，研究方向为统计学方法的临床应用，围绕各类医学指标、脑电信号、医学图像等数据，应用统计分析、机器学习、影像组学等方法进行疾病危险因素分析、生存分析、疾病诊断特征挖掘与建模等。